About the volume:

Like many other aspects of seventeenth-century life, medicine cannot be understood without an appreciation of the central importance of religion in the minds of healers and their patients, and of religious attitudes in the practice of the profession.

The important developments in medical theory, practice and organization that took place in the seventeenth century were heavily influenced by the religious and politico-religious upheavals which destabilized English society throughout the entire period. Although experimental investigation, rationality and professional medical institutions rose and flourished, so too did astrology, mysticism and straightforward quackery. Further, all these contending approaches were competing and combining in a time of dynastic flux, civil war and Restoration, and, of course, plague.

This book addresses all of these matters, from the enlightened reason of Thomas Browne's *Religio Medici* to the arcana of astrological medicine, from the research dilemmas of Robert Boyle to the guile and dishonesty of the quacks of plagued London. It presents a complex and difficult story with authority and clarity and will be invaluable reading for historians of medicine and science, and students of religion and society.

About the editors:

Ole Peter Grell and Andrew Cunningham are both members of the Wellcome Unit for the History of Medicine, which is part of the Department of the History and Philosophy of Science in the University of Cambridge.

Religio Medici

For Charles Webster

Religio Medici

Medicine and Religion in Seventeenth-Century England

Edited by

OLE PETER GRELL and ANDREW CUNNINGHAM

SCOLAR PRESS

Published by
SCOLAR PRESS
Gower House
Croft Road
Aldershot
Hants GU11 3HR
England

BT
732.2
.R45
1996

Ashgate Publishing Company
Old Post Road
Brookfield
Vermont 05036–9704
USA

British Library Cataloguing in Publication Data
Religio Medici : Medicine and Religion in
   Seventeenth-Century England
   1. Medicine — England — History — 17th century.   2. Medicine —
   England — Religious aspects — History — 17th century.
   3. Medicine — England — Political aspects — History — 17th
   century.
   I. Grell, Ole Peter.   II. Cunningham, Andrew.
   610.9'42
   ISBN 1–85928–339–X

Library of Congress Cataloging-in-Publication Data
Religio Medici : medicine and religion in seventeenth-century England
   /edited by Ole Peter Grell and Andrew Cunningham.
       p.   cm.
     Includes index.
     ISBN 1–85928–339–X (cloth)
       1. Medicine—Religious aspects—Christianity—History—17th
   century.   2. Medicine—England—History—17th century.   3. England—
   Church history—17th century.
   I. Grell, Ole Peter.   II. Cunningham, Andrew, Dr.
   BT732.2.R45   1996
   610'.942'09032—dc20   96—2822
                                                                              CIP

ISBN 1 85928 339 X

Typeset in Sabon by Manton Typesetters, 5–7 Eastfield Road, Louth, Lincoln-shire, LN11 7AJ and printed in Great Britain by the Ipswich Book Company, Suffolk

Contents

Illustrations

Contributors

Harold J. Cook
Department of the History of Medicine, University of Wisconsin, Madison, USA

Andrew Cunningham
Wellcome Unit for the History of Medicine, University of Cambridge

Guido Giglioni
Faculty of Humanities, University of Macerata, Italy

Ole Peter Grell
Wellcome Unit for the History of Medicine, University of Cambridge

Anita Guerrini
Department of History, University of California, Santa Barbara, USA

David Harley
Wellcome Unit for the History of Medicine, University of Oxford

Michael Hunter
Department of History, Birkbeck College, University of London

Sarah Hutton
Wall Hall Campus, University of Hertfordshire

Mark Jenner
Department of History, University of York

Adrian Johns
Division of the Humanities and Social Sciences, California Institute of Technology, Pasadena, USA

Michael MacDonald
Department of History, University of Michigan, USA

Simon Schaffer
Department of History and Philosophy of Science, University of Cambridge

CHAPTER ONE

Introduction
Medicine and Religion in Seventeenth-Century England

Ole Peter Grell and Andrew Cunningham

Thomas (later Sir Thomas) Browne was the first to use the term *Religio Medici*, The Religion of a Physician, for the title of a book. Since its first appearance in 1642 there have been dozens who, like us, have found it irresistible to imitate the title for their own later books, either directly or indirectly.[1] This, however, is the first book since Thomas Browne's to exploit this title, which actually deals directly with the subject of the religion of physicians in the seventeenth century.

The last 30 years have seen the publication of numerous works demonstrating the importance of religion to the new investigations of nature in seventeenth-century England. In place of the old historical picture, inherited from the nineteenth century, of science advancing only as religion was beaten back to its supposedly rightful circumscribed sphere, we now have a more authentic picture of the development of natural knowledge being intimately and inseparably linked to, and inspired by, particular forms of religious belief and practice.

This historical interest has also been extended to medicine. In place of the old positivist story about the secularization of medical knowledge, and hence its advance in a simple progressive way, we have come to learn about the intimate relationship between religion and medicine at all levels in seventeenth-century England. Such historical work has made us aware of the deeply religious nature of attitudes to diseases and their causes and cures held by physicians and other practitioners, as well as by patients; this work has shown us how religious inspiration lay behind many innovations in the field of health-care provision and poor relief; it has likewise shown us the worrying religious implications to seventeenth-century man of new discoveries in anatomy. Hence it is generally accepted now that we cannot properly understand the medicine, its availability, its forms, its concerns, its social organization, unless we appreciate the deeply religious world and outlooks of seventeenth-century healers and their patients.[2] The relation of medicine and religion in seventeenth-century England is particularly important be-

cause of the dramatic changes in medical theory, practice and organization, which took place in the context of the religious and political
confrontations which destabilized English society for decades.

Hunter and Wootton have recently written that 'One of the great
differences between our world and that of our ancestors is the relatively
limited role that religion plays in modern society, and the extent to
which unbelief has come to seem rationally defensible and morally
respectable'.[3] It is certainly the case that the medical practitioner of
seventeenth-century England was terrified of atheism (in himself or
others) and greatly concerned with religion and religious orthodoxy,
both in his life and in his medicine, and it could be said that his religion
spilled over into his medicine and helped shape it. Thus while Thomas
Browne's book did not in itself make the religion of a physician into an
issue, its title certainly encapsulated a concern of all physicians and
medical men and women in seventeenth-century England.

The religious landscape of seventeenth-century England was intimately linked with political developments, from the period of the Elizabethan settlement in religion that James I inherited in the form of the
Anglican Church, to the effectual breakup of that church as the Puritan
movement flourished during the 1620s and 1630s, and right through
the Civil War and into the Commonwealth. With a restored monarchy
in 1660 came a restored Church of England, ruled by bishops of a
generally 'latitudinarian' persuasion.[4] After the so-called 'Glorious Revolution' of 1688–89, when James II was obliged to quit the throne as a
consequence of his Romanizing policies, the bishops of the Church of
England were particularly concerned (it has been argued) with accommodating Anglican doctrine to the findings of the 'new philosophy'.[5]
Physicians and other persons offering medical care were not just affected by these changes, but very much part of them.

Seventeenth-century England was also, of course, one of the European centres where the 'new philosophy' was created and developed.
Again, physicians were not just passively influenced by this, but actively
involved in it and helping shape it, and this is another theme of the
present book. One of the boldest characterizations of the developments
in natural philosophy comes from one of its participants who was a
physician, and who, as a student, deliberately sought out the advice of
Thomas Browne on how to train for medicine. Henry Power shared
Browne's views on many things, and borrows his concepts and phrases
wholesale in his work of 1664 on *Experimental Philosophy*. In particular he shared with Browne the view that God made this world to be
studied by man, and he lamented 'how few are there that perform this
homage due to their Creator'. Power claimed that such investigation is
not only desirable but also actually possible, since this world is not in

its last decline, as some people claim; how could that be, he asks, for 'he that made this great Automaton of the world, will not destroy it, till the slowest Motion therein has made one Revolution'. Our age, he claims, is not a decayed age but a most lively one:

> And this is the Age wherein all mens Souls are in a kind of fermentation, and the spirit of Wisdom and Learning begins to mount and free it self from those drossie and terrene Impediments wherewith it hath been so long clogg'd, and from the insipid phlegm and *Caput Mortuum* of useless Notions, in which it has endured so violent and long a fixation.
>   This is the Age wherein (methinks) Philosophy comes in with a Spring-tide; and the Peripateticks [that is, the followers of Aristotle] may as well hope to stop the Current of the Tide, or (with *Xerxes*) to fetter the Ocean, as hinder the overflowing of free Philosophy: Me-thinks, I see how all the old Rubbish must be thrown away, and the rotten Buildings be overthrown, and carried away with so powerful an Innundation. These are the days that must lay a new Foundation of a more magnificent Philosophy, never to be overthrown: that will Empirically and Sensibly canvass the *Phaenomena* of Nature, deducing the Causes of things from such Originals in Nature, as we observe are producible by Art, and the infallible demonstration of Mechanicks: and certainly, this is the way, and no other, to build a true and permanent Philosophy.[6]

Henry Power is speaking here, in explicitly Platonic and Paracelsian alchemical language, about the soul in its search for knowledge being freed from the natural philosophy built on the works of Aristotle (the 'old Rubbish'), and of it thus being able to begin to build new and more certain knowledge, 'a more magnificent' natural philosophy, one which will seek the causes of natural phenomena in nature, rather than in scholastic logic, and one which is confirmed by human ingenuity and experiment. He places all this within a view of the Christian's responsibility to God, and the working-out of the divine plan for the universe: for the Christian, natural knowledge is very much related to God. Power's statements here are of course as much propaganda as prophecy, but it certainly was the case that by the end of the seventeenth century the natural philosophy built on Aristotle had been challenged and replaced by a variety of alternatives. The alchemical and chemical natural philosophies of Paracelsus, Van Helmont and Robert Boyle, and the mechanist natural philosophies of René Descartes and then Isaac Newton, were each dominant for a while, and were adopted as the basis of one or other reformed versions of medicine in the course of the century. The adoption of each of these natural philosophies entailed particular religious positions.

A comprehensive account of the interrelation of medicine and religion in seventeenth-century England would almost be equivalent to a complete history of medicine in the period, and is obviously impossible here, but many facets of this constant, and constantly changing, relationship are explored in the chapters which follow. Our intention is that taken together these chapters will show something of the liveliness and diversity of the current state of studies of the multiple issues which were involved in the relation of religion and medicine in seventeenth-century England.[7]

We begin in the obvious place, with the views of Sir Thomas Browne himself. The literature on Browne is enormous but surprisingly there has hitherto been no study dedicated to Browne's views on nature and medicine and their relation to his religion. Sir Thomas was a firm member of the Church of England, and expressed his views on the proper religion of a physician at a time when that church was under great pressure from its Puritan wing. In investigating Browne's views of reason, nature and religion, Andrew Cunningham argues in Chapter 2 that the grounds on which Browne concluded that the Church of England was the true and best church for a Christian, are the same grounds on which he argued for the active involvement of the Christian in investigating nature, and in particular in questioning the *dicta* of authority. In both domains, Browne's quest was for the grounds of 'sure rational belief', and in both domains he called for the free deployment of one's God-given reason. Browne remained a member of the Church of England through the long dark days of the Civil War and Commonwealth, and his loyalty to the royal cause was eventually rewarded by a knighthood. *Religio Medici* has had an exceptionally enduring afterlife as an influential text, and the persistence of Browne's reputation as a physician who could be a model of tolerance in religion and an advocate of free investigation in nature, in particular as promoted by Sir William Osler, is traced by Cunningham into the nineteenth and twentieth centuries.

Astrology, which to the modern mind involves superstitious or at least non-rational belief, had been part of medicine for centuries, and indeed the academic physician had been routinely trained in assessing the past and future of disease from the moment when the patient took to his or her bed. In Chapter 4 Michael MacDonald shows how in the seventeenth century the horoscope was a tool in diagnosis and prognosis, just like uroscopy; it was acceptable to patients because it helped reassure them by relating their illnesses to the workings of the cosmos. But it was also always on the edge of being a black art, potentially invoking the devil himself, and thus subject to condemnation by the religiously orthodox. MacDonald looks at the flourishing of astrological medicine in the first half of the century, when it became a route to making a good living for practitioners who had not received a university degree, and at the range of complaints for which it was most employed. However, the Civil War and religious opposition led to the decline of astrological medicine (though not its disappearance) in the second half of the century, and its 'crumbling respectability', as MacDonald describes it, meant that this type of medicine was effectively finished by the 1720s.

The élite, university educated, physicians of the College of Physicians of London used astrology in their medicine to a greater or lesser degree, and considered themselves competent to examine astrological physicians. The College was essentially conservative in outlook, as befitted an institution established to police good medical practice. Although the membership of the College held a range of religious positions, Hal Cook's study of this institution and the religious affiliations of its members shows that they did not belong to the religious sects. Thus the College was vulnerable to attack from the sectarian radical practitioners such as the astrological and herbal practitioner Nicholas Culpeper, in the Civil War and Commonwealth periods. The generally conservative instincts of the physicians of the College made them more at home in the post-Restoration climate, though even then they were liable to have physicians intruded into the membership by the king on the grounds of their religious affiliation.

The practitioner of anatomy could find that his investigations led him into dangerous areas with respect to faith. In the Galenic system of medicine generally practised by university-trained physicians, the body was considered as the servant of the soul, and the presence of the soul was what conferred life (vitality) on the body and its parts. The question of quite what the relationship was between this somatic soul and the immortal soul of Christian man, was usually delicately sidestepped.[8] Nevertheless it was quite clear that if one proposed that life was *not* something imposed on the human body from outside, but was a characteristic or property of the parts themselves, or an emergent property of their interrelations, then one was liable to be accused of impiety or even heresy. Guido Giglioni, in Chapter 5 shows that such conclusions were drawn from his anatomical work by William Harvey, and that he was followed in such thinking by the celebrated anatomist of mid-century, Francis Glisson, who was not only the Regius Professor of Medicine at Cambridge but also the leading light in promoting anatomical investigation in the College of Physicians in the 1640s and 1650s. Both men came to such conclusions from considerable experience of practical anatomizing. Giglioni finds that, although Glisson produced his theory in order to confute the apparent Godlessness of Descartes's view of the body, yet his own view that matter – all matter – was alive was correctly perceived as heretical by the Cambridge

Platonists Henry More and Ralph Cudworth, and duly criticized by them.

Sir Thomas Browne was called to court in 1664 as an expert witness in a case of witchcraft. His opinion was that witches certainly exist, and that the evidence in the case showed the workings of witchcraft. Partly as a consequence of Browne's testimony the two accused women were found guilty and put to death. Physicians were often called on to give an opinion on whether extreme mental states were physical or spiritual in origin and, if spiritual, whether they were good or evil, the result of the prompting of the divine spirit or 'the deceiving spirit' (as Browne called the devil). In an age when many were claiming that their religious warrant came from an inner light, divinely installed, this was a problem. For how was one to tell in religious matters who was speaking the truth? The physician's knowledge of anatomy and of the workings of the mind could be used to resolve such issues. Of course the claim to have inner inspiration as authority for one's beliefs and actions, functions to circumvent the book or tradition as the primary source of authority, both directly in religion and also in medicine. In the first half of the seventeenth-century England Paracelsian and Helmontian physicians tended also to be 'enthusiasts' in their religion, and radical and egalitarian in their politics. The inner light, rather than traditional book learning, told them what the truth was. For those who adopted the Paracelsian or Helmontian approach, it was the spiritual forces at work in nature which the physician – divinely chosen – was harnessing in his medical activity, itself conceived of as assisting in completing God's work, especially in chemically drawing on the spiritual forces of vegetable and mineral ingredients to make drugs with active properties.

The dangers of 'enthusiasm' are Adrian Johns's theme in Chapter 6. The religious enthusiasts he studies claimed that their inspiring visions began from reading the Scriptures. How, in the eyes of their critics, could enthusiasts be correctly reading the Scriptures, if the effect was for them to hallucinate false visions? Were they suffering the 'distempers of a disaffected brain'? Johns therefore explores seventeenth-century arguments for the relation between the reading of scripture, the human body and the soul, all of which centred on theories of the passions. He draws attention in particular to the work of the Anglican physician and anatomist Thomas Willis and his research on the structure and functioning of the brain, of the nerves, and of the relevance of this research to the question of enthusiasm.

Miracles, Thomas Browne had written in *Religio Medici* (hereafter *RM*) are

> the extraordinary effect of the hand of God, to which all things are
> an equal facility; and to create the world as easy as one single

creature. For this is also a miracle, not only to produce effects
against, or above Nature, but before Nature ... I hold that God can
do all things, how he should work contradictions I do not understand, yet dare not therefore deny.

(*RM*, I.27)

Had the age of miracles passed? Did God still convey special messages
to the faithful through miraculous phenomena? Did the physician have
a role in accounting for or caring for people undergoing miraculous
interventions? Simon Schaffer, writing in Chapter 7, discusses the case
of a young girl who, during the Restoration crisis of enthusiasm and
dissent, went without food or drink for months at a stretch, with her
abstention being monitored by relays of observers. Was this the evidence of divine energy in her? Was it a simple fraud? Physicians were
called on to give their opinion, and their right to give an opinion was
also disputed, for it was maintained by some that this was a phenomenon of spiritual, not physical, origin. The central body of the new
philosophy, the Royal Society, was also co-opted. As Schaffer writes, 'a
range of commentators turned Taylor's case into their own'. Schaffer
explores the local political and religious context of the controversy –
how the interpretation of the girl's condition was contested by spokes-
persons of different religious persuasions – and shows that the passionate responses to the fasting girl indicate that even if this episode of
prodigious abstinence was not a miracle it was clearly a wonder.

The precise correlation between particular religious commitment and
medical philosophy did not necessarily remain constant as the political
and religious complexion of the country changed in the course of the
century. After the Restoration the Helmontian position, hitherto almost
exclusively the province of radical Puritan practitioners, could be taken
up by royalist, Anglican physicians, as the example of George Thomson
shows. Ole Peter Grell (Chapter 8) shows that even after the Restoration the issue was still about different medical philosophies, different
physical remedies, different religious ideologies. The great plague of
London during 1665 gave the Helmontian physicians the ideal occasion
for a trial of their 'chymical physick' against that of the Galenist physicians of the College of Physicians. It was a contest between those seeing
themselves as true Christian physicians against those they portrayed as
heathens whose medical interventions were part of Satan's plot to destroy mankind. Grell examines the dissection that Thomson undertook
of a body which had died of plague, in order to find the cause of the
disease, and shows how this act of dissecting was as religiously oriented
an event as it was a medical one, especially since Thomson both caught
and cured himself of plague in the course of it, using remedies prepared
by his godly chemical physic. For Thomson, the adoption of the correct

medical approach could serve to make men more religious; even atheism could be lessened in this way. Moreover, in his Anglicanism and his
eirenicism Thomson's religious attitudes in the Restoration period are
unexpectedly reminiscent of those of Thomas Browne in the 1640s,
even though their attitudes to the College of Physicians and medical
authorities were quite different. Grell discovers a link between the two
medical and religious worlds of Browne and Thomson in the Arminianism
of Thomson's patron, Bishop Sheldon.

Francis Mercurius van Helmont, the son of the great Jan Baptista van
Helmont, was active as a physician in England in the 1670s, when he
attended Lady Anne Conway, one of the most highly educated, intelli-
gent and philosophical women of the period. In Chapter 9 Sarah Hutton
shows that, whether or not he was successful in alleviating her pain, Van
Helmont was the most successful, and certainly the most *sympathique*
of the long roster of famous physicians who attended her in her pursuit
of treatment for her chronic head pain. The younger Van Helmont was
recommended to Lady Anne by her relative Henry More, the Cambridge Platonist. Van Helmont believed that 'whatever is, is a Spirit'.
Van Helmont's influence was such as to convince Lady Anne to convert
to Quakerism, and to study the Kabbala. Hutton argues that Van
Helmont, her medical attendant, profoundly influenced Lady Anne's
philosophical opinions as expressed in her posthumous book, such that
she came to embrace monistic vitalism, and that her own experience of
continual pain may have contributed to her rejection of both dualism
and materialism in understanding the relation of God to the operations
of the universe He created.

Amongst those many people, both physicians and laypersons, from
whom Lady Anne Conway had desperately sought medicine was Robert
Boyle. Boyle was the dominant figure in the early Royal Society, and his
concerns with the making of matters of fact and with the appropriate
relation between private and public knowledge in the development of
the new philosophy, have been of great recent interest to scholars.
Michael Hunter's chapter on the man he terms 'The reluctant philan-
thropist' discusses Boyle's long-term interest in medicine, in the making
of new medicines and in making them public for the common good. But
Boyle was not a physician, and Hunter explores Boyle's resultant ambivalent attitude to the members of the medical profession and their
claimed monopoly of medical innovation, and contrasts it with his deep
religious conviction that for the true Christian one of the central duties
was to engage in the Christian act of mercy of helping heal the sick, as
Christ himself had done. Boyle proves to be an ideal figure to study the
issues involved and the anxiety aroused at the intersection between
religiously inspired attitudes towards medical charity on the one hand,

and the demands of the new philosophy on the other. Moreover, the issues of social class, of how it was proper for a gentleman to behave and what it was proper for a gentleman to do for the vulgar, are shown, in the case of the Honourable Robert Boyle, to cut across these other concerns with religious charity and the development of natural knowledge, just as they had done earlier in the case of Sir Thomas Browne.

The existence of disease and suffering in a world regulated by a benign and providential God has repeatedly been a thorny point for Christians. What was the function of disease when it struck the godly, what was God's message to the godly, and what should be their response? Moreover, did the particular religious affiliation of patients affect their attitudes to disease and healing? David Harley argues that it was crucial. In Chapter 11 he portrays the attitudes and experiences to health and disease of two Presbyterian families, the Henrys and the Newcomes, over a period of some 60 years from 1650. For these Presbyterians, affliction was sent by God as a correction for sin, even to the godly, and it was their view that the soul needed affliction for its own improvement and discipline. Harley quotes Philip Henry as writing 'Take away the cause, and the effect will cease. When the patient becomes a penitent, see what a blessed change follows'. Yet the godly patient also had an obligation to care for his or her health and to seek secular remedies once he or she was visited by disease. Medicines worked by God's grace, and were the means not the cause of recovery. In tracing the intricacies of the Presbyterian attitude to illness, Harley draws attention to the shift, late in the century, from viewing God as afflicting the individual personally, to seeing Him as ruling through a more general providence, which was to bring with it a change in the perceived immediacy of the relation of the afflicted individual to God's correcting and admonishing hand.

On the publication of his *Principia* in 1687, Isaac Newton found that his work was immediately applied to explaining the functioning of the human body and to medicine. Most of those involved in applying Newtonian theory to medicine and anatomy, and who between them produced a great deal of new work, were Scots living and working in England, followers of the Scottish Episcopalian physician Archibald Pitcairne. Unlike historians of the last century or so, Newton's contemporaries and successors recognized that, for Newton, force was God's means of action in the world, and that Newton's system of the universe was an account of the constant and immediate operations of God – not of the operations of the God-less universe, as it was later to be transformed into. The physicians who adopted it also recognized its theological implications. Anita Guerrini, in Chapter 12, argues that those studying Newtonian physic as well as those studying Newtonian physics had by the 1720s transformed this into an essentially deist position, in which God is neither constantly active in His universe, nor does this deity necessarily have the attributes of the Christian God. George Cheyne was the most religious-minded of such followers, but the religious dimensions of his synthesis were largely ignored. The Newtonianization of anatomy and medicine may thus, perhaps, be seen as the dying gasp of providentialism.

In the 1720s an eccentric clergyman, the Reverend John Hancocke, said that the new theories of the Newtonian physicians had not replaced the efficacy of a little innocent experiment in medicine. In the last years of the seventeenth century Hancocke had accidentally performed such an experiment by drinking cold water in a fever and thus curing himself. Years later he revealed this secret to the world. This irresistibly entertaining story is told by Mark Jenner in the final chapter. Hancocke's claims proved very popular, and hence had to be disposed of by the medical profession. What they claimed was that the well-being of the body is no business of the guardians of the well-being of the soul: a clergyman speaking about medicine is no better than a quack. Indeed, reaching for *ad hominem* invective, they derided him as an 'enthusiast', one deluded by false visions. In his conclusions, Jenner draws our attention to the significance of this continuing association of (religious) enthusiasm with (medical) quackery into the eighteenth century, and underlines how, in our search to understand the changes in the practice, availability, delivery and nature of medicine in seventeenth- and eighteenth-century England, we need to give at least as much attention to the role of religion as to that of the medical market-place. These make suitable conclusions for the present volume too. The links between medicine and religion continued strongly into the eighteenth and nineteenth centuries, and we hope to explore these in subsequent volumes.

Notes

1. For a listing of these see Geoffrey Keynes, *A Bibliography of Sir Thomas Browne Kt., M.D.*, Oxford, Clarendon Press, 1968, Appendix I, 'Religio Medici: Imitators', pp. 231–58.
2. Among the most important such works are: Charles Webster, 'English Medical Reformers of the Puritan Revolution: A Background to the "Society of Chymical Physitians"', *Ambix*, 1967, 14, 16–41; Charles Webster, *The Great Instauration: Science, Medicine and Reform, 1626–1660*, London, Duckworth, 1975; Piyo Rattansi, 'Paracelsus and the Puritan Revolution', *Ambix*, 1963, 11, 23–32; Piyo Rattansi, 'The Helmontian-Galenist Controversy in Restoration England', *Ambix*, 1964, 12, 1–23; Walter Pagel, *Paracelsus: An Introduction to Philosophical Medicine in the Era of the Renaissance*, (2nd edn) Basle, Karger, 1982; Allen G. Debus, *The English*

Paracelsians, London, Oldbourne, 1965; many of the essays in Roger French and Andrew Wear (eds), *The Medical Revolution of the Seventeenth Century*, Cambridge, Cambridge University Press, 1989, make significant contributions to the issues. On the sixteenth-century background to the religious basis of health-care provision for the poor, including England, and to the effect of different confessional positions on medicine respectively, see Ole Peter Grell and Andrew Cunningham (eds), *Health Care Provision and Poor Relief in Northern Protestant Europe, 1500-1700*, London, Routledge, 1996, and Ole Peter Grell and Andrew Cunningham (eds), *Medicine and the Reformation*, London, Routledge, 1993.

3. Michael Hunter and David Wootton (eds), *Atheism from the Reformation to the Enlightenment*, Oxford, Clarendon, 1992, Introduction.

4. D.R. Hutton, *The Restoration: A Political and Religious History of England and Wales 1658–1667*, Oxford, Clarendon Press, 1985.

5. James R. Jacob and Margaret C. Jacob, 'The Anglican Origins of Modern Science: The Metaphysical Foundations of the Whig Constitution', *Isis*, 71, (1980), 251–67.

6. H. Power, *Experimental Philosophy, in Three Books: Containing New Experiments Microscopical, Mercurial, Magnetical* ... , London, 1664, repr. 1966, M.B. Hall (ed.), New York, Johnson Reprint Corporation. All quotations are from the Conclusion, pp. 183, 189 and 192.

7. As the editors, we are all too aware that there are many other relevant themes that it was not possible to include in the present volume. Among those that come immediately to mind and on which there has been recent scholarly work are midwifery and man-midwifery; popular medicine; magic and medicine; faith healing; charitable medical institutions; Poor Law provision; the physician role forced on the ministers ejected in the 1660s; and amongst individuals, Greatrakes the Stroker, and Thomas Sydenham.

8. On this issue see Vivian Nutton, 'The Anatomy of the Soul in Early Renaissance Medicine', in G.R. Dunstan (ed.), *The Human Embryo: Aristotle and the Arabic and European Traditions*, Exeter, University of Exeter Press, 1990, pp. 136–57.

CHAPTER TWO

Sir Thomas Browne and his *Religio Medici*: Reason, Nature and Religion

Andrew Cunningham

The man, his mind and his brain

Sir Thomas Browne was the first to use the expression *Religio Medici* for the title of a book. Ever since its first publication in 1642 his little book has claimed an attention out of all proportion to its size. It made the religion of physicians an issue, and made Browne himself the most famous physician to have had a religion. It has in recent centuries generally been interpreted as a brave and laudable call for toleration in religion, put forward in a period of great religious strife, and simultaneously as an argument for the compatibility of devout Christian faith with the free investigation of nature. Thus in the twentieth century Sir Thomas is presented as a physician who on the one hand was tolerant in the domain of religion, and who on the other also claimed that faith and reason – for which people have read religion and science (in the modern sense of that term) – are separate domains which can and should take their proper, complementary roles in one's understanding of the structure and functioning of the universe. This view of *Religio Medici*, and of its author's attitudes to reason, nature and religion will all be explored in this chapter.

Browne has fascinated many scholars, and there are many possible legitimate ways of exploring his thinking and writing to bring out different facets of this complex man. By far the greatest scholarly interest in Browne's writings today is sustained by students of English literature, and he is by some considered to possess one of the best styles of any writer of the seventeenth century: one modern critic has suggested it is 'possibly the most beautiful English prose that has been written'.[1] The Romantics loved his style. Charles Lamb described it as 'obscure but gorgeous'; Coleridge wrote that 'the style throughout is delicious';[2] De Quincey thought his rhetoric was 'deep, tranquil, and majestic as Milton'.[3] Browne's writing is fantastical, rhetorical, complex, ornate, baroque, extravagant, exquisite, paradoxical (very), devious, ecstatic, playful, whimsical even. These qualities were deliberate, for Browne worked hard at his prose style. In his own age his style and literary mannerisms meant he was taken as a writer of great *wit*, meaning primarily not humour but a sort of admirable cleverness.[4] Although Stanley Fish managed to put the cat amongst the pigeons with his dismissive remarks on Browne's literary achievement a few years ago, Browne's reputation has since been retrieved by literary scholars.[5] I mention these literary qualities at the beginning, because although Browne's prose will appear frequently in the course of the chapter its merits *as* prose will not be a direct concern of mine here. It is important to acknowledge that in the case of Browne above all, the medium is a great part of the message (which is very appropriate for the man who coined the English term 'literary').[6] But it is also important to remember that the medium is not the whole message. What Browne is saying about the religion of a particular physician – himself – in the England of the early seventeenth century is at least as significant as the sonority of the language in which he says it.

It is irresistible when discussing Thomas Browne to quote him constantly, both in and out of context, and thus catch his voice which says such quotable things and in such quotable ways. But although the persona is dominant, Browne is actually rather elusive as a person-in-the-text, for even though it is written largely in the first person it nevertheless remains tantilizingly 'open but inscrutable',[7] and perhaps deliberately so, Browne believing that it is not open to the vulgar to see inside the minds of the wise.[8] So it is also irresistible with Thomas Browne to start by trying to catch his image. The portraits, one hopes, might give one a view of Sir Thomas which is solid and dependable. But, even in his portraits he may be elusive too. For as Joseph Heller has taught us in *Picture This*, paintings can have many afterlives. This picture (Figure 2.1), now in the National Portrait Gallery, has had a number of identities in the twentieth century alone, portraying at least two different sets of people, and painted by three different artists. In 1922 it was a picture of Charles I and his queen, Henrietta Maria, and was by Van Dyck. Later it was of Sir Thomas Browne and his wife, painted from life by Joan Carlile. Now it is of Sir Thomas Browne and his wife, and the painter has become anonymous. *If* this is Thomas Browne then, as he wrote in *Religio Medici*: 'The face reveals the soul; there are mystically in our faces certain characters which carry in them the motto of our souls, wherein he that cannot read A.B.C. may read our natures'. But Browne also wrote, and in the same book, it is different in pictures: 'in a portrait, things are not truly, but in equivocal shapes' (*RM*, I.12).

But there is another way for us to see Browne in, one might nearly say, the flesh, and that is through his death. Death is a great concern of

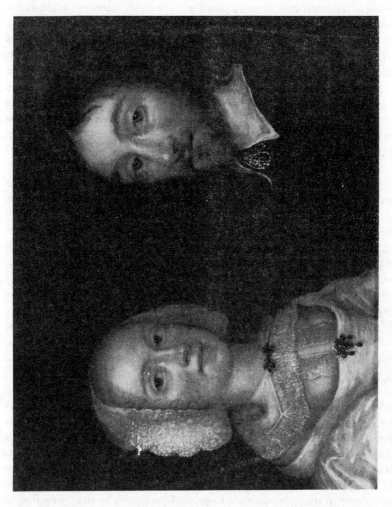

2.1 Portrait of Sir Thomas Browne and his wife Dorothy.

Browne's, and he writes about it a great deal in *Religio Medici*. Indeed, as we shall see, that book is in part a meditation upon death, and the Christian's response to it. Browne calls himself 'as wholesome a morsel for the worms as any' (*RM*, I.40), and he talks about wanting to quit the world and leave no memorial behind him. 'At my death', he writes, 'I mean to take a total adieu of the world, not caring for a monument, history or epitaph, not so much as the bare memory of my name to be found anywhere but in the universal register of God' (*RM*, I.41). In *Urn Burial* he asked rhetorically 'Who knows the fate of his [own] bones or how often he is to be buried?' In his own case the answer to this curious question was, twice; for his fate was to have his skull removed from his grave and at large in the world for almost 80 years, long after he had died. And the consequence of this, in turn, was that his skull and the fantastical brain which had been within it came to be investigated more thoroughly and more scientifically than, perhaps, that of any other seventeenth-century figure, in order, in part, to investigate the seat of his genius. The results were, as he might have liked, paradoxical in the extreme. As we shall see later, Sir Thomas's skull in its afterlife would again serve as a focus of the question of the relationship of religion and physicians, by serving as a quasi-religious icon for physicians in the early twentieth century.

What happened was this.[9] Sir Thomas Browne was buried in the church of St Peter Mancroft in Norwich in 1682 and for 158 years his body, like that of a later Brown, lay a-mouldering in its grave. Then, in 1840, the coffin was accidentally disturbed. His coffin-plate was found to say, in Latin, that 'sleeping in this coffin, by the dust of his alchemical body he converts the lead into gold',[10] and one of those who saw it claimed that the lead of the coffin had been 'completely decomposed and changed into a carbonate which crumbled at the touch', so there might indeed have been an alchemy of some kind at work here. When the coffin was opened, a local paper reported that the features of Sir Thomas Browne 'were perfect, and especially the beard'. But the next week a witness begged to correct this: 'such was not the case, nothing more was found than in ordinary instances, the bones being perfectly bare; the skull was of the finest conformation, the forehead being beautifully developed'. But the next week another witness claimed that the beard *had* been in a good state of preservation 'and of a fine auburn colour'; moreover, the forehead was not 'beautifully developed' as it had been the week before, but 'remarkably small and depressed; the head unusually long'. The editor of the rival Norfolk weekly paper reported that the beard did indeed exist 'profuse and perfect', while the forehead 'was remarkably low, but the back of the cranium exhibited an unusual degree of capaciousness'. Quite remarkably it was also reported that the brain was still present, 'considerable in quantity but changed to a state of *adipocere* – resembling ointment of a dark brown hue'. This is remarkable, because *adipocere*, 'grave wax', is the one thing Sir Thomas Browne supposedly was the first to discover (he discusses it in *Urn Burial*). The obsessive concern of local observers with the shape of the skull seems to have been due to a recent visit to Norwich of a lecturer on phrenology.

Meanwhile someone filched the skull, and the coffin was resealed before it could be returned. After spending five years in mysterious circumstances, the skull was presented to the Norfolk and Norwich Hospital Museum in 1845. There it stayed for many years. The church-wardens of St Peter Mancroft continued to be anxious to rebury the skull with the body. In 1922 the authorities at the Norfolk and Norwich Hospital Museum decided that before they gave the skull back they wanted it scientifically investigated. So they sent it by special messenger to the Royal College of Surgeons in London. Sir Arthur Keith, Conservator of the Surgeons' Museum, and forger of Piltdown Man, was to do the job. Sir Arthur was still hoping for a scientific – an evolutionary – science of phrenology. 'It was my ambition', Sir Arthur said, 'to make the skull of Sir Thomas Browne a text from which I might preach a sermon concerning the forces which mould the skull and brain into their several forms, and to illustrate the methods I had devised to measure and elucidate the nature of the forces which are involved'.[11] He was indeed to speak about this issue a couple of years later (though rather inconclusively), but illness meant Sir Arthur had to pass the investigative task to a student of Karl Pearson, Miriam Tildesley. She had, according to Keith, 'been trained in the exact methods of the Biometric Laboratory of University College [London], and had already made an excellent contribution to the literature of racial craniology'.[12]

Miriam Tildesley was interested in the study of skulls in order to study racial characters. But she also thought that the study of the skull of someone like Sir Thomas Browne might tell us something about the mind of the man, and in such a case 'we know the cranial cavity from our casts, and the mind of the man from his books'.[13] Are there valid correlations between, for instance, a receding chin and weak character or between a receding brow and low mentality? This was the problem Tildesley confronted: the association of 'the low forehead of Sir Thomas Browne with the high intellectual capacity he evidences'.[14] Sir Thomas might be said to have been prophetically sympathetic to such an experiment, for in *Urn Burial* he had written that 'the dimensions of the head measure the whole body, and the figure thereof gives conjecture of the principall faculties; Physiognomy outlives our selves, and ends not in our graves'.[15]

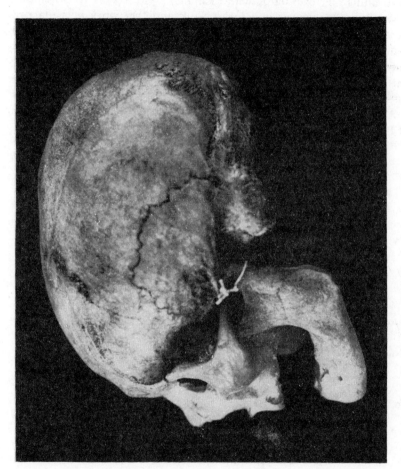

2.2   Lateral profile of the skull of Sir Thomas Browne.

Detailed measurement of Sir Thomas Browne's skull, and comparison
with the skulls of series of seventeenth-century males led Tildesley to
conclude that yes, the forehead of Sir Thomas's skull was somewhat
low by comparison with other males, and yes again the back of the
head was significantly broader than usual (Figures 2.2 and 2.3). Thus
her conclusion ultimately had to be that 'the correlation of superficial
head and brain characters with mentality is so low as to provide no
basis for any prognosis of value'.[16] So after all the work in the laboratory, Sir Thomas Browne, paradoxically, remains a man of intellect and
genius – a highbrow – even though in cranial terms he was unmistakably a lowbrow. As Coleridge wrote about Browne in a slightly different context: 'In short, he has brains in his head, which is all the more
interesting for a *little twist* in the brains'![17]

After this last adventure in the laboratory, the skull was reinterred in
St Peter Mancroft, where it remains today.

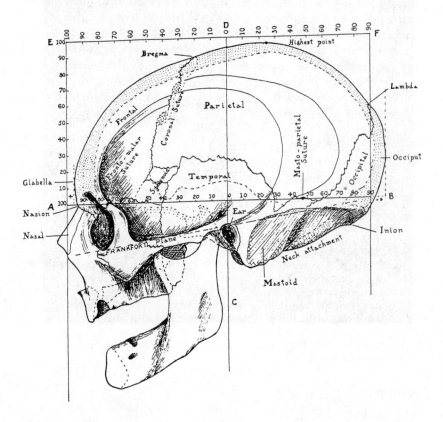

2.3   Drawing of lateral profile of the skull of Sir Thomas Browne.

'A miracle of thirty years': the life and the book

Was Sir Thomas Browne's life as interesting as his afterlife? Not according to Lytton Strachey, who wrote that 'Everyone knows that Browne was a physician who lived at Norwich in the seventeenth century; and, so far as regards what one must call, for want of a better term, his "life", that is a sufficient summary of all there is to know'.[18] But other commentators have seen Browne's life, though short on incident, as nevertheless full of interest.[19]

Thomas Browne was born in London, son of a mercer and his wife, in 1605. He had very early memories of simpling for plants and seeing a comet. Tom Browne's schooldays were spent at Winchester, and he was an undergraduate at Broadgates Hall, Oxford – transformed while he was there into Pembroke College – where, as part of the necessary study for the degree he would have read natural philosophy from Aristotelian texts. He took his BA in 1626, his MA in 1629. Then, in 1630, he started the peregrinations necessary to construct an up-to-date medical education for himself, going (it is believed) to Montpellier, then Padua, and finally to Leiden where he graduated in medicine in 1633. He took the opportunity to acquire languages on his journeys: 'besides the Jargon and Patois of several provinces, I understand no less than six Languages', he says in a passage celebrating the fact that he has escaped 'the first and father sin ... Pride' (*RM*, II.7). The languages were French, Italian, Spanish, Portuguese, Dutch and Danish (the Danish was to be very important), not to mention Latin which he spoke fluently, and he also had Greek and Hebrew. These travels Browne really seems to have enjoyed. As he wrote in *Religio Medici*:

> I am of a constitution so general that it consorts and sympathises with all things; I have no antipathy, or rather Idiosyncrasy, in diet, humour, air, anything; I wonder not at the French for their dishes of frogs, snails and toadstools, nor at the Jews for locusts and grass-hoppers [presumably he is here referring to the occasional diet of the Jews mentioned in the Old Testament], but being amongst them, make my common viands; and I find they agree with my stomach as well as theirs ... [Similarly] national repugnances do not touch me, nor do I behold with prejudice the French, Italian, Spaniard or Dutch; but where I find their actions in balance with my countrymen's, I honour, love, and embrace them in the same degree ... All places, all airs, make unto me one country; I am in England everywhere and under any meridian ...
>
> (*RM*, II.1).

Returned to England, Browne seems first to have gone into medical practice in Oxfordshire. It is here that he is thought to have composed *Religio Medici*, as it seems to have been finished before October 1635, since he wrote in it 'as yet I have not seen one revolution of Saturn, nor hath my pulse beat thirty years' (*RM*, I.41), and he makes reference to visiting patients (*RM*, II.6).

He incorporated MD at Oxford in 1637; by which time he had already moved to Norwich, at the exhortation of his old Oxford tutor, Dr Lushington, recently appointed chaplain to the Bishop of Norwich, and Browne settled in practice there, where he could 'imbibe the pure Aerial Nitre' of East Anglian air,[20] and here he was to remain for the rest of his life. Norwich, of course, was at that date the second city of the kingdom after London. In 1641, aged 36, Browne took a 19-year-old bride, and although in *Religio Medici* he had expressed the wish that humans could procreate like trees – without coition – he nevertheless immediately proceeded to start a family of 12 children, of whom six survived to adulthood.

At this point, in 1642, a London printer, Andrew Crooke, printed, without Browne's knowledge, a first edition and a second (corrected) edition of *Religio Medici*, from a manuscript copy circulating amongst and beyond Browne's circle of friends. The work was put out without an author named, and the printer gave the work an entirely appropriate engraved title-page. Even before Browne knew about this publication the Catholic virtuoso, Sir Kenelm Digby, under arrest by the Parliamentary army in Southwark, was recommended to read it by his patron, the Earl of Dorset, and in two amazing feats he read the book in a sitting (having already gone to bed), and then wrote a 124 printed-page (16 pp. MSS) commentary or Animadversions on it the next day and night.

When Browne learnt of the publication of his work, he produced a corrected, or at least authorized, version which was put out by the same printer in 1643. The title-page was the same (except for the date) (see Figure 2.4). It shows what is probably an Icarus-figure seeking to reach heaven by his own efforts, and in his fall being rescued by the hand of God.[21] The man calls out: '*a caelo salus*': 'salvation from heaven'.[22] The hand of God and His fingers – most especially His little finger[23] – feature largely in *Religio Medici*, guiding the life of the true Christian and divine providence. Ardolino points out that reference is probably also being made to the healing capacities of God's hand: 'In short, the numinous Hand of God represents divine providence, healing, and salvation'.[24] In particular, and this is significant in Browne's case, falling from the rock has an ancient Stoic meaning: to plummet from tranquillity, steadfastness and self-control into the storms of tempestuousness and despair; Christian symbolism used the same image of falling from the rock to express the loss of salvation by falling from God's church.[25] All in all the picture makes a nice summary of many of the themes of the book.

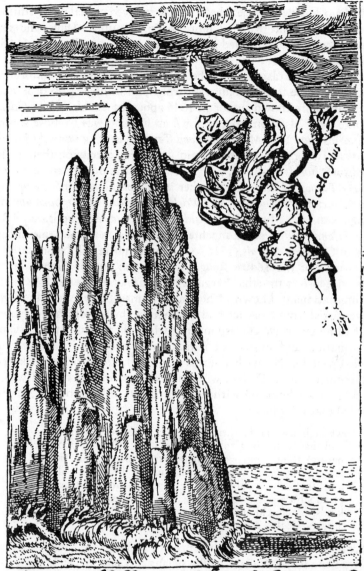

2.4   Title-page of the first edition of *Religio Medici*.

Religio Medici became a bestseller. It received a total of 12 editions in Browne's life-time, with 62 more in English up to 1966, and several since. It was first translated into Latin in 1644, into Dutch in 1665 and into French in 1668.[26]

Having had a taste of published authorship thrust upon him, Browne published three further significant works, all in English, and became an internationally known author. In 1646 appeared *Pseudodoxia Epidemica*, a large work also commonly known as *Vulgar Errors*, whose subtitle is *Enquiries into Very Many Received Tenents, and Commonly Presumed Truths*. Two rather more esoteric works appeared together in 1658: *Hydriotaphia: Urne-Burial or, a Brief Discourse of the Sepulchral Urnes Lately Found in Norfolk*, together with *The Garden of Cyrus or, the Quincunciall, Lozenge, or Net-Work Plantations of the Ancients, Artificially, Naturally, Mystically Considered*. Posthumously appeared *A Letter to a Friend* (1690), and a much extended version of the same under the title of *Christian Morals* (1716). Our concern here will be primarily with the works of the 1640s: *Religio Medici* and *Vulgar Errors*, but with reference also to the ethical arguments of *Christian Morals*.[27]

Internationally known as he was, Thomas Browne hardly seems to have stirred from Norwich and Norfolk for the rest of his life. However, he had an extensive correspondence with other learned men, swapping information and objects of natural-historical interest. Moreover, he built up at his Norwich home a large collection and a workshop of experiments. John Evelyn, who had been in correspondence with him over his own book on gardens, visited him in October 1671. He recorded that Browne's

> whole house and Garden being a Paradise and Cabinet of rarities, and that of the best collection, especially Medails, books, Plants, natural things, did exceedingly refresh me ... Sir Thomas had amongst other curiosities, a collection of the Eggs of all the foule and birds he could procure, that Country (especially the promontorys of Norfolck) being (as he said) frequented with severall kinds, which seldome or never, go farther into the Land, as Cranes, Storkes, Eagles, &c, and variety of Water foule.[28]

Through his fame as an author Browne received the Honorary Fellowship of the Royal College of Physicians in London 1664. Towards the end of his life Browne's quiet support of the royalist position had its accidental reward. In 1671, after the Restoration, Charles II made a visit to Norwich, where a dolphin was dissected in his honour.[29] It occurred to the king to mark his visit by conferring an impromptu knighthood on some worthy and loyal citizen. The mayor declining the honour, Thomas Browne was lighted on as Norwich's internationally famous author, and knighted.

Religio Medici is a personal document, 'an exercise to myself' as Browne says in the Preface, written for the eyes of its author and, as its highly wrought style indicates, written with the expectation that it would reach the eyes of others too. It is a personal credo, a musing on what the author believes with respect to the Christian religion, and on the grounds on which he believes it. Since Browne was the master of the linguistic conceit we can expect the title to have had multiple meanings. The first phrases of the long opening sentence of the book show Browne drawing attention to the double theme of the book: the fact that he could be held doubly guilty of atheism. So this book on the religion of a physician starts by raising the issue of this physician having no religion:

> For my Religion, though there be several circumstances that might persuade the world I have none at all, as the general scandal of my profession, the natural course of my studies, the indifferency of my behaviour and discourse in matters of Religion, neither violently defending one, nor with that common ardour and contention op-posing another: yet in despite hereof I dare, without usurpation, assume the honourable style of a Christian ...
>
> (*RM*, I.1)

Yet, Browne claims, he dares assume the honourable style of a Christian, and the rest of the book concerns the grounds on which he does so. The book thus takes the reader from suspected double atheism to the author's firm Christianity.

One of its very earliest readers, Sir Kenelm Digby, correctly remarked to Browne that *Religio Medici* 'is of so weighty subjects, and so strongly penned, as requireth much time and sharp attention but to comprehend it'.[30] Many commentators have even despaired of locating any principle of structure in the text. It is probably impossible adequately to summa-rize *Religio Medici* (I have tried). For it is not a closely argued treatise, nor a piece of polemic, but a sequence of linked thoughts. However, it is recognized nowadays by some historians that the book is organized round the successive themes of faith, hope and charity.[31] As a cluster of themes these were, of course, first brought together by St Paul in I Corinthians 13: 11–13. St Paul's context is a discussion of charity and of the veils, or dark glass, of knowledge in this life, compared to the afterlife, all of which is highly pertinent for Browne's message in *Religio Medici*:

> When I was I child, I spake as a child, I understood as a child, I thought as a child: but when I became a man I put away childish things. For now we see as through a glass, darkly; but then face to face: now I know in part; but then shall I know even as also I am known. And now abideth faith, hope, charity, these three; but the greatest of these is charity.
>
> (I Corinthians 13: 11–13)

For a good Christian like Browne, of course, hope is about death and the prospect of an afterlife; hence death takes up a great deal of *Religio Medici*. This faith-hope-charity structure of *Religio Medici* is itself part of Browne's argument: for it announces that these are the proper concerns of the good Christian. That in this world we see only 'as through a glass darkly', is in particular a key to his view of the roles of reason and faith, of authority and experiment, in religion as much as in the exploration of nature.

The Religion ...

Browne's Christian philosophy

Interpretations by historians of Browne's religious position have been extraordinarily diverse, with the most common views being directly contradictory: that he either had *no* serious religious commitment, or that *everything* was religious for him, including the supposed 'science'. One commentator, Dewey Ziegler, has suggested that Browne had an 'indifference to truth', that he did not really believe anything about religion: he couldn't, because 'the science Browne was practising cut off nature from the divine'. Thus Browne has only a 'religious imagination' severed from dogma and hence severed from the real problems of his day. His religious position is thus, in Ziegler's opinion, purely 'aesthetic', and Browne is simply amused by the paradoxes evident in religion. Hence Ziegler can take literally Browne's phrase about living in 'divided and distinguished worlds', and read one of them as a world of *both* reason and belief (nature, science), and the other as mere amused aesthetics (religion).[32] By contrast, Stanley Fish claims the opposite: that 'Browne's commitment to the devaluing of rational thought and the subsequent exaltation of knowledge through faith is evident on every page'.[33]

It is also particularly striking how frequently commentators have chosen to see Browne as making some kind of out-of-time or eternal statement. Joan Webber, for example, has suggested that *Religio Medici* is a work so personal that it is remote from the religious and political concerns of the day. She says:

> Written in 1634 and published in 1642, the *Religio Medici* has civil war for its context, but we only know that because we know its dates ... Active in the world though [its first readers, the Earl of Dorset and Sir Kenelm Digby] were, these good Royalists saw nothing to criticize in Browne's abstraction from the world.[34]

Yet it is in fact quite clear that Browne has a position on religious and political matters – not a non-position – and the exigencies of religious and political affairs called his expression of this position into being. It was certainly clear to contemporaries that *Religio Medici* dealt with controversial issues, and that it took strong positions on a number of important matters. In their instant responses, both the Catholic virtuoso Sir Kenelm Digby and the Protestant Alexander Ross (schoolmaster, pedant and anatomy writer) thought it needed taking down a peg or two. Ross in particular attacked Browne's apparent tolerance of Catholics: 'if our faith be all one with that of Rome: this may indeed be *religio Medici*, the religion of the House of *Medicis*, not the Church of *England*'.[35]

All three of the organizing themes of *Religio Medici* (faith, hope and charity) were potentially controversial, since what Browne said about hope and death, and of the fate of the soul and body after death, and about man's duties of charity in this world, was of as great interest to the atheist-hunters as what he said about faith. The figures assembled by D.C. Allen, the genial historian of intolerance, indicate that, taking Europe as a whole, throughout the sixteenth and seventeenth centuries there was an average of one published attack on atheists every 30 days. Browne was to be accused of expressing atheistic opinions in *Religio Medici* in his own time and in later years of the seventeenth century by self-appointed atheist-hunters, but he was usually let off with a caution.[36]

This period when Browne was writing his *Religio*, up to and including the time (1643) it was published with his collaboration, was when the struggle was at its height between the 'high' Church of England and the Puritans: between the extremes of the Roman Catholic Council of Trent and the Calvinist Synod of Dort, as Browne saw it. William Laud had been made Archbishop of Canterbury in 1633, and the Puritans in England were vociferous against his policy of 'thorough', that is, of purging Puritans from clerical livings, and ensuring that Puritan practices in church arrangement (such as removing the altar from the east end) and worship (the rejection of the cross in baptism, etc.) were rooted out, and the uniformity of Church of England practices followed. To Puritans this threatened the restoration of popery. In 1641, in the early meetings of the Long Parliament, the members, heavily Puritan and Presbyterian, were talking passionately about abolishing the bishops and the Book of Common Prayer, basic elements of the Church of England. Laud, guiding star of the Church of England, was impeached in 1641, eventually to be executed in 1645; the Civil War began in 1642.

To find the elements of Browne's actual religious position we can start from the sketch of his life by John Whitefoot, his first biographer, who was his friend for 50 years. There are three short passages from Whitefoot's biographical note which are significant.[37] In the first, Whitefoot associates Browne's views with those of Hugo Grotius (who did indeed, as Whitefoot claims, think that the Church of England was the best model of a church in Christendom, as we shall discuss further below):

> In his religion he continued in the same mind which he had de-clared in his first book, written when he was but thirty years old, his *Religio Medici*, wherein he fully assented to that of the church of England, preferring it before any in the world, as did the learned Grotius.

Then, on his deathbed Whitefoot heard Browne submit himself to God's Providence with a courage both *rational* and *religious*:

> His patience was founded upon the christian philosophy, and a sound faith in God's Providence, and a meek and humble submis-sion thereunto, which he expressed in few words ... when his own turn came, he submitted with a meek, rational, and religious cour-age.

In the third pertinent passage Whitefoot reports that Browne was able to make the rational faculty dominant over the affections and passions; this was to behave like a true Greek philosopher of the Stoic school.

> He had no despotical power over his affections and passions ... but as large a political power over them, as any Stoick, or man of his time, whereof he gave so great experiment, that he hath very rarely been known to have been overcome with any of them. The strong-est that were found in him, both of the irascible and concupiscible, were under the controul of his reason.

It is clear from these comments by Whitefoot that what Browne was trying to do was to fulfil the role of a true Christian philosopher in the modern age. His position was *philosophical*, in the ancient Greek sense, in that he was seeking the true goal of philosophy: peace of mind, *ataraxia*, by placing his passions beneath the control of his reason. The position was typically *Stoic*, amongst the various forms of Greek phi-losophy, in that tranquility of soul is what is being sought, through an *active* process of philosophizing, with positive submission of the self to fate, and in that the investigation of nature, seen as something rational rather than irrational, plays a significant role in understanding and reaching the divine for a Stoic. The position was *Christian* in that Christianity was taken by Browne to be the fulfilment of Greek philoso-phy; and hence the peace of mind which philosophy seeks can be found through the *revealed* religion of Christianity, as interpreted through the judicious use of *reason*.

The essential thing to notice is that Browne's position as a philosopher was one which we have now lost. It involved the whole of life and how one led one's life. Thus for Browne the issues of passion against reason and reason against faith (*RM*, II.9), were intimately involved with living the ethical life – which is the whole of one's life. For in *Religio Medici* Browne is teaching what he elsewhere calls 'the Divine Ethics of our Saviour': a Christianized Stoic ethics.[38] And in this divine ethics, *reason* and *conscience* are intimately linked. For Christian ethics demands the right use of reason, enabling one to master one's unruly passions:

> And therefore while so many think it the only valour to command and master others, study thou the Dominion of thy self, and quiet thine own Commotions. Let Right Reason be thy *Lycurgus*, and lift up thy hand unto the Law of it; move by the Intelligences of the superior Faculties, not by the Rapt of Passion, not merely by that of Temper and Constitution. They who are merely carried on by the Wheel of such Inclinations, without the Hand and Guidance of Sovereign Reason, are but the Automatous part of mankind, rather lived than living, or at least underliving themselves.[39]

And in actively living the life of the true Christian philosopher, this right use of reason is linked with the proper deployment of one's *conscience*:

> Mean while there is no darkness unto Conscience, which can see without Light, and in the deepest obscurity give a clear Draught of things, which the Cloud of dissimultation hath conceal'd from all eyes. There is a natural standing Court within us, examining, acquitting, and condemning at the Tribunal of our selves, wherein iniquities have their natural Theta's, and no nocent is absolved by the verdict of himself.[40]

Thus the life of the proper Christian for Browne involves control over the self, not being swayed by the world, cleaving to virtue for its own sake, not for earthly reward. One should be calm, quiet, satisfied with one's own lot and thankful for it, envying no one, exercising virtue, a model of fortitude and resilience, hearkening to one's conscience, giving to those in need.

> He who is thus his own Monarch contentedly sways the Scepter of himself, not envying the Glory of Crowned Heads and Elohims of the Earth. Could the world unite in the practise of that despised train of Virtues, which the Divine Ethicks of our Saviour hath so inculcated unto us, the furious face of things must disappear, Eden would yet be found, and the Angels might look down not with pity, but Joy upon us.[41]

Browne finds this Stoic Christian philosophy, this view that true Christian charity consists in the practice of the highest personal virtue sup-

ported by reason and conscience, in St Paul's writings on charity.[42] It is
to that same chapter of the first *Letter to the Corinthians* in which Paul
uses the faith-hope-charity metaphor, that Browne is referring when he
writes:

> where Charity is broke the Law it self is shattered, which cannot be
> whole without Love, that is the fulfilling of it. Look humbly upon
> thy Virtues, and tho thou art rich in some, yet think thy self poor
> and naked without that crowning Grace, which thinketh no Evil,
> which envieth not, which beareth, believeth, hopeth, endureth all
> things.[43]

But while this attitude is unmistakably Stoic, it has been fully Christianized by Browne, with the Stoic rules of living adopted, but their doctrines rejected:

> Rest not in the high strain'd Paradoxes of old Philosophy supported
> by naked Reason, and the reward of mortal Felicity, but labour in
> the Ethicks of Faith, built upon Heavenly assistance, and the happi-
> ness of both beings. Understand the Rules, but swear not unto the
> Doctrines of *Zeno* or *Epicurus*. Look beyond *Antoninus* [i.e. Marcus
> Aurelius], and terminate not thy Morals in *Seneca* or *Epictetus*. Let
> not the twelve, but the two Tables be thy Law ... Be a moralist of the
> Mount, an *Epictetus* in the Faith, and christianize thy Notions.[44]

The 'ethics of faith' need to be adopted over the ethics of reason: one
should be not just a philosopher, but a Christian philosopher.[45]

So if we return to the issues of faith, hope and charity, which consti-
tute the immediate themes of *Religio Medici*, it is now clear that Browne
is interpreting St Paul as saying that if you have faith (which comes
through God's grace), then faith gives you hope of salvation and eternal
life. And the expression of having faith and hope is nothing less than
the practical exercise of Christian charity through correct living.

And, even more important for our present purposes, the proper Christian should deploy *faith* where he cannot see, and *reason* where he can.
Reason is constantly contrasted with faith by Browne, but not opposed
to it: they complement one another, they do not contradict one another.
They are both necessary. Each has its role in the life of the Christian
philosopher, and each has not just a role for which it is suitable, but a
role for which it is necessary:

> How the dead shall arise, is no question of my faith; to believe only
> possibilities, is not faith, but mere Philosophy; many things are
> true in Divinity, which are neither inducible by reason, nor con-
> firmable by sense, and many things in Philosophy conformable to
> sense, but not inducible by reason. Thus it is impossible by any
> solid or demonstrative reasons to persuade a man to believe the
> conversion of the Needle to the North; though this be possible, and
> true, and easily credible, upon a single experiment unto the sense. I

> believe that our estranged and divided ashes shall unite again, that our separated dust after so many pilgrimages and transformations into the parts of minerals, plants, animals, elements, shall at the voice of God return unto their primitive shapes, and join to make up their primary and predestine forms.
>
> (*RM*, I. 48)

It can hardly be sufficiently emphasized that this distinction between faith and reason on Browne's part is not the same as the distinction between faith and reason we might make today. For in making such a distinction today we would be unavoidably invoking a conflict (or, at the very least a contrast) between *religion* and *science*. These are not the categories within which Browne is thinking. The contrast is not a seventeenth-century one. The discipline category 'science' as used by us in such a contrast was unknown to Browne, since it was a creation of the nineteenth century, when indeed the supposed age-old historical conflict between religion and science was also brought into existence. The intellectual domain analogous to our 'science' was, for Browne, natural philosophy, itself a branch of philosophy.

So in religion we should expect to find Browne making distinctions between those issues of doctrine (belief) and of discipline (practice) which are or ought to be matters of *faith*, and those which are matters of *reason and conscience*; we should also expect him to be distinguishing between those matters of doctrine and discipline which are essential to good Christian belief and ritual, and those which are *adiaphora* (as Erasmus called them), things indifferent. And this we find. This resorting to reason and conscience (wherever appropriate) is a God-given duty, for 'there is a natural standing Court within us, examining, acquitting, and condemning at the Tribunal of our selves'.

> In brief, where the Scripture is silent, the Church is my text; where that speaks, 'tis but my comment: where there is a joint silence of both, I borrow not the rules of my religion from *Rome* or *Geneva*, but the dictates of my own reason.
>
> (*RM*, I.5)

Thus, in Browne's view, the Christian has a duty to use his own reason and conscience to enquire into the truth of his religion and its foundations, and into the grounds on which he should trust authority. In querying the tenets of one's faith, reason is for Browne a natural (and God-given) resource to use; this put Browne's position at odds with both Catholics and Calvinists. Thorough querying of the tenets of faith allows one to focus on the essentials: you end with a nucleus of faith, which is true, which has to be believed. Having distinguished between what is essential in faith and what is not, you are able to tolerate those who disagree with you on 'things indifferent'.

For our purposes here, the most important distinction between a Christian philosopher of Browne's persuasion and a Christian *tout court*, is that the Christian philosopher allows a great role to reason and reasoning in coming to his understanding of divine truths and in his concept of what the proper practice of Christianity should be: he does not lean on authority in either area. For authority is mere authority. As Browne was to point out: in both religion and nature, to lean on authority without the use of reason and conscience, leads many times not to truth but to its opposite.

Reason and faith have distinct roles for Browne. In the domain of religious mysteries, reason is misplaced; such was the case, says Browne, when scholastic logic was used to illustrate and defend Christian mysteries 'by syllogism'. But religious mysteries are there to be experienced *as* mysteries:

> Methinks there be not impossibilities enough in religion for an active faith ... I love to lose myself in a mystery, to pursue my reason to an *oh altitudo*.[46] Tis my solitary recreation to pose my apprehension with those involved enigmas and riddles of the Trinity, with Incarnation and Resurrection. I can answer all the objections of Satan, and my rebellious reason, with that odd resolution I learnt of Tertullian: *Certum est quia impossibile est* [It is certain because it is impossible]. I desire to exercise my faith in the difficultest point, for to credit ordinary and visible objects is not faith, but persuasion ... and this I think no vulgar part of faith to believe a thing not only above, but contrary to reason, and against the arguments of our proper senses.
>
> (*RM*, I.9)

It has to be said also that when it came to religious experience itself, Browne was an adherent of a mystical, a neo-Platonic, version of spirituality, and the term 'mystical' constantly recurs in positive contexts in *Religio Medici*. In neo-Platonic vein Browne bursts into verse (*RM*, I.32) in order to lament

> O how this earthly temper doth debase
> The noble soul, in this her humble place!
> Whose wingy nature ever doth aspire
> To reach that place whence first it took its fire ...

The last words of his *Christian Morals* clearly locate what Browne regarded as the highest religious experience:

> And if, as we have elsewhere declared [in *Hydriotaphia*], any have been so happy as personally to understand Christian Annihilation, Extasy, Exolution, Transformation, the Kiss of the Spouse, and Ingression into the Divine Shadow, according to Mystical Theology, they have already had an handsome Anticipation of Heaven; the World is in a manner over, and the Earth in Ashes unto them.[47]

Indeed, for Browne, nature itself presented 'mystical letters' for the Christian with eyes to see and who cared to 'suck Divinity from the flowers of nature' (*RM*, I.16).

The position of Christian philosopher was not easy. Exercising this duty, and finding the right balance for the Christian between passion, reason and faith, created much inner turmoil for Browne, which he relished: 'Let me be nothing if within the compass of myself, I do not find the battle of Lepanto, passion against reason, reason against faith, faith against the Devil, and my conscience against all. There is another man within me, that's angry with me, rebukes, commands and dastards me' (*RM*, II.9). The significance of the 1571 battle of Lepanto in this simile is that it had looked like the ultimate battle between defensive Christendom and offensive unbelief, and in which, after great loss of life, the united Christians were ultimately victorious over the Turks. While the Christian philosopher was, Browne believed, thus morally obliged to concern himself with the respective roles of reason and faith, yet Browne experienced a constant inner dialogue within himself over them: 'Thus the Devil played at chess with me, and yielding a pawn, thought to gain a queen of me, taking advantage of my honest labours; and whilst I labour'd to raise the structure of my reason, he striv'd to undermine the edifice of my faith' (*RM*, I.19).

The Church of England is best

The position of Christian philosopher, with its combination of reason and faith, had been available for over a millenium and a half, but it was resorted to only from time to time over that period, and only by certain individuals. Thus while it was far from new with Browne, it was still a relatively unusual position to take. It is clear that Browne's particular formulation and application of this position, and the reasons why he adopted it, lie in his personal responses to the religious crises of his own day, both in England and on the Continent. By looking at this response, we will also be able to see why the ideal Christian philosopher could see the Church of England in particular as the ideal form of church, if it were only free from its current troubles.

It was on the grounds of reason and conscience (not passion or prejudice) that Browne favoured Anglicanism: there is no church, he wrote, 'whose every part so squares unto my conscience, whose articles, constitutions, and customs seem so consonant unto reason; as the Church of England (*RM*, I.5). The issue of the grounds of authority in religion exercised many Englishmen's minds in the 1630s, though they were a minority who found in favour not of authority, but of reason and conscience. Amongst such men were a number who flirted with – or

were believed to be flirting with – those difficult-to-define but danger-
ous-to-hold religious positions: Arminianism and Socinianism. And these
were amongst the firmest Anglicans of the period. Browne was one of
them.

In the 1630s the 'Arminians' in England were the remnant of the
liberal 'Erasmian' Protestants of the sixteenth century, and who took
(or were given) their name after the Dutchman Jacob Harmensen (or
Hermanzoon, or Hermandszoon, d. 1609).[48] 'Arminianism' was a reaction to strict Calvinism, and especially to its doctrines of predestination
and election. Its essence, according to Hugh Trevor-Roper, 'was that
God's grace was universal, that Christ died for all men, and that all
men, therefore, were capable of salvation; by the exercise of their free
will, they could benefit by that freely offered grace'.[49] As none had the
guarantee of election, the Arminians claimed, none had the monopoly
of truth, and hence none had a divine mandate to impose their religion
on others. Thus persuasion, not persecution, should be the approach
toward other religions. Hugo Grotius, a follower of Arminius, preached
the universal application of Arminius's views as a way of reuniting the
Protestant churches. As Trevor-Roper describes the situation, Grotius

> believed that it could provide a basis upon which liberal Calvinists
> in the Netherlands, Anglicans in England, Gallicans and liberal
> Hugenots in France, could unite leaving the extremists of popery
> and Puritanism to wither gradually away. He also believed that the
> leadership in such a movement naturally belonged to England ...
> To Grotius, the court of James I offered hopes comparable with
> those which the court of Henry VIII had offered to Erasmus.[50]

In 1613 Grotius visited England where, he believed, the learned King
James would lead the Protestant princes in reuniting Christendom, at
the head of a centralist, comprehensive church, situated in both doctrine and discipline between Rome and Geneva, returned to true primitive Christianity.[51] With its peculiar compromise of Catholic and Reformed Protestant doctrines and discipline, and headed by a monarch,
the Church of England was indeed uniquely appropriate for this purpose. As Grotius wrote to his own brother in 1645, 'Liturgia Anglicana
ab eruditis omnibus habita semper est optima', the Anglican liturgy has
always been held by all learned men to be the best. At the end of his life,
Grotius even said that he wanted to die, and his wife to live, in the
Anglican communion.[52]

However, it is typical of compromise institutions that times of stress
lead to one or other of the parties coming to the fore, and finding the
other wing insupportable. And this was the case in the early decades of
the seventeenth century with the Anglican Church. A turning point came
with the victory of the Dutch Calvinists at the Synod of Dort in 1618.

For this condemnation of all the Arminian positions led, in England, to the Calvinists of the Anglican Church becoming highly wary of the 'Arminians' in their midst. With their openness to church ornament and ceremony and their view that grace was available to all, these 'Arminians' now looked, to the eyes of the church Puritans, as though they were half-way to popery. As the Puritan wing came under increasing pressure in the 1630s from the Laudian leadership of the church in its campaign for uniformity in discipline and doctrine, so the Puritans came to see the 'Arminians' in their midst as authoritarian and absolutist, while the association of some of these 'Arminians' with Archbishop Laud made them also seem tyrannical and episcopal if not actually papist.

Browne held similar views to these 'Arminians'. For instance he deals with questions dividing Calvinists from others, questions as vexed as predestination, more particularly of 'double predestination', the doctrine that some have been elected by God to eternal salvation, the rest to eternal damnation. 'I believe', Browne says, 'many are saved who to man seem reprobated, and many reprobated who in the opinion and sentence of man, stand elected' (*RM*, I.57). Thus, as we cannot know who are to be ultimately saved, we have no sanction for using election to decide who the saints are in this life. And Browne clearly believes equally in the saving grace of God.[53]

Socinianism is the other half of this pairing of difficult and abusive terms which became associated with the position that Browne held. Socinianism, named after Faustus Socinus (d. 1604), was regarded as an arch-heresy – as bad as Anabaptism – by both Catholic and Protestant, including as it did denial of the Trinity, of the divinity of Christ, of predestination and of Christ's atonement for sin. Socinians were opposed to the punishing of heretics and against the alliance of Church and State. The approach that Socinus and his followers had taken in reaching these positions was particularly striking. For they had founded themselves on the twin bases of scrupulous biblicism and the right to reason in religion. Without scriptural support no belief was mandatory on a Christian (as with the case of the Trinity). Scripture was revealed truth, but, as a modern scholar has written, 'in order to perceive the truths of revelation a man had of necessity to seek the guidance of reason, without which revelation was not self-evidencing ... Right reason and divine truth must, of necessity, agree'.[54] Insisting on the necessity of deploying one's reason when reading scripture, and of refusing to persecute those of other beliefs, came to be taken as the two marks of Socinianism. In an anxious age, anyone advocating either or both of these *approaches* to ascertaining religious truth, could be held guilty (rightly or wrongly) of holding Socinian *doctrines* as well, of adhering to what Laud called 'that foul heresy and the most dangerous that ever

spread itself since the beginnings of Christianity'.[55] 'Socinian' was therefore a very handy term of abuse to be used against anyone who claimed
in matters of religious faith that reason and conscience were to be
preferred over adherence to authority. As we have seen, Browne's views
on the use of reason and his apparent toleration of Catholics could look
remarkably like Socinianism in the eyes of a hostile observer.

Very few persons in England actually were thorough-going Socinians,
but many were charged with it. Thomas Browne, however, may have
come closer to it than most. For his tutor at Oxford, whom he followed
to Norwich, was Thomas Lushington, who actually translated two
genuine Socinian works from Latin into English, *The Expiation of a
Sinner* (1646), which he distributed widely round Norwich, and *The
Justification of a Sinner* (1650); however, Lushington took care to keep
his identity hidden.[56]

Both Arminian and Socinian views would generally lead one to
being in favour of toleration in religion. It was in the England of 1642
still invidious and potentially dangerous to call for toleration. Although a modern historian of toleration such as Nicholas Tyacke can
find the occasional English person calling for toleration before this
date – such as Thomas Helwys, a Baptist, arguing in 1612 that 'men's
religion is betwixt God and themselves' and there should be no com-
pulsion yet, Tyacke concludes, 'Intolerance remained the English order of the day'. It remained so until the later 1640s, when some of the
sectaries of the New Model Army, and especially the Baptists, called
for every man to have 'the free liberty of their own conscience in
matters of religion, or worship, without the least oppression or persecution, as simply upon that account'.[57] But even then, the Baptists
were a minority voice, and what most Christian denominations and
sects continued to want was uniformity of belief – uniformity of
everyone, that is, with themselves.

The view that toleration was desirable in religion, and reason is
essential to faith, were particularly dangerous in the period when *Religio
Medici* was published, for toleration seemed to many to mean atheism.
Francis Cheynell, a Puritan minister and academic, had appointed himself as the scourge of Arminians and Socinians, whom he saw as equivalent to atheists and papists. He found them everywhere, including on
the Archbishop of Canterbury's throne, but especially in and around
Oxford. Cheynell did not sleep in his persecuting rage. Such persons
had, be believed, created obstacles to him getting a theology degree, and
had obliged him to leave his fellowship at Merton College. In the 1630s
some of them were gathered around the young Lucius Cary, Lord
Falkland, in a grouping known to historians as the 'Great Tew Circle',
after Falkland's country house near Oxford.[58] While Browne was not a

member of this circle, for he was seeking his continental education during the years of its flourishing, the characterization of their opinions that has been made by Hugh Trevor-Roper reveals that Browne's views were virtually identical to theirs. They too sought a church founded on reason as well as faith, in which points of controversy were subjected to the test of reason, a church which sought a middle way between the extremes of Catholics and Calvinists, a church with room for both altar and pulpit. Like Browne, they saw Hugo Grotius as their presiding genius, and like Browne and Grotius, saw the Church of England as the embodiment of such an ideal church.

In Oxford and Great Tew there were (amongst others) Lord Falkland himself, Christopher Potter, Provost of Queen's College, John Hales, Henry Hammond and Thomas Lushington, who could all plausibly be accused of Arminianism and Socinianism. But Cheynell's special wrath was reserved for William Chillingworth (1602–44) whom Cheynell pursued, literally, to the grave.

Chillingworth's major work, dedicated to Charles I, was *The Religion of Protestants a Safe Way to Salvation* (1636) in which he called for free judgement, toleration in religion, support of the Church of England as the church of uniformity and not contrary to truth or to the Bible, and in which he indicated that relative certainty is the best we can hope for:

> Let all men believe the Scripture and that only, and endeavour to believe it in the true sense, and require no more of others, and they shall find this not only a better, but the only means to suppress Heresy, and restore Unity ... And if no more than this were required of any man, to make him capable of the Churches Communion, then all men so qualified, though they were different in opinion, yet notwithstanding any such difference, must be of necessity one in Communion.[59]

Chillingworth's case was indeed somewhat unusual, and almost intentionally calculated to rouse the ire of a zealous Presbyterian minister. For Chillingworth had converted from the Church of England to Catholicism in 1630, then had instantly became a 'doubting papist', and reconverted to the Church of England![60] Obviously, from a Puritan point of view, Chillingworth had held several damnable opinions, but the last is the worst, the call for toleration and the use of reason.

> *Mr Chillingworth* (your friend) [Cheynell wrote] did run mad with reason, and so lost his reason and religion both at once. He thought he might trust his reason in the highest points; his reason was to be judge, whether or no there be a God; whether that God wrote any book; whether the books usually receiv'ed as canonical be the books, the scriptures of God: what is the sense of those books; what religion is best; what church purest.[61]

As if playing out some awful Greek tragedy, in his last days Chillingworth, injured fighting for the royalist forces, fell into the hands of his greatest enemy, both personal and theological, Francis Cheynell, now fighting for the Parliamentary cause. Cheynell harangued Chillingworth for days to get him to recant, but without success. Cheynell published a record of the deathbed exchanges, and of his attendance at Chillingworth's funeral, in a book on 'The last days of Chillingworth', which John Locke described as 'one of the most *villanous* Books that ever was printed'. Cheynell was particularly proud of the fact that he buried Chillingworth's book, throwing it into the grave with a dreadful curse and a half: 'Get thee gone then, thou cursed book, which hast seduc'd so many precious souls; get thee gone, thou corrupt rotten book, earth to earth, and dust to dust; get thee gone into the place of rottenness, that thou mayst rot with thy author, and see corruption.'[62] This was in 1644, the year after the authorized edition of *Religio Medici* was published.

Chillingworth advocated reason in religion in two differing senses, according to the analysis of Robert Orr.[63] First, in the traditional Thomist sense of the mind being a receptacle of divinely implanted truths plainly written for all to see: when we consult our reason, we discover divine truths within, on which we all agree. And second in a novel sense, as a *critical* faculty which scrutinizes and appraises the evidence for propositions; this sense of the term calls for the weighing of evidence and of authorities, it is 'right reason' (in Chillingworth's words), the God-given safeguard against 'prejudices and popular errors'. The rational and reasonable in scripture and church practice can be accepted. The *irra*tional can be discovered and discarded; while the *supra*rational, things above reason, in a word religious *mysteries*, can be recognized for what they are, and be accorded the faith they deserve. Chillingworth invoked this new sense of reason as he argued simultaneously against extreme Puritans who believed that the things one should believe are plainly revealed (via 'private revelation') directly in reading the scriptures, and against Jesuits and other Catholics who believed they are plainly revealed by the infallible Church.

These positions on reason and its use in religion are identical to those of Thomas Browne in *Religio Medici*, though no direct connection between Browne and Chillingworth is known. So it is no surprise to find that the scourge of Chillingworth, Francis Cheynell, attacked Browne's *Religio Medici* too, for what looked to him like its learned atheism, characterizing it as a work fit to corrupt the religion and morals of the gentry and aristocracy, and by implication a Socinian work. He condemned it in a fast sermon to the House of Lords in March 1645, reproving their lordships for not knowing what constitutes proper honourable life and belief for Christian lords and gentry. In the course of his sermon Cheynell turned to attacking Archbishop Laud as an Arminian, Socinian, papist and atheist:

> *Machiavel* himself could not but censure, such grosse corruption, and abominable contempt amongst those that call themselves Christians. *Summopere vituperandi sunt Religionis contemptores & corruptores, Disp. de repub. I.c.10.* Take heed of such Chaplains which poyson Noble Families with Socinianism, leaven them with Atheism, or corrupt them with Prophanenesse: Beware of them that have no more Religion, then is to be found in that unworthy Book, called *Religio Medici, A Book too much applauded by No-ble-men.*[64]

Cheynell also saw the dangers to Christianity of the Platonist position that Browne favoured, for Cheynell saw this as merely another veil for atheism. In his work on *The Rise, Growth and Danger of Socinianism* (1643), again attacking Archbishop Laud, Cheynell wrote:

> I know the *Socinians* doe talk much of the offices of Christ, but they receive nothing from the Scripture, concerning Christ's offices, but what is as they say agreeable to Reason ... Reason by its own light did discover unto them that the good and great God had prepared eternall happinesse for our immortall soules: if this then be enough (as the *Socinians* say it is) to receive all the things as Principles of Religion which Reason by her own light can discover to be true, (and how neer the *Arch-Bishop* comes to them, let the Reader judge) then the *Philosophers*, especially the *Platonists*, were in an happy condition, & it will be lawfull for a man to cry out aloud, *Sit anima mea cum Philosophis*, and he shall never be thought an Atheist, nay shall passe for a good Christian ...[65]

One can see what a narrow path Browne walked in *Religio Medici* in calling for the application of reason and conscience in religion, while avoiding the accusation of being a Socinian or atheist.

So in what sense is Browne an advocate of toleration in religion in *Religio Medici*? The modern sense of religious toleration is based on a view of rights: every individual has a right to his or her own opinion, and therefore should not be forced against their will to profess or practise any particular religion. In this sense, Browne was certainly not tolerant. But he was tolerant in a seventeenth-century sense, which may perhaps (in contrast) be described as based on a view of duties: on each person lay the duty of discovering and practising true Christianity. In Browne's view, this meant that all men had an obligation to investigate the grounds of Christian religion for themselves, and to seek its validity using reason and scripture. In arguing that the difficulty – even the impossibility – of gaining certitude in religion means that no one has a divine mandate to persecute anyone else in the name of religious belief or practice, Browne was saying that it is the Christian's duty to be tolerant over 'things indifferent'. But that does not mean that he was particularly open-minded or forgiving with respect to either Catholics or Puritans.

Nor indeed did his toleration extend to him thinking that all men had a right to their own point of view on the grounds that all men are equal. Indeed he thought the opposite, holding to what one might call a doctrine of the two comprehensions. For he made a distinction between the *wise*, on the one hand, and *rude heads* – the vulgar – on the other, and this runs like a refrain through *Religio Medici*. It is something of an obsession for Browne, this distinction between the wise and the un-learned, between the reasonable and the unreasoning, between the gen-tleman and the mob. It is a traditional Stoic viewpoint; and it is a distinction, of course, about social hierarchy, and politics.

> If there be any amongst those common objects of hatred I do contemn and laugh at, it is that great enemy of reason, virtue and religion, the multitude, that numerous piece of monstrosity, which taken asunder seem men, and the reasonable creatures of God; but confused together, make but one great beast, and a monstrosity more prodigious than Hydra.[66]
>
> (*RM*, II.1)

This distinction between the wise and the rude is also about belief and the right role of reason. And Browne regards the extreme Protestant sects – the Puritans – as the product of vulgar enthusiasm and vulgar (that is, inadequate) reasoning.

Michael Wilding has shown that, in producing the 'authorized' ver-sion of 1643, Browne made many small alterations to the text to adjust his position to the present circumstances.[67] He shows that, if one reads the text in the context of 1643, then Browne is actually extending his famous toleration *only* to Catholics: he dislikes the sects, he dislikes the religious/political radicals. Even one of the 'ancient heresies' which Browne claimed to have suffered as a young man, mortalism, Wilding shows was hardly obsolete, but current in the 1640s, and in particular associated with the radical sects. That Browne had rejected it is signifi-cant. Browne's view on the Antichrist (that he doesn't exist, and cer-tainly hasn't been identified) and the dating of the millenium (it can't be dated, so is not just round the corner) both place him squarely against the radical millenarians.

Indeed, in contrast to the views of some modern commentators on Browne such as Joan Webber, it is clear that *Religio Medici* is a strongly conservative work in political terms, as well as religious ones, with Browne's views being expressed in a vocabulary atuned to the troubled times in which he was writing, and critical of current changes toward a less hierarchical society. For instance, Browne speaks of social hierarchy as natural: there is a 'natural dignity, whereby one man is ranked with another, another filed before him, according to the quality of his desert, and pre-eminence of his good parts' (*RM*, II.1). Today, alas, this natural state has been perverted:

> Though the corruption of these times, and the bias of present practice wheel another way, thus it was in the first and primitive Common-wealths, and is yet in the integrity and cradle of well-ordered polities, till corruption getteth ground, ruder desires labouring after that which wiser considerations contemn, every one having liberty to amass and heap up riches, and they a license or faculty to do or purchase anything.
>
> (*RM*, II.1)

And again: 'Statists [political theorists] that labour to contrive a Commonwealth without poverty, take away the object of charity, not understanding only the Commonwealth of a Christian, but forgetting the prophecy of Christ [i.e. 'the poor you shall have always with you']' (*RM*, II.13). And in this context Browne mentions medicine as a necessary and honourable profession, speaking of 'Those three Noble professions which all civil Commonwealths do honour' (*RM*, II.9), theology, law and medicine. As Charles Webster has taught us in *The Great Instauration*, some Puritans were at this period planning to abolish all professions in the cause of making a better and more egalitarian society. From such comments Browne's social and political conservatism should be evident. Browne's famous tolerance was very limited.

We can conclude about Browne's religious commitment that it seems to have started, logically or chronologically or both, from philosophy, searching for the role of Christian philosopher. It ended in Anglicanism, to which he was persuaded by reason and conscience, those two great tests. His Anglicanism is a response to the situation of his life, and perhaps some of his devotion to it had been learnt abroad, particularly in that hotbed of Arminianism, Leiden.

So the religion of this particular physician does not come down to a matter of simple toleration; this is to make Browne far too much of a modern. And, as has been shown, the explicit rationality of his standpoint was an integral part of his religious position: we are not entitled to separate his religious beliefs and practices from his rational standpoint, and make him into a modern in our own image. His religion was thoroughgoing, it was a way of life, a commitedly Christian way of life, an attempt to practise 'the Divine Ethicks of our Saviour'.

... of a physician

The opening words of Religio Medici discussed the double dangers for
Thomas Browne the physician of being suspected of atheism. Now we
need to explore the other side of the problem: the danger of someone
educated specifically as a *physician* being suspected of having no religion, and yet having the strongest Christian faith. 'For my Religion',
Browne wrote, 'though there be several circumstances that might persuade the world I have none at all, as the general scandal of my
profession, the natural course of my studies ...' (RM, I.1). Like Browne's
apparent toleration of those of other Christian persuasions, this too
involves the potential charge of atheism, and is equally resolved into
strong Christian faith. What Browne is claiming is that the physician is
not doomed to atheism, but his natural studies should lead him to God,
as much as his religious studies will do. This is the other side of the
religion of a physician, the other meaning of the title of the book. It is
certainly striking that Browne constantly talks about God via the mysteries of both scripture and nature *at once*: they are God's two books, in
that familiar expression: 'Thus there are two books from whence I
collect my divinity; besides that written one of God, another of his
servant Nature, that universal and public manuscript, that lies expansed
unto the eyes of all; those that never saw him in the one, have discovered him in the other ... ' (RM, I.16). This does not involve substituting
the 'natural' path to God for the religious path: the two routes run to
the same goal. Religio Medici, the religion of a physician, thus constitutes a double route to God.

But nature is always a potential problem for the good Christian. For
in considering, contemplating, investigating or admiring nature one
always runs the risk of attributing to nature the characteristics or the
identity of God.[68] To claim that God was present everywhere in nature
was heretical; to claim that nature had all the properties and qualities,
such as goodness and providence, that Christians attributed to God was
atheistical. Passion and misplaced reason were to blame for such confu-
sions of God with nature, wrote Browne, in a matter where faith should
be trusted: 'The bad construction and perverse comment on these pair
of second causes [i.e. nature and fortune], or visible hands of God, have
perverted the devotion of many to Atheism; who, forgetting the honest
advices of faith, have listened to the conspiracies of Passion and Reason' (RM, I.19). It is essential to recognize, Browne urges, that nature is
simply the hand or instrument of God, it is 'that settled and constant
course the wisdom of God hath ordained the actions of his creatures,
according to their several kinds' (RM, I.16). Then we can read it aright
and use it as an additional route to God. This, Browne implies, will take

one on a route away from the dangers of atheism, and toward true religion.

It was indeed the case in this period that the relation to faith of rational discussion of natural knowledge was being fervently discussed. Schoenveld has shown, for instance, that in Leiden, where Browne had graudated in medicine and possibly learnt his Arminianism, the appearance of Descartes's *Discourse on Method* (1637), especially its Latin verson of 1644, led to theological issues being put to methodical doubt. Later (1656) the members of the university had to be warned that there was a proper distinction of roles:

> matters and questions which are proper to Theology and become known only by revelation through God's Holy Word – as being entirely separate from those questions that can and should be investigated and be known from nature through reason – should be left to Theologians alone, without allowing others, especially Philosophers to arrogate these to themselves in lectures and disputations in any way.[69]

The physician was in a peculiar position in all this, due to his necessary exposure to the study of nature. There was indeed a popular belief that physicians were natural atheists, expressed in a medieval tag: *ubi tres medici, duo athei* – where there are three physicians there are two atheists. Physicians were all taken to be followers of Galen, the Greek physician of the second century AD. The Galenic soul of the physicians was thought to be not immortal. Browne gives an instance of a doctor he met in Italy 'who could not perfectly believe the immortality of the soul, because Galen seemed to make a doubt thereof' (*RM*, I.21). Paul Kocher, writing on 'The physician as atheist' has shown that the character of the atheistic physician was sometimes represented in print, even by physicians, as for example, by William Bullein in 1564. Kocher points out that Galen's irreligion came to attention because of doctors' actual irreligion in the sixteenth century. But he also shows that it was the case that in the sixteenth and seventeenth centuries adherents of Paracelsianism, conceived as a *Christian* medicine, used Galen's (and Aristotle's) 'irreligion' – i.e. the fact that they were not Christians – to attack their Galenic rivals. As one such Paracelsian wrote: 'surely such naturall Philosophie is the next way to make men forget thee, O God, and to become Atheists: for it teacheth men to cleave and sticke fast unto the nature of thinges, not ascending [to] nor considering the Creator'.[70]

But what Browne is arguing in *Religio Medici* is that the physician is actually in an exceptional position to guide others, and that, properly managed, the studies of the physician lead not towards but away from atheism. For the physician has learnt natural philosophy, and studied the microcosm – man himself – at first hand. Browne himself has personally engaged in anatomizing, yet 'by raking into the bowels of the deceased, continual sight of Anatomies, Skeletons, or Cadaverous reliques, like Vespilloes, or Grave-makers' (RM, I.38) he has not, he says, been hardened against apprehension about his mortality, nor has he abandoned Christian hope. Rather, the reverse. 'Without further travel', he says, we can each contemplate God's wonders in miniature in the cosmography of ourselves: 'we carry with us the wonders we seek without us: There is all *Africa* and her prodigies in us, we are that bold and adventurous piece of nature, which he that studies, wisely learns in a *compendium*, what others labour at in a divided piece and endless volume' (RM, I.15). Indeed, we are the masterpieces of the Creator, we alone are 'the amphibious piece between a corporal and spiritual essence, that middle form that links those two together, and makes good the method of God and nature, that jumps not from extremes, but unites the incompatible distances by some middle and participating natures' (RM, I.32). Hence the physician is in a privileged position to appreciate divinity in nature, and also man's special pivotal role in the chain of being. Thus the investigation of nature is desirable on religious grounds and, for this, the use of reason is essential, indeed it is our duty. For

> the world was made to be inhabited by beasts, but studied and contemplated by man: tis the debt of our reason we owe unto God, and the homage we pay for not being beasts ... The wisdom of God receives small honour from those vulgar heads, that rudely stare about, and with a gross rusticity admire his works;[71] those [people] highly magnify him whose judicious enquiry into his acts, and deliberate research into his creatures, return the duty of a devout and learned admiration.
>
> (RM, I.13)

On this theme Browne lyricizes:

> It is thy maker's will, for unto none
> But unto reason can He ere be known ...
> Teach my endeavours so thy works to read,
> That learning them, in thee I may proceed ...
>
> (RM, I.13)

Thus not only will nature lead us to God, but the exercise of reason in this domain will confirm our faith.

What the physician in his role as natural philosopher is looking for in nature is 'final' causes, 'final' because they express the final purpose of a thing, the explanation of why it is as it is, the purpose for which, as the Christian saw it, a thing had been created just as it is by the Creator himself, either directly, or indirectly through His servant, nature.

> Every essence, created or uncreated, hath its final cause, and some positive end both of its Essence and operation: This is the cause I grope after in the works of nature, on this hangs the providence of God; to raise so beauteous a structure, as the world and the creatures thereof, was but His Art, but their sundry and divided operations with their predestined ends, are from the treasury of his Wisdom. In the causes, nature, and affections of the eclipse of sun and moon, there is most excellent speculation; but to profound further, and to contemplate a reason why his providence hath so disposed and ordered their motions in that vast circle, as to conjoin and obscure each other, is a sweeter piece of reason, and a diviner point of Philosophy; therefore sometimes, and in some things there appears to me as much divinity in Galen his books *De Usu Partium*, as in Suarez *Metaphysics* ...
>
> (RM, I.14)

The first cause is God; nature and fortune are the second causes, through which God works.[72]

What was Browne's position with respect to medicine? He had enjoyed a conventional education on the Continent, and was certainly a mainstream Galenic physician, as his university degrees and honorary membership of the College of Physicians indicate. Moreover, his son Edward followed him into medicine, and his father encouraged him to travel and study on the Continent; Edward rose to being President of the College of Physicians, the height of institutional conformity. Sir Thomas's many letters to Edward in London, in which diagnosis, prescriptions and other medical matters are discussed, seem conventional for the time in their language and content, with Browne favouring Peruvian bark (cortex) in fevers, and diagnosing from the urine etc.

Yet from *Religio Medici* and from elsewhere in his published writings and letters, it is clear that Browne had a sympathy – at the very least a strong interest – in neo-Platonic and especially Paracelsian explanations. He also put this into practice: a series of chemical experiments on blackness that Browne pursued on Paracelsian principles has been studied by Allen Debus.[73] It is also clear, given Browne's belief in the presence and activity of spirits in the world, that adherence to Paracelsian medicine could have been seen as more religiously correct than adherence to the medicine of the pagan Galen. Moreover, Paracelsian medicine can be deeply mystical, and together with Browne's interest in Hermetic mysteries, his interest in mysticism in religion could have been perfectly complemented by an equivalent mysticism in medicine.[74]

There is also a celebrated letter of Browne to Henry Power, son of an old friend, who was beginning the study of medicine.[75] Browne says that it is not possible to become a doctor out of books, so he will recommend authors 'as tend less to ostentation than use, for the directing a novice to observation and experience'. The basic 'fathers of the faculty' are

Hippocrates and Galen. Power should read anatomy, especially Harvey on the circulation; the knowledge of plants, animals and minerals should be pursued in gardens, fields and apothecary shops, while reading Theophrastus, Dioscorides, Matthiolus, Doedens, the English herbalists, Spigelius. 'See chemical operations in hospitals, private houses ... Be not a stranger to the useful part of chemistry. See what Chymistators do in their officines'. From the diversions of chemistry and surgery, turn to the business of medicine, that is to the institutes of medicine, reading Sennert.

> This done, see how Institutes are applicable to practice, by reading upon diseases in Sennertus, Fernelius, Mercatus, Hollerius, Riverius ... But in reading upon diseases satisfy yourself not so much with the remedies set down ... as with the true understanding the nature of the disease, its causes, and proper indications for cure.

This is a balance of classical authors and modern writers. Everything should be turned to use and to medical practice. Chemistry should be studied, at least its useful part. But here Browne does not recommend Paracelsus or Van Helmont, but says: 'begin with *Tyrocinium Chymicum*, Crollius, Hartmannus, and so by degrees march on'. Olivier Leroy, a twentieth-century commentator on Browne, cites this letter to Henry Power and asks: if this letter had not been known, which writers would we assume Browne would recommend for medicine, from the evidence of *Religio Medici*? Our list would include Cardan, Paracelsus, Van Helmont and Agrippa, but possibly not Galen![76] So our first assumptions would be misplaced. The advice to Power might, however, have been given by Browne simply as to a beginner in medicine, and a more innovative and radical list of medical authorities might have been offered by him in other circumstances. At all events, this letter makes plain Browne's concern with observation and experience in medicine, while not rejecting ancient and more modern authority.[77]

We have an extended published example of Browne applying reason, observation and experience to nature, and this is his *Pseudodoxia Epidemica*, the *Vulgar Errors* of 1646, (hereafter *VE*), with several enlarged editions issued by him in the course of his lifetime. It has been claimed that this work was conceived by Browne following a suggestion by Francis Bacon that the advancement of learning needed 'a calendar of falsehoods and of popular errors now passing unargued in natural history'.[78] Browne wrote this very large work, he says, 'as medical vacations, and the fruitless importunity of Uroscopy would permit us', and it must have taken up a lot of his spare time in his twenties and thirties, indicating the extent of his identification with the new learning of the seventeenth century.

As with *Religio Medici*, Browne is here concerned with the need to base truth on reason and experience. It is desirable for us, he says, to

'timely survey our knowledge, impartially singling out those encroach-
ments, which junior compliance and popular credulity hath admitted.
Whereof at present we have endeavoured a long and serious *Adviso*,
proposing not only a large and copious list, but from experience and
reason attempting their decisions' (*VE*, p. 3). This work is aimed at the
advancement of learning:

> Nor can we conceive it may be unwelcome unto those honoured
> Worthies, who endeavour the advancement of Learning: as being
> likely to find a clearer progression, when so many rubs are levelled,
> and many untruths taken off, which passing as principles with
> common beliefs, disturb the tranquillity of Axioms, which might
> otherwise be raised ...
>
> (*VE*, p. 6)

The title of this work links it immediately to Browne's concerns in
Religio Medici about the vulgar: the common people believe what is
only pseudo-true. But the work is addressed not to the mob but to the
gentry, although unfortunately vulgar thinking is not absent even from
here, for amongst the gentry too there is a 'rabble', a sort of 'Plebian
heads'. If the gentry can be stopped from believing these vulgar errors,
the erroneous beliefs will 'wither of themselves', for the gentry will be
an example to the vulgar, and true knowledge will flow out from
them.[79]

Browne begins the book with an extensive section in which he in-
spects the grounds on which the vulgar, and indeed mankind in general,
are subject to false belief. First, there is the common infirmity of human
nature, which led Adam to sin and which we all inherit. The vulgar
people are further characterized as suffering from feeble understanding,
being incompetent to judge between the true and the false: 'For the
assured truth of things is derived from principles of knowledge, and
causes which determine their verities. Whereof their uncultivated
understandings, scarce holding any theory, they are but bad discerners
of verity ...' (*VE*, p. 26). The vulgar are dominated by their brute
appetites, and disdain 'strict and subtle reason' (ibid.); they are both
credulous and incredulous, which is 'not only derogatory unto the
wisdom of God, who hath proposed the World unto our knowledge,
and thereby the notion of Himself; but also detractory unto the intellect, and sense of man expressedly disposed for that inquisition'. (*VE*,
pp. 37–8) Their supinity or neglect of enquiry means they 'neither make
Experiment by sense, or Enquiry by reason; but live in doubt of things,
whose satisfaction is in their own power ... ' (*VE*, p. 39). People are too
willing to rest on authority, especially that of the ancients, even though
the ancients were so often and so obviously wrong, which we can
recognize 'not only by critical and collective reason, but common and

country observation' (*VE*, p. 42). Arguments from authority have no special virtue; by contrast 'our advanced beliefs are not to be built upon dictates, but having received the probable inducements of truth, we become emancipated from testimonial engagements, and are to erect upon the surer base of reason' (*VE*, pp. 47–8).

What is most striking to the modern reader in this catalogue of human weaknesses and this call for the investigation of nature to be based on reason, observation and experiment, is the central role played in it by God and His arch-foe Satan. This should warn us again against interpreting Browne either as someone trying to separate 'science' from religion, or as a proto-scientist, even in this book of his which deals so largely with nature and calls for observation and experiment. Browne repeatedly speaks here, as he had done also in *Religio Medici*, of it being a God-given duty for man to take up the role of natural philosopher and to investigate God's creation. But further, Browne places the intellectual weaknesses and fallibility of man firmly within the historic divine story: man is naturally intellectually weak because he is descended from Adam who fell; and the greatest incitement today to false belief is still the activity of Satan as the promoter of false opinion. Not only does Satan incite us constantly to atheism, the greatest form of false belief, by suggesting to us that God does not exist, or that He has no providential care for mankind, or that there are many gods, or that he himself (Satan) is God, or that he himself does not exist (and that therefore there is no evil in the world), but Satan also exploits nature itself both to deceive us with false miracles, and to interpret as natural his own perversions of nature. Only from a proper understanding of the hidden or secret workings of nature will we be able to distinguish the workings of the devil.

> For many things secret are true: sympathies and antipathies are safely authentic unto us, who ignorant of their causes may yet acknowledge their effects. Beside, being a natural Magician he [Satan] may perform many acts in ways above our knowledge, though not transcending our natural power, when our knowledge shall direct it.
>
> (*VE*, p. 67)

There is thus no separation here for Browne between the pursuit of truth in nature and the Christian's practice of true religion: the investigation of nature is literally an investigation of God, of 'the notion of Himself', of His creation, of His providence and His final causes. Experiment and observation, together with the deployment of our God-given reasoning faculty, are our tools in this investigation. God 'hath proposed the world unto our disputation' (*VE*, p. 20). The religion of a physician thus naturally, by his duty to God, leads him away from reliance on authority and toward experiment and observation: 'In Natural Philosophy, more generally pursued amongst us, it [i.e. authority] carrieth but slender consideration; for that [i.e. natural philosophy] also proceeding from settled Principles, therein is expected a satisfaction from scientifical progressions, and such as beget a sure rational belief' (*VE*, p. 48). That is to say, natural philosophy starts from settled principles and then proceeds by building firm knowledge on firm knowledge, thus making a progression in knowledge ('scientifical progressions'), the kind of progression which begets 'a sure rational belief'.

Browne's attitude here to authority needs comment, for he has been judged, for all his fine words, to be firmly in thrall to ancient authority figures in *Vulgar Errors*, and to have a very bookish approach to learning, which would seem inappropriate for someone talking about the investigation of nature. Browne was indeed highly academic by inclination, possessing a large library, and he was acquainted with an enormous range of writers ancient and modern on the most diverse and recondite of subjects. Many of his own minor writings are on the obscurest and the most antiquarian of topics. His own writing style is the most artifical and literary of anyone of his century. So Browne is obviously passionate about writers and writing, and thus deeply concerned with authors/authorities and their texts. But Browne was in no way in thrall to authors/authorities. Nor is he rejecting authority, especially not the classical authorities. The situation is this: authority/authors are for Browne a *starting-point* of research, indeed his favourite starting-point. As Marie Boas Hall has pointed out, Browne's 'vulgar errors' are all errors in books: 'this work is in fact a natural history of learned error'.[80] Sometimes authorities are right, sometimes they are wrong. The only way to tell is to assess them by critical reason and, when it comes to questions about nature, by observation and experiment. For instance much of Browne's work on nature was a sort of commentary on Aristotle's *History of Animals*, a book Browne regarded as very erroneous (as his comments in his letters to his son Edward testify), but one which he also regarded as singularly important. A whole chapter of the introduction to *Vulgar Errors* is devoted to listing the most untrustworthy of the ancient writers 'who, though excellent and useful Authors' unfortunately were particularly prone to copying out errors from other writers without checking (*VE*, p. 52). So Browne does not follow authorities slavishly; but nor does he jettison them wholesale. Instead he subjects what they say, item by item, to critical reason, to observation and experiment: 'Nor is only a resolved prostration unto Antiquity a powerful enemy unto knowledge, but any confident adherence unto Authority, or resignation of our judgements upon the testimony of any Age or Author whatsoever' (*VE*, p. 47).

This is what we must avoid, Browne says: any 'resignation of our
judgements upon the testimony of any Age or Author whatsoever'. The
parallels, the continuity, of Browne's views here in *Vulgar Errors* with
his position in *Religio Medici* should require no underlining. In religion
and in investigating nature – itself a duty given us by God – we should
not follow authority blindly, but question it; we should instead rely on
our reason and on our sense, on experience and experiment. In short,
we should use our God-given judgements to attain 'a sure rational
belief' in both areas. The expression 'sure rational belief', which sounds
so odd in modern ears, neatly encapsulates Browne's aim in the pursuit
of truth both in religion and in God's creation.

There is one particular area where the coherence of Browne's views of
truth in both nature and religion has threatened to make his historical
reputation notorious. Browne wrote in *Religio Medici* that he believed in
witches: 'I have ever believed, and do now know, that there are Witches'.
His argument was that witches are spirits and are necessary to fulfil the
Great Chain or Ladder of Being, from God down.[81] It is a perfectly
conventional argument for the time, and one which is both religious and
natural-philosophical/medical: it typifies the religion of a physician that
Browne advocated. We know that in his capacity as a physician Browne
was called in to at least one witch trial to give an expert opinion. On 13–
14 March, in 1664, at the assizes in Bury St Edmunds, Rose Cullender
and Amy Duny of Lowestoft were tried and convicted for bewitching
children, and put to death. Dr Browne of Norwich, 'a Person of great
knowledge' (as a contemporary report called him), testified,

> And his opinion was, That the Devil in such cases did work upon
> the Bodies of Men and Women, upon a Natural Foundation, (that
> is) to stir up, and excite such humours super-abounding in their
> [the victims'] Bodies to a great excess, whereby he did in an ex-
> traordinary manner Afflict them with such Distempers as their
> Bodies were most subject to, as particularly appeared in these
> Children; for he conceived, that these swouning Fits were Natural,
> and nothing else but that they call the Mother [i.e. hysteria], but
> only heightned to a great excess by the subtilty of the Devil, co-
> operating with the Malice of those which we term Witches, at
> whose Instance he doth these Villanies.[82]

Apparently Browne cited fresh instances of witchcraft from Denmark
(and this is where it was significant that Danish was one of his languages), where there had recently been 'a great discovery of witches
who used the very same way of afflicting persons, by conveying pins
into them'. An eighteenth-century sceptic of witchcraft, Frances
Hutchinson, was to write, 'This was a case of blood, and surely the
king's subjects ought not to lose their lives upon the credit of books
from *Denmark*'.[83]

This incident has been a great trial for admirers of Browne in all his historic disguises: Browne the apparent liberal proponent of toleration and moderation in religion, Browne the timeless exquisite writer, and Browne the open-minded proto-scientist jettisoning superstition in favour of cool rationality. Even Patrides, his most recent editor, calls Browne's statement of belief here 'an astonishing utterance; but I think intentionally so', and puts it down to Browne's sense of necessary cosmic order.[84] But it is actually at a more profound level of belief for Browne, a level we cannot share in our usual attempts to make Browne a modern liberal. For Browne claimed that it is an act of the devil to propagate in us the *un*belief in witches – it is an instance of how the devil tries to make us interpret the natural as unnatural, it is a devilish encouragement to atheism.[85] And Browne is perfectly explicit in *Religio Medici* about the existence – the necessary existence if the great chain of being is to be complete – everywhere in this material world, of spirits, good and bad (*RM*, I.35), and hence of witches. Good spirits are our guardian angels (*RM*, I.33); possibly, as the Platonists say, there is a world spirit (*RM*, I.32); certainly there is the spirit of God active within us 'the fire and scintillation of that noble and mighty Essence, which is the life and radical heat of spirits' (*RM*, I.32). Witches are amongst the devil's scholars, and they delude us by making natural effects look like magic. 'Thus', he writes, 'I think at first a great part of Philosophy was Witchcraft, which being afterward derived to one another, proved but Philosophy, and was indeed no more but the honest effects of Nature: What invented by us is Philosophy, learned from him [the devil] is Magic' (*RM*, I.31). This is precisely what Browne also later maintained in *Vulgar Errors*, and what he is reported as arguing 20 years later at the trial in Bury: that these swooning fits were natural, 'but only heightened to a great excess by the subtility of the Devil, co-operating with the malice of those we term witches'. The devil, through his pupil witches, uses natural means to achieve perverted, devilish ends, intending thus to undermine our 'sure rational belief' in God and His workings. Given Browne's general favouring of experiment to test authority and testimony, it is interesting to find that Browne did not join with some of the more cynical gentlemen at the trial who insisted on performing what they called 'experiments' to test the veracity of the children, as a result of which they concluded that 'the whole transaction of this business was a mere Imposture'.[86]

What I have been presenting above is a different picture of Browne's view of nature than that presented by some twentieth-century commentators who have suggested that Browne's predeliction for reason, experiment and the 'new philosophy' of the seventeenth century put him in a quandry with respect to religious belief – that he had, somehow, to justify the one if he wanted still to believe in the other, and that this is what he was doing in *Religio Medici*. Using John Donne's words they have asked: did the new philosophy 'call all in doubt' for Browne?[87] Or did he resign himself to a fideist position with respect to religion, believing what he was told to believe, without subjecting doctrine to the test of reason, and did he meanwhile conduct his natural philosophy wearing, as it were, another hat? The most common way in which historians have resolved this problem of their own making has been to argue that Browne was an early scientist or proto-scientist and, though he was manifestly religious, yet he managed to keep his religion and his science separate, and that this is to be admired in him. Gordon Chalmers, for instance, has claimed that we can legitimately distinguish in Browne's writings his 'reasons for research', which were clearly often religious, and 'the reasons he uses in order to draw inferences from his observations', which were not demonstrably religious, and Chalmers concludes from this that 'on the whole Sir Thomas Browne did keep his particular scientific speculations free of theology and ethics ... [which indicates] that in his scientific practice Sir Thomas Browne was really scientific'.[88] This whole problem, however, is predicated on the assumption that the science-religion antithesis of the nineteenth and twentieth centuries can be read back on to the religious-minded natural philosophers of the seventeenth century, as they went about investigating the creation as a God-given duty. Thomas Browne was not arguing for making any kind of separation between religion and natural investigation, but quite the reverse: he was arguing that the one reinforced the other, that exploration of nature was an appropriate and worthy undertaking for a Christian and led him ever closer to his creator. Both were to be conducted using our God-given reasoning faculty.

However, we need to bear in mind that in pursuing this argument Browne was not engaged in the exercise of 'natural theology'. Some of his contemporaries were beginning to engage in such natural theological arguments in order to counter and win over the atheists that they were convinced were all around them seeking to undermine society and true religion. For instance in 1676, Thomas Tenison, later Archbishop of Canterbury but at this date minister at Browne's church, St Peter Mancroft in Norwich, wrote a poem '*contra hujus saeculi Lucretianos*' [Against the Lucretians of our age], illustrating Gods wisdom and providence from anatomy, and the rubric and use of parts in a manuscript ... in Latin after Lucretius his style' and dedicated it to Thomas Browne himself and to a Dr Lawson.[89] This is the key natural theology argument: it starts from the findings of natural philosophy, in this case from anatomy, and uses them to show that nature reveals the actions (and hence the existence) of a providential designer, the Christian God; hence atheism is misguided, and all the evidence of creation is against it. But in *Religio Medici* Thomas Browne by contrast is arguing that the study of nature is an *additional and complementary* route to God, rather than being a route to atheism. Both this argument and the natural theological argument are concerned with God, atheism and nature, but they are different arguments and we should not confuse them. However, we would certainly be correct to conclude that Browne wrote *Religio Medici* primarily because he was, like so many men of his age, obsessed with the dangers of atheism.

The religion of physicians: the skull, the man and the book

Today there are three kinds of general response to *Religio Medici*. Two we have already touched on: that of the English literature scholar; and that of the historian of science and medicine, who uses Browne as a touchstone for the state of the supposed dispute between science and religion in seventeenth-century England. But there is a third continuing interest, one which is in a way more important than either of these two, and it is one which, unusually, links the world of the historian of medicine with the world of medicine itself. I am referring to the still-living response of certain physicians wanting some sort of model or ideal for their professional and private lives. This image of Browne as a model physician derives from the real dispute between the respective supporters of science and religion, which took place of course not in the seventeenth but in the nineteenth century, in the wake of the publication of Darwin's *The Origin of Species* (1859).

This image of Browne was created by the most famous modern Brownian,[90] Sir William Osler, a physician who was very influential in setting his own life as a model for the ideal life of a physician and whose legacy is still with us, although he died as long ago as 1919. Osler rose to become successively professor of the Institutes of Medicine at McGill, of Clinical Medicine at Pennsylvania, Physician-in-Chief to the Johns Hopkins Hospital in Baltimore, and Regius Professor of Medicine at Oxford, and his book *Principles and Practice of Medicine* (1892), in which he sought to unite two discordant medical realms of his day – clinical medicine and laboratory medicine – became a classic and, in a modern guise, was still in print until recently.

Osler was introduced to Browne and *Religio Medici* while still at school. *Religio Medici* turned Osler to becoming a bibliophile and collector. He resolved to collect every edition of *Religio Medici*.[91] But the book had a far greater significance for him than this. At 49 years of age, Osler could say of *Religio Medici*:

no book had has so enduring an influence on my life. I was introduced to it by my first teacher, the Rev. W. A. Johnston, Warden
and Founder of the Trinity College School [in Toronto], and I can
recall the delight with which I first read its quaint and charming
pages. It was one of the strong influences which turned my thoughts
towards medicine as a profession, and my most treasured copy –
the second book I ever bought – has been a constant companion
for thirty-one years – *comes viae vitaeque* ... [92]

Johnston, Osler's teacher, was a High Church Anglican, with strong
sympathy for the Oxford Tractarians, and he might have moved over to
Rome with Newman had he stayed in England.[93] Osler too was Church
of England when he was a young man, for his father was an Anglican
clergyman and missionary, sent to Canada by the Society for the Propa-
gation of the Gospel in Foreign Parts.

Born in 1849, Osler was a young man making his life choices at the
very time when the furore resulting from the publication of Darwin's
Origin of Species was at its height. The Church of England of his father
and his father's clerical colleagues was not only 'high' and ritualistic,
but with respect to the issues raised by Darwin it was highly defensive,
doctrinally rigid, and anti-science. Osler was introduced to *Religio
Medici* at a moment when he was uncertain whether to become a
minister of religion or a doctor, and he felt the book turned him to
medicine. It thus enabled him, in his adolescent spiritual crisis, to take a
first step away from the anti-science rigidities of the Church of England
that he knew. But *Religio Medici* of course held for him still much
religion, and thus permitted him to conclude that religion and an
interest in nature could be compatible: that is, in nineteenth-century
terms, that religion and science were really compatible, not incompatible.
Gradually, Osler moved further and further away from mainstream
Church of England Christianity, and in 1872 even spent 18 months as a
student in the 'godless' environment of University College, London,
which proved to be a 'dangerous school' for him.[94] Ultimately Osler
became an agnostic, but he never rid himself completely of God and the
religious mission: as late as 1910 he was still producing what he called
'lay sermons', such as the one of that year on 'Man's redemption of
man'. The relatively open and tolerant Church of England that Browne's
Religio Medici presented to Osler's young eyes was obviously far more
attractive to him than the Church of England that Osler knew from his
own home environment. Browne's apparent tolerance presumably meant
to Osler that one could be spiritual in a gentle, non-dogmatic way
without being of an exclusive religious persuasion, or indeed even a
Christian.

Osler learnt the text of *Religio Medici* off by heart. He frequently
called Browne 'my life-long mentor', and recommended Browne's wis-

dom in many lectures. He described Browne as 'that most liberal of men and most distinguished of general practitioners', and 'an even-balanced soul', and called him one of his 'old friends in the spirit'.[95] For Osler, Browne 'presents a remarkable example in the medical profession of a man who mingled the waters of science with the oil of faith. I know of no one in history who believed so implicitly and so simply in the Christian religion, yet it is evident from his writings that he had moments of ardent scepticism'.[96] That is to say, in Osler's view, Browne had succeeded in mixing those two unmixables, science and faith, which Osler himself had found so hard to reconcile, and like Osler he had suffered ardent scepticism while retaining a core of simple faith (though Browne's faith was more explicitly Christian than Osler's). Osler's interpretation of Browne's religious position was always at this imprecise but idealized level. As he told students, Osler felt that the book was a moral guide to life: 'Mastery of self, conscientious devotion to duty, deep human interest in human beings – these best of all lessons you must learn now or never: and these are some of the lessons which may be gleaned from the life and from the writings of Sir Thomas Browne.'[97] It obviously required the ear of someone who had himself struggled with the relation of science and religion to hear Browne teaching these lessons of aChristian morality in *Religio Medici*.

Osler's identification with his Sir Thomas Browne was as total as he could make it. He had discovered that Sir Thomas had written 'On my coffin when in the grave I desire may be deposited in its leather case or coffin my pocket Elzevir's Horace, "Comes viae vitaeque dulcis et utilis" worn out with and by me'.[98] The *Religio Medici* had been Osler's own 'gentle and valued companion of his way and life'. So in his turn, when he was laid out in the cathedral of Christ Church, Oxford in 1919 Osler lay, in the words of his biographer, 'in the scarlet gown of Oxford, his bier covered with a plain velvet pall on which lay a single sheaf of lilies and his favourite copy of the "Religio", *comes viae vitaeque*'.[99]

In 1901, in anticipation of the Norwich celebrations of the three hundredth anniversary of Browne's birth, Sir William Osler presented a glass case in which to keep and display the skull of Sir Thomas, still out of its grave, with quotations from *Religio Medici* on the theme of death, mortality and immortality, engraved around the case (see Figure 2.5). The transformation was now complete: Sir Thomas's skull had been turned into a full religious relic and object of pilgrimage of the adherents of the Christian religion which Osler believed that Browne had taught in *Religio Medici*.[100]

In his love of Browne and of *Religio Medici* in particular, Osler has been notably followed in modern times by another physician-bibliophile, practitioner-historian, Geoffrey Keynes, physician to the Bloomsbury

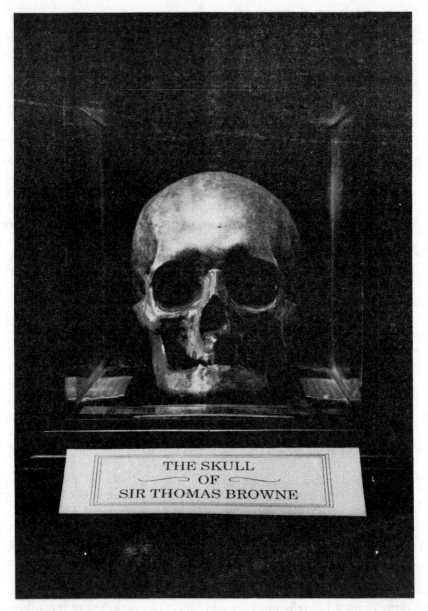

2.5 Cast of the skull of Sir Thomas Browne, in a case presented by Sir William Osler.

Group, modern pioneer in blood transfusion, and brother of Maynard (though he hated being identified like that). Keynes was to produce the modern complete edition of Browne's works. Like everyone else in our story, he was to receive a knighthood. However, the initial religious dimension was absent in this case: Keynes was an agnostic from an early age. When at Cambridge as a student in 1908, Keynes was introduced to the poetry of John Donne by Rupert Brooke, and Keynes started to collect. Then Keynes 'fixed on' Sir Thomas Browne 'as one of the greatest literary artists, as well as being a doctor, and therefore to be collected'.[101] Keynes and another student, Cosmo Gordon, boldly wrote to Osler, then Regius Professor of Medicine at Oxford, who welcomed them. Keynes became a lifelong fan and promoter of what he described as 'the Oslerian tradition' – a particular attitude to life, responsibility, history in medicine, and centred round the clinician's task.[102] As we have seen, Osler for his part thought this was an attitude he had discovered in the life and religion of Thomas Browne – tolerant, international in outlook, being at once sceptical and full of simple faith, allowing equal legitimacy to the spiritual and the scientific, and deeply ethical. For a spiritually minded but sceptical physician of the scientific age, it was the perfect religion of a physician.

Notes

Acknowledgement: I am very grateful to Ole Grell for his advice on matters theological and historical.

1.   Hardin Craig, writing in 1950, cited in Frank Livingstone Huntley, *Sir Thomas Browne, a Biographical and Critical Study*, Ann Arbor, University of Michigan Press, 1962, p. 105.
2.   Letter of 1804, cited in Huntley, *Sir Thomas Browne*, p. 134.
3.   From 'Rhetoric' in De Quincey's *Collected Writings*, D. Masson (ed.), Edinburgh, Black, 1890, vol. 10, p. 105.
4.   William Petty said to Pepys in January 1664 that *Religio Medici* was one of the three books that during his life had been 'most esteemed and generally cried up for wit in the world'. This was not a compliment: Petty went on to say that the wit lay 'in confirming some pretty sayings, which are generally like paradoxes, by some argument smartly and pleasantly urged which takes with people who do not trouble themselfs to examine the force of an argument which pleases them in the delivery, upon a subject which they like ... ' (Robert Latham and William Matthews (eds), *The Diary of Samuel Pepys*, 11 vols, London, Bell, 1970–83, vol. 5, p. 27).
5.   For detail on this see Frank J. Warnke, 'A Hook for Amphibium: Some Reflections on Fish', in C.A. Patrides, (ed.), *Approaches to Sir Thomas Browne: The Ann Arbor Tercentenary Lectures and Essays*, London, University of Missouri Press, 1982, pp. 49–59.
6.   Huntley, *Sir Thomas Browne*, p. 169.
7.   Joan Webber, 'Sir Thomas Browne: Art as Recreation', in her *The Elo-*

quent 'I': Style and Self in Seventeenth-Century Prose, Madison, Milwaukee, University of Wisconsin Press, 1968, pp. 151, 153. As Browne says in the Preface, 'there are many things to be taken in a soft and flexible sense, and not to be called unto the rigid test of reason'.

8. Browne writes that wise and prudent men 'so contrive their affairs that although their actions be manifest, their designs are not discoverable ... for vulgar eyes behold no more of wise men than doth the Sun: they may discover their exterior and outward ways, but their interior and inward pieces he only sees, that sees into their beings' (*Vulgar Errors*, Book III, ch. 20).

9. I follow the reconstruction presented by M.L. Tildesley, in her article, 'Sir Thomas Browne: His Skull, Portraits, and Ancestry', *Biometrika*, XV, (1923), 1–76.

10. Anthony Batty Shaw, *Sir Thomas Browne of Norwich*, Norwich Browne 300 Committee, 1982, caption to illustration 30. The inscription was by Sir Thomas's son, Edward.

11. Sir Arthur Keith, *Phrenological Studies of the Skull and Brain Cast of Sir Thomas Browne of Norwich, delivered at Edinburgh, 9th May 1924*, The Henderson Trust Lectures, no. III, Edinburgh, The Trustees, 1924, p. 2.

12. Tildesley, 'Sir Thomas Browne', p. 1, Introductory Note by Sir Arthur Keith.

13. Tildesley, 'Sir Thomas Browne', p. 4. Tildesley is such an amusing writer that one suspects her tongue was at times in her cheek.

14. Tildesley, 'Sir Thomas Browne', p. 41. She found that none of the artists of the putative portraits of Sir Thomas 'had been *quite* candid about the depressed forehead of the subject': that is, the low forehead does not seem to be represented in any of the supposed portraits (ibid., p. 53). The current authentic portrait of Sir Thomas (Figure 2.1) was not available to her as a possibility.

15. C.A. Patrides (ed.), *Sir Thomas Browne: The Major Works*, Harmondsworth, Penguin Books, 1977, pp. 296–7. All quotations are from this edition, with the spelling modernized; references to *Religio Medici* are to the numbered paragraphs of the text.

16. Tildesley, 'Sir Thomas Browne', p. 68.

17. 1804 letter, quoted in Huntley, *Sir Thomas Browne*, p. 134.

18. 'Sir Thomas Browne', in his *Books and Characters, French and English*, London, Chatto and Windus, 1922, see p. 31.

19. I base my account of Browne's life on a number of works, including: Jeremiah S. Finch, *Sir Thomas Browne: A Doctor's Life of Science and Faith*, New York, Schuman, 1950; Joan Bennett, *Sir Thomas Browne: 'A Man of Achievement in Literature'*, Cambridge, Cambridge University Press, 1962; Huntley, *Sir Thomas Browne*.

20. *Letter to a Friend*, in Patrides, *The Major Works*, p. 392.

21. See Carlo Ginzberg, 'High and Low: The Theme of Forbidden Knowledge in the Sixteenth and Seventeenth Centuries' *Past and Present*, no. 73, 1976. My thanks to Dr S. Kusukawa for bringing this to my attention.

22. Professor Michael McVaugh has kindly assured me, on the basis of a computer search, that this is not a quotation from classical sources. But he suggests that there might be an allusion being made to Psalm 19: 7, in

the Vulgate version (Psalm 20: 6 in the Authorized): 'Now I know that the Lord saveth his anointed: for he will hear him from his holy heaven with the saving strength of his right hand', 'Nunc cognovi quoniam salvum fecit Dominus christum suum. Exaudiet illum de caelo sancto suo, in potentatibus salus dexterae eius'.

23. See especially *RM*, I.21.

24. Frank Ardolino, 'The Saving Hand of God: The Significance of the Emblematic Frontispiece of the *Religio Medici*', *English Language Notes*, 15 (1977) 19–23.

25. Ardolino, 'The Saving Hand of God', p. 21.

26. On these see Sir Geoffrey Keynes, *A Bibliography of Sir Thomas Browne Kt. M.D.*, 2nd edn, Oxford, Clarendon Press, 1968. The Latin, French and Dutch versions were all first published in Holland; on which see Cornelis W. Schoneveld, *Intertraffic of the Mind: Studies in Seventeenth-Century Anglo-Dutch Translation with a Checklist of Books Translated from English into Dutch, 1600–1700*, Leiden, Leiden University Press, 1983, ch. 1, 'One Book: Sir Thomas Browne's *Religio Medici* in Holland'.

27. Editions used: for convenience, Patrides's edition of *Religio Medici*, *Letter to a Friend* and *Christian Morals*; all in *Sir Thomas Browne: The Major Works*. For the complete *Pseudodoxia Epidemica*, the letters and the miscellaneous writings, I have used Sir Geoffrey Keynes's edition of *The Works of Sir Thomas Browne*, 4 vols, 1977, London, Faber and Faber.

28. *The Diary of John Evelyn*, John Bowle, (ed.) Oxford, Oxford University Press, 1983, p. 241.

29. Letter, Browne to his son Edward, 14 June 1676, printed in Keynes, *Works*, vol. 4, p. 61.

30. Letter, Digby to Browne, 20 March 1642/3; printed in Keynes, *Works*, vol. 4, p. 236.

31. This triple theme is pointed out by Patrides, *The Major Works*, p. 133, but not explored by him; it has also been noticed by Joan Webber and Frank J. Warnke.

32. Dewy Kiper Ziegler, *'In Divided and Distinguished Worlds': Religion and Rhetoric in the Writings of Sir Thomas Browne*, Cambridge, Mass., Harvard University Press, 1943, pp. 72, 35, 98; this rather silly thesis is, one should note, the work of a very young man.

33. Stanley Fish, 'The Bad Physician: The Case of Sir Thomas Browne', in *Self-Consuming Artifacts: The Experience of Seventeenth Century Literature*, Berkeley, University of California Press, 1972, pp. 353–73, see p. 363.

34. Webber, 'Sir Thomas Browne: Art as Recreation', p. 164.

35. *Medicus Medicatus, or the Physicians Religion Cured by a Lenitive or Gentle Potion*, 1645, p. 2. In a medical analogy, Ross wrote that he had written this criticism 'to let green heads and inconsiderate young Gentlemen see, that there is some danger in reading your Book, without the *spectacles* of judgement; for, whilst they are taken with the *gilding* of your phrase, they may swallow unawares such *pills* as may rather kill then cure them' (ibid., p. 80).

36. Don Cameron Allen, *Doubt's Boundless Sea: Skepticism and Faith in the Renaissance*, Baltimore, Johns Hopkins University Press, 1964, pp. 7–8.

Tobias Wagner in 1677, and D. Colberg in 1680 were to be troubled by
Browne's doubts, Colberg calling him 'a doctor who writes in contempt
of God's Word' (ibid., pp. 12–13 and notes); J.F. Reimann, writing in
1725, was to excuse Browne as a man 'who confessed himself a skeptic
in philosophy but not in religion', whose 'life and words are pure piety'
(ibid., p. 19).

37. Virtually the whole of Whitefoot's 'Some Minutes for the Life of Sir
Thomas Browne', originally prefixed to Browne's *Posthumous Works* of
1712, are reproduced in Patrides, *The Major Works*, pp. 502–5; for the
quotations below see pp. 504, 504–5, and 503 respectively.

38. *Christian Morals*, Patrides, *The Major Works*, p. 424.

39. *Christian Morals*, Patrides, *The Major Works*, p. 427.

40. *Christian Morals*, Patrides, *The Major Works*, p. 426.

41. *Christian Morals*, Patrides, *The Major Works*, p. 424.

42. This is somewhat surprising, at least if one thinks of Paul's sermon to
the Stoics and Epicureans in the *Acts of the Apostles*, ch. 17.

43. This is 1 Corinthians 13; *Letter to a Friend*, Patrides, *The Major Works*,
p. 411–12.

44. *Christian Morals*, in Patrides, *The Major Works*, p. 464. The 'twelve
tables' are the tables of the Roman law, drawn up by the decem viri in
451 BC. The 'two tables' are the tablets of stone on which the Ten
Commandments were given to Moses by God: in Christian exegesis,
following Philo, the first tablet contained the religious commandments
(love the lord thy God), the second the moral commandments (love thy
neighbour), as characterized by Christ. The point Browne is making is
that one should follow the Christian law rather than mere human law,
as a basis for ethical living.

45. On these issues in general, see Roger French and Andrew Cunningham,
Before Science: The Invention of the Friars' Natural Philosophy, Aldershot, Scolar Press, 1996, ch. 1.

46. Short for 'O altitudo sapientiae et scientiae Dei', O, the height of the
wisdom and knowledge of God; see Romans 11: 33, the Vulgate reading
(Authorized gives 'depth' rather than height).

47. Patrides, *The Major Works*, p. 472.

48. Here I follow Hugh Trevor-Roper, 'Laudianism and Political Power', in
his *Catholics, Anglicans and Puritans: Seventeenth Century Essays*, London, Secker and Warburg, 1987, pp. 40–119.

49. Trevor-Roper, 'Laudianism', p. 93.

50. Trevor-Roper, 'Laudianism', p. 53.

51. See Hugh Trevor-Roper, 'Hugo Grotius in England', in his *From Coun-
ter-Reformation to Glorious Revolution*, London, Secker and Warburg,
1992, pp. 47–82.

52. Trevor-Roper, 'Laudianism', p. 98 and note on p. 98.

53. J. van den Berg, 'Sir Thomas Browne and the Synod of Dort', *Sir
Thomas Browne M.D. and the Anatomy of Man*, Leiden, Brill, 1983,
pp. 19–24.

54. H. John McLachlan, *Socinianism in Seventeenth Century England*, Oxford, Oxford University Press, 1951, p. 12.

55. Letter of 1639, quoted in McLachlan, p. 43.

56. *The Expiation of a Sinner. In a Commentary upon the Epistle to the
Hebrewes. By G.M.*, London, 1646; and *The Justification of a Sinner:*

Being the Maine Argument of the Epistle to the Galatians. By a Reverend and Learned Divine, London, 1650. McLachlan, ch. 7, 'Two Oxford Socinians'.

57. Nicholas Tyacke, 'The Rise of "Puritanism" and the Legalizing of Dissent, 1571–1719', in Ole Peter Grell, Jonathan I. Israel and Nicholas Tyacke (eds), *From Persecution to Toleration: The Glorious Revolution and Religion in England*, Oxford, Clarendon Press, 1991, pp. 17–49, see p. 23–30.

58. See Hugh Trevor-Roper, 'The Great Tew Circle', in his *Catholics, Anglicans and Puritans: Seventeenth Century Essays*, London, Secker and Warburg, 1987, pp. 166–230.

59. *The Religion of Protestants a Safe Way to Salvation ...* , Oxford, ?1638 edn, the final words of the first preface, 'The Preface to the Author of *Charity Maintained ...* '.

60. On Chillingworth, see J.D. Hyman, *William Chillingworth and the Theory of Toleration*, Cambridge, Mass., Harvard University Press, 1931.

61. Francis Cheynell, *Chillingworthi Novissima: or, the Sickness, Heresy, Death, and Burial of William Chillingworth ...* , London, Noon, 1725, (originally published 1644), p. 27.

62. Francis Cheynell, *Chillingworthi Novissima*, p. 60.

63. This paragraph derives from Robert R. Orr, *Reason and Authority: The Thought of William Chillingworth*, Oxford, Clarendon Press, 1967, ch. 6, 'The law of reason'.

64. Francis Cheynell, *The Man of Honour, Described in a Sermon, Preached Before the Lords of Parliament, in the Abbey Church of Westminster, March 26, 1645. The Solemn Day of the Publique Monethly Fast*, London, Gellibrand, 1645, p. 65; emphasis as in original. I am indebted for this reference to David Harley.

65. Francis Cheynell, *The Rise, Growth, and Danger of Socinianisme. Together with a Plaine Discovery of a Desperate Designe of Corrupting the Protestant Religion, Whereby It Appeares that the Religion Which Hath Been so Violently Contended for (by the Archbishop of Canterbury and His Adherents) Is Not the Pure Protestant Religion, but an Hotchpotch of Arminianisme, Socinianisme and Popery ...* , London, Gellibrand, 1643, p. 41.

66. This dislike of the multitude Browne may have got from his tutor, Lushington. In a celebrated sermon at Oxford in 1624 Lushington criticized the king for seeking a Catholic marriage for Prince Charles, and also referred to Parliament as 'Now the peasant thinks ... '. He was obliged to recant publicly on both counts. See Huntley, *Sir Thomas Browne*, pp. 43–4.

67. Michael Wilding, '*Religio Medici* in the English Revolution', in Patrides, *Approaches to Sir Thomas Browne*, pp. 100–14.

68. On this recurrent problem see French and Cunningham, *Before Science*, ch. 4.

69. Schoneveld, *Intertraffic*, p. 4.

70. 'R.B.', 1585; P.H. Kocher, *Science and Religion in Elizabethan England*, New York, Octogon Books, 1969 (orig. publ. 1953), p. 251. On the general issue in England at this time, see John Henry, 'The Matter of Souls: Medical Theory and Theology in Seventeenth-Century England',

in Roger French and Andrew Wear (eds), *The Medical Revolution of the Seventeenth Century*, Cambridge, 1989, pp. 87–113.

71. Compare Joseph Glanvill, *Essays on Several Important Subjects in Philosophy and Religion*, London, 1676, p. 5: 'His works receive but little glory from the rude wonder of the ignorant, and there is no wise man that values the applauses of a blind admiration'. I am indebted to Guido Giglioni for this reference.

72. William P. Dunn, *Sir Thomas Browne: A Study in Religious Philosophy*, Minneapolis, University of Minnesota Press, 1951, is particularly valuable on the Platonic dimensions of Browne's argument here and in *RM*, I.14–I.16; see ch. 3, 'The art of God', esp. pp. 104–7.

73. Allen G. Debus, 'Sir Thomas Browne and the Study of Chemical Indicators', *Ambix* **10** (1962), 29–36.

74. See Charles Webster, 'English Medical Reformers of the Puritan Revolution: A Background to the "Society of Chymical Physitians"', *Ambix*, **14** (1967), 16–41; see esp. p. 27.

75. The letter is printed in *Works*, vol. 4, pp. 255–6, and is dated to 1646 by Keynes. Charles Webster has studied the relation of this advice to the career and investigations of young Power in 'Henry Power's Experimental Philosophy', *Ambix*, **14** (1967), 150–78.

76. Olivier Leroy, *Le chevalier Thomas Browne (1605–1682) Sa vie, sa pensée et son art*, Paris, Gamber, 1931, (thèse), pp. 212–16.

77. Webster says of this letter that 'In each field of medicine a judicious selection of works by ancient, Renaissance and contemporary authors was given, together with an exultation [?exhortation] to observation and experiment'. 'Henry Power', pp. 152–3.

78. Dunn, p. 17, and others. In *Vulgar Errors* Browne does not claim that the concept of the book was built on Bacon's suggestion.

79. I have written in English rather than Latin, writes Browne, 'Nor have we addressed our pen or stile [i.e. stylus] unto the people, (whom books do not redress, and are this way incapable of reduction) but unto the knowing and leading part of learning; as well understanding (at least probably hoping) except they be watered from higher regions, and fructifying meteors of knowledge, these weeds must lose their alimental sap and wither of themselves; whose conserving influence, could our endeavours prevent, we should trust the rest unto the scythe of Time, and hopeful dominion of Truth' (*Vulgar Errors*, To the Reader).

80. 'Sir Thomas Browne Naturalist', in Patrides, *Approaches*, pp. 178–87, see p. 180.

81. Arthur O. Lovejoy, *The Great Chain of Being: A Study of the History of Ideas*, New York, Harper, 1960 (first published 1936).

82. *A Tryal of Witches, at the Assizes Held at Bury St Edmonds for the County of Suffolk ... Before Sir Mathew Hale, Kt ...* , London, Longman, 1835 (reprint of 1682 original), see p. 16. See also R.D. Stock, *The Holy and the Daemonic from Sir Thomas Browne to William Blake*, Princeton, Princeton University Press, 1982, p. 62; and *Works*, vol. 3, p. 293, from Browne's commonplace books.

83. Stock, *The Holy and the Demonic*, p. 62.

84. Patrides, *The Major Works*, Introduction, p. 27.

85. *Vulgar Errors*, Book 1.

86. *A Tryal of Witches*, p. 17.

87. And new philosophy calls all in doubt,/The element of fire is quite put out;/The sun is lost, and th'earth, and no mans wit/Can well direct him where to look for it./ ... 'Tis all in peeces, all cohaerence gone;/All just supply, and all Relation/ ... ' (Donne, *The First Anniversary*, 1611).

88. See Gordon K. Chalmers, 'Sir Thomas Browne, True Scientist', *Osiris* (1936), 2, 28–79, for quotation see p. 78; Almonte C. Howell, 'Sir Thomas Browne and Seventeenth Century Scientific Thought', *Studies in Philology*, 22 (1925), 61–80.

89. *Works*, vol 4, p. 57; Browne to his son Edward, 25 February ?1676; Browne mentions this in the context of warning Edward against reading Lucretius' poem, 'there being divers impieties in it, and tis no credit to be punctually versed in it'. Tenison's poem was not published. Given that the argument is against that arch-atheist Lucretius, it is a nice joke that it is in his poetic style. In *Vulgar Errors* Browne also mentions that Raymund Sebund 'hath written a natural theology, demonstrating therein the Attributes of God, and attempting the like in most points of Religion'; *Works*, vol. 2, p. 49.

90. I use this term in hope to distinguish admirers of Sir Thomas from 'Brownists', a sixteenth-century sectarian position, and Brunonians, followers of the eighteenth-century physician, John Brown.

91. See Osler's essay, 'Sir Thomas Browne', an address delivered and first published in 1905; reprinted in *Selected Writings of Sir William Osler 12 July 1849 to 29 December 1919*, G.L. Keynes (ed.), London, Oxford University Press, 1951, pp. 40–61.

92. Harvey Cushing, *The Life of Sir William Osler*, 2 vols, Oxford, Clarendon Press, 1925, vol. 1, pp. 504–5; the first antiquarian book Osler ever bought was the Globe Shakespeare.

93. Cushing, *Life*, vol. 1, p. 27.

94. As Johnston warned his own son in 1876: 'Suffice it to say if you go there [University College] you will find many excellent opportunities you can not find elsewhere most particularly *infidel* ideas. What would I give to be well versed in such ideas: but only to disprove them in other people. Probably it is a dangerous school for you my son. Unquestionably W. Osler shews it was so to him ... Would that you had time to read Mivarts "Lessons from Nature" & you would say "woe to Darwin Huxley and Co"'. Quoted in Cushing, *Life*, vol. 1, p. 148.

95. The quotations are from 1902; Cushing, *Life*, vol. 1, p. 589; and vol. 2, p. 455. Osler's other 'old friends in the spirit' were Plutarch, Montaigne, Browne, Fuller, and Izaak Walton.

96. Cushing, *Life*, vol. 2, p. 25.

97. Osler, *Selected Writings*, p. 61.

98. Cushing, *Life*, vol. 2, p. 681. The quotation is not from Horace.

99. Cushing, *Life*, vol. 2, p. 686.

100. Though the skull was reinterred in St Peter Mancroft, a cast of it is still in the glass case, now in the Sir Thomas Browne Library of the Norfolk and Norwich Hospital.

101. Sir Geoffrey Keynes, *The Gates of Memory*, Oxford, Clarendon Press, 1981, p. 54. Keynes resolved to make a complete collection of Browne's works and prepare a bibliography, which he eventually completed. Keynes's collection of Browne's works is in the Cambridge University Library.

102. Keynes, *The Gates of Memory*, see esp. p. 51 and the Appendix 'The Oslerian Tradition'.

CHAPTER THREE

The Career of Astrological Medicine in England

Michael MacDonald

When they mentioned them at all, historians used to have fun writing about early modern astrologers. They enlivened their panoramas of life in a more superstitious, prescientific age with colourful characters that seemed (and sometimes were) drawn straight out of the pages of Jonson, Butler and Swift, and the pictures of Hogarth. To them once famous figures like John Dee, Simon Forman, William Lilly and John Partridge were master charlatans who preyed gleefully on a gullible public, vending their bogus learning alongside mountebanks hawking their worthless nostrums. They were streetwise quacks like Jonson's Subtle; they cluttered their consulting rooms with absurd magical bric-a-brac, like Sidrophel's stuffed alligator in Hogarth's satire of astrology.[1] Until the 1970s the main historical problem posed by the early modern astrologers was why in the world anyone fell for them. But since the publication of Keith Thomas's *Religion and the Decline of Magic* (1971), it has become impossible to see astrologers simply as objects of ridicule. For he showed that astrology was actually a central – if controversial – feature of the intellectual and social history of the early modern period, especially of the history of medicine, which has become a branch of both. Belief in the principles of astrology was widespread and became more so as the period progressed.[2]

For the historian A.T. (after Thomas) the problem has become more complex and significant, if less amusing. The problem for us is to explain why astrology's prestige declined as its popularity grew. To solve that puzzle, we must be able to grasp the attractions of astrology and to see its strengths and weaknesses from the perspective of our ancestors, rather than from the point of view of modern science and medicine. Our effort to imagine our way back into the distant past is complicated in the first instance by the very different nature of early modern society. England was a small but highly stratified nation, in which the gap between the learned and the unlearned was greater than it is today. The culture of the élites had a Latin base that connected it to other élites on the Continent and to the past but excluded the great majority of men and more women, despite the increasing use of English in fields that had been vernacular-free zones. Élite culture changed at a very different pace from that of the common people, and between 1500 and 1800 they grew further apart in many ways. To make any progress at all in understanding the career of astrology, we have to keep that dichotomy constantly in mind.[3]

Astrology and medicine

Astrology had always had a place in medicine in the West, and medicine was anciently an aspect of astrological practice. Its principles were developed in texts that predated the classical age, and they were refined during the Middle Ages as Arabic learning introduced old texts and new ideas into the Latin world. In late medieval England as on the Continent astrology was a learned art. Some astrologers taught at Oxford or Cambridge, and the chief practitioners were clients of the crown and high nobility. Almost all were clerical intellectuals; a few had been educated in medicine in Italian universities. The astrologers' most lofty pursuit was casting horoscopes for the king and greater magnates, but they were employed primarily as court physicians. The most famous amongst them were the royal astrologer and doctor, John Argentine, who served Edward IV and his doomed sons, and William Parron, who was Henry VII's physician and figure-caster. The Italian John Baptista Boerio was chief physician to both Henry VII and Henry VIII. By the early sixteenth century, the link between astrology and medicine at the royal court 'had become something of an institution', according to Hilary Carey, the most recent historian of medieval English astrology.[4]

Knowledge of astrological principles and symbols steadily expanded in the late medieval and Tudor periods. Educated laymen such as Chaucer displayed a sophisticated grasp of the art in the fourteenth and fifteenth centuries, and astrological symbolism was woven into the fabric of cathedrals in their stained glass and sculpture programmes.[5] After a period of apparent decline, astrology revived in a burst of vernacular publication during the reign of Elizabeth I. Elizabethan literature is full of astrological reference and allusion, and most of the leading authors were sympathetic to the art, despite contemporary doubts about its legitimacy.[6] Many physicians, including men in the first couple of generations of Fellows of the London College of Physicians, studied astrology and some of them practised it or published astrological treatises or almanacs. The College's examinations of Simon Forman are instructive in this context. In his first interrogation Forman admitted that his expertise in medicine was based primarily on astrology, rather than the classical texts set by the College. The examiners agreed thereafter to limit their questioning to his knowledge of astrological medicine. They not only presumed their own competence in that field, but found his abilities sadly wanting, in their opinion. 'He answered so absurdly and ridiculously', they noted in their Annals, 'that it caused great mirth and sport amongst the Auditors'.[7] It was still more common for astrologers to style themselves as physicians: roughly one-third of the known British authors of almanacs between 1485 and 1700 were medical men, 91 in all.[8] Many more astrological doctors published nothing.

The most celebrated astrologer of the sixteenth century was John Dee. A fabulous polymath with a marvellous library, he inspired a large and talented band of acolytes to study mathematics, navigation, physics, alchemy, astrology and angelic magic. To them, Dee was a demigod. Perhaps he was so to himself, for his overweening intellectual ambition led him to practise magic in a search for religious truths. Inevitably, in an age of religious reform and confessional war, he found himself in deep trouble. When Dee returned from an adventurous sojourn in Europe where he conjured archangels with the help of his scryer, a suspect character called Edmund Kelly, he was attacked as a master of the black arts. His home was sacked and despite the Queen's loyalty, he was exiled from London to Manchester. His notoriety was amplified by references to him by writers hostile to magic, or its abuses. He is named in Ben Jonson's devastating satire *The Alchemist* and other plays. To such detractors, he was a virtual devil, the English Faustus, and all of the mystical and scientific pursuits he stood for were tainted by irreligion and imposture. The darker side of Dee's reputation did not deter those who had fallen under his spell, but it cast a shadow of suspicion on them and their work.[9]

Although Dee himself seems not to have practised medicine, except perhaps on his family and himself, there is a direct line of descent from him to the most prominent Elizabethan and Jacobean medical astrologers, Simon Forman and Richard Napier. Both knew Dee and were strongly influenced by his work.[10] Like him, they studied magic as well as alchemy and astrology, but unlike him, they also established huge medical practices. Forman soon became almost as notorious as Dee himself. His popularity as a physician and fortune-teller brought him patients from every stratum of London society and from the court, but it also excited the envy and hostility of the College of Physicians, who harried him for years for practising medicine without their approval, imprisoning or driving him into hiding on several occasions. Forman was an unforgettable personality: mercurial, mesmerizing, combative, sexually rapacious. He was that rare thing, a paranoid with platoons of real enemies.[11]

Richard Napier was an altogether different kind of man. Pious and scholarly, he had been educated as a theologian at Oxford. In 1597 he consulted Forman about some lost property and became fascinated by the man and his practice. Napier learned practical astrology from Forman and acquired a copy of his remarkable textbook of astrological medicine.[12] He established a practice of his own at Great Linford, in Buckinghamshire, which he continued until his death in 1634.[13] Measured in terms of the number of their clients, Forman and Napier were probably the most popular astrological physicians of the age, and their surviving manuscripts certainly make them the best documented. Together they treated between 1,000 and 2,500 clients a year, submitting all kinds of illnesses and problems to astrological analysis. Their papers provide the richest and fullest insight into the methods and attractions of astrological medicine.[14]

Both Forman and Napier believed fervently in the truth of astrology. Both cast figures for themselves, Forman to help guide him through an especially dangerous love affair, for instance, Napier to assess the perils posed by his illnesses and resolve family problems. But neither regarded astrology as a perfected system or infallible art. They collected and studied the available authorities, and Napier especially demonstrated an interest in the evolving discoveries in astronomy.[15] They also insisted on accuracy in stellar observations, patient interviews and record-keeping. Forman and Napier kept meticulous notebooks that included astrological calculations, patients' complaints and prescriptions, which they reviewed regularly, recording the actual outcome of their treatments. And in fact, both were more systematic in observing and recording them than the regular physicians whose papers have survived, with the possible exception of the celebrated Theodore Mayerne.[16]

From their practice books it is apparent that for Forman and Napier astrology was above all a tool, like uroscopy. Napier contrasted the two in a remark to George Atwell that is notably modest in its claims. Experience had shown him, he told the young man, that inspection of the patient's urine led him to false conclusions ten times more frequently than his horoscope.[17] Astrology certainly did not supplant the clinical assessment of the patients' symptoms, which remained the most important factor in diagnosis and treatment.[18] Forman's textbook insists that the astrologer begin consultations by eliciting and noting essential information about patients, including sex, age, place of residence and, of course, the time of the consultation. He was to enquire carefully about the relationship of the patient's representative, if he or she had not come in person.[19] He should then erect a map of the heavens for the moment and elicit the patient's description of his or her own complaints, carefully noting them down for future analysis in light of the course the illness took and the patient's history. Finally, when all of this data had been recorded, the physician analysed the illness in light of *both* the figure and the clinical signs, made a diagnosis and pre-scribed remedies. These last were usually the standard battery of purges, emetics and phlebotomy, although both Forman and Napier also occa-sionally dispensed magical amulets.[20]

The main features of these practices were identical to those employed by regular physicians. Both relied on clinical observation and used the same remedies. Both made diagnoses and prescriptions in light of vital information such as the age and sex of the patient.[21] The main differ-ence was that astrologers cast a horoscope, and it is worth asking (rather than merely assuming) what the significance of that additional step was. At this level of astrological practice, analysis of the stars did not pre-empt clinical evidence, as I have already stressed. It was a flexible tool, and the horoscope could be evaluated to different degrees of specificity. In simple cases involving ordinary patients, analysis might include just a brief consideration of the position of the moon and sun and the configuration of the first and eighth houses of the heavens, the houses of illness and death, respectively. In more mysterous afflictions and when clients were wealthy enough to pay for additional pains, the astrologer went on to assess the significance of more planetary and stellar relationships. In practice, because of the complexity of astrologi-cal forces, the horoscope did not produce an unambiguous diagnosis nor foreordain an appropriate therapy. The horoscope, in other words, did not and could not *impose* a significance on the patient's illness. It had to be interpreted.[22]

Why, then, did astrologers cast figures and analyse them at all? To answer that question, we have to attend to their conscious and uncon-scious or semi-conscious motivations. Consciously, astrologers at this level of expertise used figures to guide their analysis of symptomatic complaints in a manner analogous to the way doctors today employ laboratory tests like, for instance, a blood series. If a patient presents lassitude, jaundice and weight loss nowadays, his physician orders blood tests that include a liver spectrum. If the liver enzymes are elevated, he might then go on to question the patient about his drinking habits and order a more specific battery of tests to determine whether he has cirrhosis or cancer of the liver (or both). In a similar way, the astrologer analysed the pattern of stellar influences interactively, eliciting further information from the client when the horoscope had particular, sinister features. The range of these secondary signs was broader than it would be today, but it was not dissimilar. The client's diet and exercise habits were important, as Galenic orthodoxy insisted, and so were psychologi-cal factors, such as marital stress or abnormal moods or thoughts.[23]

On a conscious level, therefore, astrological analysis provided a means to focus the attention of the clinican on significant symptoms, and gave him greater confidence in his diagnosis. On an unconscious or semi-conscious level, it encouraged and indeed required him to approach each consultation in an unusually systematic way. The best astrologers were obsessed with both the accuracy of their stellar calculations and the information they received from their patients or their representatives. In Forman's textbook, the author's anxiety about the latter borders on a paranoid fear that he will be deceived by false tales designed to test or embarrass him, but as excited as his language sometimes is, the underlying concern is still with clinical accuracy.[24] The best astrologers were also interested in perfecting their diagnostic skills by reviewing and correcting their mistakes. Napier recorded the outcome of his treatments when he learned it and cross-referenced case notes, practices recommended by Forman. A fascinating exchange between Napier and Arthur Dee, John Dee's son and also an astrological physician, shows the process of self-criticism in action. Recalling two cases they had discussed earlier and analysed astrologically Dee wrote:

> Concerning the other question I propounded in Moorfields, ... we were both deceived, for it proved not so. I have sent you the figures to consider of it, and I have found it by experience that it is not sufficient to find the lord of the fifth house with another planet, unless it be in the ascendant ... I pray you to send me some receipts of worth found by your own practice.[25]

It is hardly surprising that both Forman and Napier probably were excellent clinicians. But how many astrological physicians were so scrupulous? That question is as difficult to answer for them as it is for early modern physicians. Most astrological and non-astrological case books have perished, and given the acute erosion of astrology's prestige after the Restoration, it is remarkable that any of the former have survived at all. But there are two reasons for believing that Forman and Napier were typical in this respect of the best of their breed. The surviving notebooks of their contemporaries and successors display less concern for recording clinical data, but they are similarly meticulous.[26] Finally, in the medical market-place competition for patients was keen, and it is surely significant that throughout the seventeenth century the most famous astrologers treated armies of patients over many years. Satisfied customers were their best advertisements.

One reason why astrological physicians were popular was because they were in all likelihood good doctors by the standards of the time. In an age when experience was the critical factor in learning to diagnose disease and treat it, astrologers had an unusual amount of experience that they were trained to organize systematically. But there were other factors as well. A practical one was that they were comparatively cheap. Astrological practice was structured much like general practice today:

patients came to the doctor for short visits and a prescription. They could and did treat a lot of clients, sometimes as many as four or five an hour. The practice of élite physicians, by contrast, was still modelled on a patron–client relationship. They often spent long periods of time on their patients, sometimes attending them in their homes, and gave them extensive advice.[27] In crass economic terms, this meant that MDs tried to limit their practices to relatively few rich people, whereas astrological physicians grew rich treating the masses for small sums. The astrologer John Case no doubt had this in mind when the famous John Radcliffe offered him the taunting toast, 'Here's to all the fools, your patients, brother Case'. Case replied, 'I thank you good brother, let me have all the fools and you are heartily welcome to the rest of the practice'.[28] The fees Napier charged in 1600 were usually 2 shillings, and he treated a substantial number of patients for free. Regular physicians charged 10 shillings or more; a pound a day was not unheard of.[29]

There was, however, another reason why patients flocked to astrological physicians, an immaterial one. All medical practitioners sold information, advice and hope: information about what afflicted their patients, advice about how to treat their maladies and hope that their illnesses could be healed or, at the very least, that they would follow a probable course to recovery or death. But astrologers also sold meaning, as Ron Sawyer has argued persuasively.[30] Astrology added a cosmological and social dimension to healing. The horoscope was more than a map of the heavens; it was a chart of man's relationship to the higher bodies in the universe and to the forces that controlled them and everything on earth around him. Medieval and Renaissance scholars had elaborated the ancient model of the observable cosmos, adding supernatural realms, linking together the beings and things that inhabited the visible and invisible worlds in a chain of being and, finally, identifying correspondences that linked things and events on the levels of existence with forces of sympathy and antipathy.[31]

The astrologer's charts situated an individual client in this universe. They showed that the individual's physical or mental affliction was detectable in the motions of the heavens: that there was a correspondence between events in macrocosm, the universe, and the microcosm, his own body. In other words, astrology rationalized the ill person's profoundly egocentric experience of disease and related it to the physical and social context in which it occurred, indeed to the whole pattern of motion, change and events in the world. Similarly, it provided guides for re-establishing the balance of the humours in the form of specific instructions for the administration of therapeutics at propitious times, harmonizing the process of healing with heavenly motion. In the social realm the astrologer used his charts to call attention to conflicts that also needed healing, through reconciliation, for instance, or in extreme cases actions against a witch.[32] As schematic and fragmented as the notes of astrological consultations look splayed upon the pages of a manuscript, they are in fact diagrams of a ritual as rich in transcendent significance as the healing rites described by modern medical anthropologists.[33]

Small wonder that astrological medicine had a strong appeal in an age of faith and ancient science. But, one might object, most men and women were unlettered, and few had the intellectual training fully to grasp the theological and scientific complexities of contemporary cosmology. This is surely true. And yet the principles of that cosmology were widely taught in literature, in sermons, in illuminations and prints and, most pertinently, in the diagrams and epigrams of cheap, simple astrological almanacs which outsold every other kind of publication in the seventeenth century.[34] The fundamental facts would have been hard to avoid. Moreover, it was no doubt unnecessary to grasp the whole picture to understand the significance of the astrological-medical ritual. Anthropologists have taught us that very few people understand fully all of the significances of rituals amongst twentieth-century peoples with cosmologies and ritual lives as complex as that of early modern England. Nevertheless, the participants in healing rites in those cultures accept them as vehicles of meaning and as means to effect physical and social atonement.[35]

By this point, it should be easy to see why inaccuracies of prediction and even outright failures were insufficient to shatter faith in astrology. Astrologers never claimed to achieve absolute accuracy using their complex instrument, and their customers got more from them than just medical treatment.[36] Moreover, the prognostic inaccuracies of non-astrological medicine were just as great or greater and its remedies were mostly the same. And despite the addition of Paracelsian drugs to the therapeutic arsenal, most medicines were duds; there were no magic bullets. The ineffectiveness of contemporary medicine was a prominent theme in all kinds of literature, and it was echoed in the opinions of private individuals. The radical intellectual John Toland spoke for many when he swore of regular physicians, 'I shall never more put my self under the management of such, whose art is founded in darkness, and improv'd by Murther'.[37] Nothing like a clinical trial of either diagnostics or therapeutics comparing the success rates of astrologers and general physicians was possible or even imaginable. It mattered not at all that astrological doctors had little academic training in medicine; newly degreed academics had little practice in treating patients, and astrologers acquired experience at a faster rate because of the greater numbers of their clients. At its best, astrological physic was regular medicine with a greater symbolic significance and probably a greater psychological impact.

Astrologers and their clients

How widespread was the practice of astrological medicine? It is impossible to answer that question with exactitude because of the nature of medical practice and the sparse and fragmentary evidence that survives for both astrological and non-astrological healers. There were certainly many more London astrologers than those caught up in the College's sporadic sweeps.[38] Some, such as William Lilly's teacher, John Evans never got into trouble for their astrology, and so do not appear as astrologers in the College Annals. Lilly mentions a dozen or so who were practising in the city in the 1630s, some of whom he taught.[39] The picture is the same, but more blurred, outside of London. Any examination of the medical personnel in a particular diocese turns up medical men whom we know from other sources to have been astrologers. In Napier's diocese of Lincoln, for instance, his pupils Sir Richard Napier (the elder Napier's nephew), Ralph Wallis, Gerance James, and William Marsh were astrological physicians. A practitioner who was not one of his students, William Bredon, rector of Thornton in Bedfordshire, achieved considerable celebrity.[40] Investigations of Norwich have also turned up doctors who were astrologers and astrologers who were doctors. The former included the Harveys, Sir Thomas Browne and Arthur Dee, the latter Nicholas Fiske.[41]

Their enemies complained that astrologers had hung out their signs in every town in England by the early seventeenth century.[42] They doubtless exaggerated. Astrology was not part of the formal curricula of the universities, although students continued to learn it from sympathetic scholars. Before 1640 there were distinguished astrologers at both Oxford and Cambridge – Thomas Allen and Richard Burton at the former, for example – and some of the graduates they trained practised physic.[43] Most medical astrologers learned their trade, however, by informal apprenticeship and the study of texts that were increasingly easy to obtain, especially after 1640.[44] Very little capital was necessary to establish a practice, and it is striking that almost all of the major figures in the 'profession' were social upstarts. For a time in the late sixteenth and seventeenth centuries, astrological medicine offered a lucrative way for a bright, entrepreneurial lad to better himself. The ease with which people could learn astrological physic and begin practising it meant that there were a great many lesser figures in the trade who were scarcely different from cunning men and women. Some were certainly out-and-out quacks, as the critics of astrology never ceased complaining. Structurally, astrological medicine was never a 'profession' even in the limited early modern sense of the term.[45] Were the surviving evidence full of lists of medical practitioners, and it is not, we still would not be able to identify the astrologers with confidence. All we can say, lamely, is that there were a lot of them, and their numbers certainly grew during the course of the seventeenth century.[46]

What sorts of people resorted to astrologers, and what kinds of illnesses drove them to seek their help? It is a distinct exaggeration to say, as A.L. Rowse once boasted in a radio interview, that Forman's case notes are a veritable *Who's Who* of Elizabethan England, but court ladies were certainly well represented, and so were gentlemen and gentlewomen, rich London merchants and clerics. The bulk of his patients, however, were of much humbler stock: sailors and serving girls seem to have been especially numerous.[47] A half-century later, the patient profile of William Lilly was quite similar. He saw 124 members of the gentry and nobility in two years (1654–56). The majority, however, were artisans, labourers or sailors and soldiers, pretty much the average folk of seventeenth-century London.[48] Provincial practitioners naturally saw fewer wealthy merchants and worried mariners than Forman or Lilly did. But the most celebrated of them developed connections that made them fashionable amongst the gentry. About 25 per cent of Napier's clients were peers, knights, lesser gentry and their families. Professionals, meaning mainly clergymen, Oxford dons and the occasional student, formed a small but distinctive grouping amongst the rest. Most were ordinary men and women who gained their livelihoods as farmers, yeomen or husbandmen, or as artisans and labourers. Some were penniless paupers.[49] The clientele of a Dr Barker of Shrewsbury who practised at the turn of the sixteenth century also included the cream of local society and a lot of the less rich people of the town. Barker seems to have treated fewer down-and-outs than Napier did.[50] The chief difference socially beween these astrological practices and those of the regular physicians was that the astrologers treated far more people of middling and low status. The latter, while numerically the majority of the population, were the least well served by orthodox medicine. Astrologers' clients were thus more representative of the society from which they came.

The medical problems that brought them to the consulting room were also representative. Napier treated every kind of malady that afflicted his contemporaries, from the plague to pimples. Only broken bones and wounds were outside his ambit: those and similar traumas were the special province of surgeons. The most common symptoms he encountered were internal pains, gastro-intestinal disorders and women's complaints. To the extent that one can generalize about the myriad afflictions that he described, one can say that many were the signs of infectious or chronic illnesses that were difficult for laymen to identify and which had the potential to be fatal, disfiguring or plain disgusting. Social historians are always regaling us with evidence of the perils people in the past faced from mortal illness; diseases that did not kill – or did so slowly over many years – were as large or larger a danger.[51] Clients came to astrologers for a diagnosis and advice; they wanted to know if they would live or die. Napier's notebooks are littered with to-do lists of questions to be resolved astrologically or magically, asking what the outcome of someone's illness would be.[52] Patients surely hoped for a cure, but they did not *expect* it, as litigious Americans and whingeing Britons do today.

Three kinds of medical problems astrologers treated are worth sin-gling out for special attention, because their records seem to provide the fullest surviving evidence concerning them. All of the practices that have survived display an imbalance of women to men.[53] Between 55 and 60 per cent of the clients of Forman and Napier were female, and Lilly's patients included a high proportion of serving girls and young women, 37 per cent of the whole group for which he recorded status or occupation. In the first instance these figures illustrate what historians have mostly ignored: that women's health problems were a major source of misery, anxiety and occasionally death. As Edward Jorden and others recognized, women were 'subject unto more diseases and of other sortes' than men.[54] Indeed, Simon Forman was so familiar with the maladies women suffered because of their reproductive organs that he penned a treatise on the subject, as did a number of non-astrological doctors. Most of these, significantly, remained unprinted and were circulated amongst practitioners in manuscript form.[55] Progress in gynaecology was impeded by prudery or prejudice, however obvious the need for greater shared information was to male medical practitioners. It was often said that women were especially attracted to astrologers because they were less reasonable and more superstitious than men. That cal-umny should be set aside. Not only were they more frequently ill than men, they also consulted astrological physicians more often on behalf of others, especially family members. Women were the primary healers in early modern society, providing kitchen physic to their families, and they played a key but little studied role as mediators between the sick and medical practitioners.[56]

The most frequent complaints of Napier's female patients concerned menstrual irregularities. Sometimes they turned to astrologers to learn if they were pregnant or their 'terms' had stopped for another reason. Pregnancy was tricky to diagnose when amenorrhoea was commonplace due to poor diet and disease, and the stars might clarify what the midwife and friends could not determine. About 4 per cent of Napier's clients went to him specifically for pregnancy testing. The proportion may have been higher in the practices of other astrologers. Two problems that are now regarded as mainly psychological, 'green sickness' and 'suffocation of the mother' brought another 3 per cent or so of patients to Napier. Historians have made much ado about both of these diagnoses. To Napier they were terms that he applied respectively to amenorrhoea in young, unmarried women and to a disparate array of symptoms seeming linked to some discomfort in a woman's womb. He did not reserve the latter for conditions that later physicians would identify as hysteria. Neither of these maladies can be confidently diagnosed in retrospect, and their chief significance is that they were disease categories that expressed a cultural conviction that young women were subject to special, disturbing diseases that arose from sexual frustration.[57]

Contemporaries supposed that astrologers had special expertise in the related areas of supernaturally caused illnesses and mental disorders. At all levels of Elizabethan and Jacobean society, people feared witchcraft and more rarely diabolical possession. Doctors sometimes pronounced that mysterious maladies were supernatural if they could not cure them by natural means. Much more frequently laypersons made that judgement by themselves. When they did, the hapless victim could turn to an astrologer, white witch or divine. Many of the clients who trooped to Forman and Napier suspected that they were bewitched or haunted by spirits, as they put it. Astrology offered a tool for confirming or disconfirming their suspicions, and a special means, magical amulets, to counteract spiritual malevolence.

Napier probably had more such patients than any other contemporary practitioner, around 2,000 in all. As Ron Sawyer has shown, aside from their fear of supernatural harm, what the majority of these sufferers had in common were mental illness or maladies that caused them to swoon or shake or lose control of their limbs as they wasted away.[58] Often, even when the symptomatic profile fit the vague criteria of bewitchment, Napier declined to confirm his patient's suspicions. He testified in one high-profile case that a young woman was afflicted by the 'mother' rather than witchcraft, for example.[59] This kind of specific scepticism was very common.[60] But even when Napier thought his client might be bewitched, he prescribed medical treatments in an attempt to relieve the illness naturally. Similarly, he handed out magical amulets to both those whose suspicions he seems to have endorsed and those about whom he was noncommittal. These were small metal emblems, engraved with planetary signs and attached to ribbons of silk or taffeta, so they could be hung around the neck. Napier provided one for Sir Thomas Myddleton, the father of the parliamentary general and a kinsman, who feared some supernatural malevolence. Myddleton was supposed to say a prayer when he put it on, which was probably a standard instruction for his patients. The prayer in this case acted as reassurance of the religious legitimacy of the amulet and as an additional means to make it spiritually powerful.[61]

The border between the maladies of the mind and spiritual assault was notoriously indistinct.[62] Mental illnesses were a persistent problem in early modern England (as in all other complex societies), and the number of persons experiencing them was increasing at least in proportion to the rapid growth of the population. Consciousness of lesser disorders was increasing, too, as Renaissance medical texts and imaginative literature focused on melancholy as a malady rampant amongst the wealthier classes. Neither Forman nor Napier was in any sense a proto-psychiatrist, but both of them, especially Napier, treated many patients with mental disturbances that ranged from pallid melancholy to outright lunacy. Simon Forman included two striking cases of 'frantic' patients in the opening pages of his astrological textbook. He uses them to illustrate the superiority of astrological medicine in determining the causes and outcomes of such maladies.[63] About 5 per cent of Napier's patients were mentally disturbed.[64] The vast majority were afflicted with mood disorders or lesser disturbances of thought, behaviour or perception. Over 100, however, displayed signs of what he called madness or lunacy, acute mental illnesses that caused them to act violently or babble incoherent or deluded speeches.[65] For the most part, he treated all of his mentally disturbed patients in much the same way as he did his physically ill ones. Like his contemporaries he believed that mental illnesses had either physical or supernatural causes, or both. For the latter he often prescribed sigils along with remedies to restore their humoral balance.[66]

Napier was evidently a skilled part-time psychotherapist, as some of the other leading astrologers must have been. He did not record the advice he gave to his clients, but we do know that he often prayed with them and that when they could afford it they often returned for several visits with him or when they experienced a relapse. His most famous or notorious mentally ill client was the Viscount Purbeck, John Villiers, the brother of the Duke of Buckingham. The case holds special interest for us. In 1620 when the Villiers family first approached him, Buckingham had recently become the king's favourite (in every sense and implication of that word), and he was rapidly becoming the most powerful man in England, after James I himself. Napier was a pious prude, and he knew that his astrological practice and magical pursuits made him vulnerable to attack. He was extremely reluctant to become involved in the fractious faction politics that accompanied Buckingham's grab for power and his relentless attempts to advance members of his family. Purbeck himself had been ennobled and married to Sir Edward Coke's daughter, Frances, in a sordid series of manoeuvres intended to regain the king's favour towards Coke.[67] There is no evidence that Purbeck had experienced emotional disturbances before his marriage, as historians claim. But his wedding caught him up in a furious feud between Coke and his formidable wife, Elizabeth, Lady Hatton. Coke allegedly had to tie Frances to a bedpost and beat her to get her to marry Purbeck, and his wife kidnapped the girl in an attempt to frustrate the match. Lady Hatton spent the wedding in custody. After accepting the inevitable briefly, she took to the war-path again when she found out that her daughter's dowry was to include a good deal of her personal landed estate. She refused to pay, and on their side Buckingham and his mother, a woman who was Lady Hatton's equal in determination, were enraged at her and at Frances, the target of wrath closest to hand. The Duke turned her out of his household and sent her home to her parents. When he was sane and sober, Purbeck was a gentle, timorous man, hopelessly in love with his beautiful young wife. He broke down under the strain of the battle and his separation from her. At a time when his brother was treading a treacherous path between Catholic and Protestant opinion, Purbeck got into a London residence, broke the windows and shouted for everyone to hear that he was a papist.[68] His fits became worse and more embarrassing in 1623 while Buckingham was abroad with Prince Charles wooing the Spanish Infanta.

The family decided Purbeck was mad, and King James had packed him off to Napier for treatment.[69] Napier soon developed a towering contempt for Buckingham and his mother, an unusual if not unique reaction to a client's family.[70] He had the nerves of a doe and the heart of a lapdog; he needed the patience of a snake and the wisdom of an owl to deal with Purbeck. The lunatic lord was installed near Great Linford, where he was surrounded by clients of his brother and mother, many of them Catholics. The infamous Father Fisher, the Countess of Buckingham's confessor and nemesis of Bishop Laud, hung around and tugged at his spiritual sleeve in hopes of sustaining his conversion to Rome. Purbeck was almost certanly a manic depressive and an alcoholic, and Napier treated his wild oscillations between 'merry madness' and deep melancholia with medicaments, management and amulets from 1622 to 1626 and then again in 1631–32. He never recovered for very long, and each bout of Villiers' vindictiveness against Lady Purbeck precipitated another breakdown. He kept returning partly because he became deeply fond of his astrological doctor, who became fond of him in return, despite his Catholicism and his overweening relatives.[71] They on their side obviously had no objections to Napier's astrology.

This episode has been worth the space I have spent on it because it illustrates two significant facts about medical astrologers. They had a lamentable affinity for scandal, and they swarmed into the dangerous game of high politics like children running on to a football pitch. Both had calamitous effects on their reputations and occasionally for their safety. Forman became embroiled in the notorious divorce of Frances Howard from her first husband, the Earl of Essex. His death prevented him from being tried in 1613 with her and her second husband, the Earl of Somerset, for poisoning Sir Thomas Overbury, but he was named in court as an accomplice and widely accused of bewitching Essex's 'ympliment'.[72] He and his magical arts were pilloried in anti-Howard propaganda. Napier was similarly rumoured to be a witch or a necromancer during the Purbeck affair.[73] So was the despicable John Lambe, one of the most successful London astrologers. A creature of Buckingham, he offered to cure Purbeck by some fast but dubious means. If it was tried, it did not work. But Lambe's association with Buckingham continued and deepened, and after the disastrous defeat at the Isle of Rhe, he became a lightning-rod for anti-Villiers rage. Lambe was seized by a London crowd and bludgeoned so badly that he died hours afterward. The triumphant pamphlets and ballads that celebrated his murder claimed that a crystal ball had tumbled from his robes as he was assaulted and reminded readers that he had once been found guilty of witchcraft and also of raping an 11-year-old girl. The links between unpopular political policies, Catholicism, sexual transgression, witchcraft and astrology were emphasized in lurid and lampooning propaganda.[74]

The 'folkloricization' of astrology

It is notable that these scandals involved charges of illicit magic as well as services to politically controversial and widely hated courtiers. They intensified the view that astrology was irreligious and a danger to the State. Before the Civil War, the main opposition to astrology was religious, and even critics who purloined the arguments of continental humanists who objected to the scientific, logical and historical veracity of astrology included theological objections to it.[75] Ever since the thirteenth century, some theologians had attacked astrology on the grounds that it infringed on conceptions of free will that were integral aspects of soteriology. Reformation thinkers, and especially Calvinists who were less concerned about human free will, complained that astrologers taught that *God's* freedom was limited, because they presumed he must play by their rules, controlling human destiny through astral forces. They also complained that astrological prognostication was impious, because it in effect attempted to read God's mind and reveal His plans for the future, and that at the very least astrologers shifted the public's attention away from the only proper and essential concern about providence toward the secondary causes of events. In England evangelical Protestants such as William Perkins went on to claim that astrology was a kind of black magic, and that the cures astrological physicians performed were proof that their powers came from Satan, since they manifestly were not sanctioned by God. Perkins asserted that it was better to die than be healed by such means, and John Gaule was equally harsh in his condemnation of 'the Astrologian, Starre-gazing, Planetary, Prognosticating Witch'.[76] Like Dee, all of the leading astrologers before 1640 were attacked as witches at one time or another – a charge made easier to sustain by their habitual involvement in dicier kinds of magic, most of which depended on astrology to a greater or lesser extent. Despite the fact that the 1604 witchcraft statute provided a basis for capital charges for such activities, only Lambe seems to have been successfully prosecuted, and he was pardoned.[77] Aristocratic patronage and the loyalty of clerical customers shielded them from the worst.

It was the English Revolution that decisively shifted attitudes to astrology by paradoxically intensifying both public regard for it and élite suspicion of its practitioners. The flood of vernacular publishing that was unleashed by the collapse of censorship led to a rapid proliferation of medical and astrological textbooks aimed at the lay reader. The market for almanacs boomed. These always contained some basic instruction in astrology, and diagrams of astral man, showing which parts of the body and humours were influenced by various signs of the zodiac, were very common.[78] William Lilly's *Christian Astrology* (1647) became the most authoritative text of the age, rivalled only by the works of John Gadbury. Gadbury was impressively learned, as were his friends Vincent Wing, Thomas Streete and Elias Ashmole. Only the latter failed to expound astrological technicalities in print. Like Lilly, Wing issued a popular almanac. Lilly also published a handbook specifically devoted to astrological medicine, but in that arena he was eclipsed by the astrological doctor Nicholas Culpeper.[79] From his pen streamed a cascade of translations of medical books and more or less original compilations, the most famous of which is his astrological herbal, *The English Physician* (1652). More than any other writer, Culpeper popularized the principles of medical astrology.[80] All of this was good for business. A tribe of newly famous astrologers and astrological doctors set up thriving practices. John Booker's was huge: it was said that he and Lilly were the idols of the poor. Richard Saunders, Joseph Blagrave and William Salmon began to establish their reputations as astrological physicians during the Interregnum.[81] Given the numbers of books and celebrated practitioners, it is plain that many more people had become 'astrology-literate' by 1660 than ever before.

But astrologers were also drawn into the turbulent politics of the day by the irresistible pull of fame, power and money. All of the popular almanac-makers ventured predictions about the military and political fortunes of king and Parliament. Both sides employed astrological propagandists to rally support and lend confidence to their armies. Lilly became the leading parliamentarian astrologer and the State's official star-gazer after Parliament's victory. His celebrity was huge; he could even afford to intervene magnanimously to gain clemency for his royalist rival George Wharton after the latter's arrest. Representatives of every political and religious movement consulted astrologers to gauge their chances during these momentous years.[82] The establishment of the Commonwealth fired idealists with enthusiasm for all kinds of reform, including the advancement of astrology. Advocating the overhaul of the universities, John Webster called for astrology to be included in their curricula.[83] The stable of social architects Samuel Hartlib assembled for Oliver Cromwell paid scant attention to astrology, but they advocated medical reforms that would have promoted it. Their main objective was to deliver cheap, effective physic to the poor. William Petty wanted them to found a teaching hospital to be headed by a director learned in astrology. They also championed the use of chemical medicines that apothecaries could make and distribute for 'over-the-counter' use. Many astrological physicians were partisans of the same cause: Culpeper's hyperthyroid efforts dovetailed perfectly with their project.[84]

Like so many of the radical social programmes of the mid-century, medical reform achieved few of its grand aims. But it would be wrong to conclude that it was a mere sideshow that had no lasting influence. It had both positive and negative effects on the career of astrological medicine in England. Positively, it broadened knowledge and practice of astrology for several generations after the Restoration. Culpeper's efforts at popularizing astrological medicine in print were sustained by Saunders, Blagrave and Salmon.[85] Salmon and Partridge had enormous practices. By 1700 the former was receiving over 1,500 enquiries by post alone, and when the latter died in 1715 he was worth at least £2,000.[86] And, of course, Case was pulling in the 'fools': Addison said in 1710 he had earned more from the doggerel on his sign ('Within this place/Lives Dr Case') than Dryden had with all his books.[87] Provincial men like David Irish, who later became a successful mad-doctor, also did well in practice in the last years of the Stuart dynasty.[88] Negatively,

it linked astrologers in the minds of defenders of the medical establishment with political radicalism. After the revolution their spokesmen
charged repeatedly that the democratizing ideas of the medical reformers were rabble-rousing enthusiasm. Their main target were the apothecaries, or chemical physicians, but their taunts embraced popular astrologers, too.[89] David Younge, the scourge of Gadbury, claimed, for
instance, that the successors of Lilly and Culpeper aimed to destroy
'monarchy, episcopacy and nobility, and [set] up democracy in these
kingdoms'.[90] Even if readers did not swallow that hysterical charge,
their confidence in astrology must surely have been shaken by its use as
propaganda in a period of fierce partisanship and shifting political
fortunes.

The climate of élite opinion was obviously beginning to cloud omi-
nously. The Royal Society lent no suport to astrology, although Ashmole
and John Aubrey were members, and within the ranks of the astrologers
themselves a battle broke out over how to reform astrology to improve
its scientific basis.[91] The struggle was a sign of their awareness that
reform was necessary and of their talent as a group for political self-
destruction. The thrust of external attacks on astrology began to stress
its erroneous astronomical assumptions and empirical inaccuracies. The
physician Henry Power and the astronomer royal John Flamsteed both
assailed astrology on just these points. Significantly, however, their
critiques of the validity of astrology remained unpublished.[92] For the
most part, attacks on astrology came not from philosophers versed in
astronomy but from gentlemen scribblers and clerics who recycled doubts
about the accuracy of prediction that had been raised much earlier, by
Pico and others. The fact that these attacks were now so influential in
polite circles was the consequence of changing attitudes to proof, a
diffuse bias toward empiricism that became such striking feature of élite
culture in the century after the Restoration.[93] The main problem with
astrology was that it was, as the *Encyclopaedia Britannica* put it in
1771, a 'conjectural science'. Much of the antagonism to astrology was,
however, also animated by political and social prejudices. The most
successful astrologers tended to be Parliamentarians and later Whigs;
unsurprisingly, they tended also to be men of humble birth. The ridicule
that Swift and his friends brought down on Partridge in the most
famous practical joke of the age was compounded of snobbery and
partisanship as much as scepticism about his discipline. Astrology, the
Britannica's author went on to observe, 'has long ago become a just
subject of contempt and ridicule'.[94] Fewer and fewer men who saw
themselves as intellectual leaders, as John Dee had, took astrology
seriously. Earlier critics of astrology had emphasized the distinction
between 'natural' and 'judicial' astrology – the study of the stars' influ-

ence on earthly phenomena versus prediction, and the distinction was maintained in some post-Restoration attacks. This may have slowed somewhat the extension of hostility from judicial astrology to astrological medicine – or, more correctly, narrowed its scope. A few intellectuals continued to think that the heavens had some kind of influence on illnesses. Richard Mead, the most esteemed physician of the age, is the best known of these.[95] But in practice astrologers had never wished to stick to astrological theory and diagnosis; predicting the course of events and of illnesses was at the core of their trade. The medical establishment regarded the practising astrologers as crackpots who only deluded the masses and encouraged quackery.[96] Ironically, even Georgian quacks downplayed astrology in their efforts to attract wealthy and middle-class patients.[97]

The crumbling respectability of astrology took a toll on the art itself. After about 1720 no group of recognized and respected experts like John Gadbury or Elias Ashmole published new astrological theories and methods or promoted their study, and systematic astrology was too complex to thrive as a discipline or win many new enthusiasts without such stimulus. Almanacs, chapbooks and popular astrological books became cruder, less technical. The medical information in them was increasingly anachronistic and reflected the vague humouralism of folk belief.[98] Astrology and astrological medicine became increasingly 'folklorized' – to borrow Jon Butler's apt, inelegant term – a nearly complete reversal of their cultural standing in the Middle Ages and early sixteenth century.[99] But it certainly did not perish, any more than old cosmological beliefs or the needs to which astrologers addressed themselves did. Some astrological doctors practised as licensed physicians; astrological 'empircs', many of whom were women, advertised their practices in the newspapers. There was, Francis Guybon observed 'a Sort of Sympathy between Understandings' of the 'Petits Gens' and such irregular healers.[100] At a more refined level, Ebeneezer Silby, MD, and John Worsdale produced impressive new works on astrology and astrological medicine in the last decades of the century, and a Conjurer's Magazine was launched in 1791 (soon prudently renamed The Astrologer's Magazine). And as J.F.C. Harrison has shown, astrological ideas formed an integral part of the millenarian movements that formed around the demotic prophets Joanna Southcott and Richard Brothers in the same period.[101] Despite these signs of survival and even revival, astrology had nevertheless lost forever the central place it had achieved in English culture during the late sixteenth and seventeenth centuries. It persisted and occasionally thrived as an enthusiasm of occultists and radicals and as an element of folklore and folk medicine amongst the lower classes.

From the perspective of the historian of medicine, the relegation in modern times of astrology to folk culture may seem irrelevant or laudable. But one wonders if it did not signal a divergence between lay notions of sickness and healing, at least amongst certain groups, and the ideas of health-care providers. Roy Porter is no doubt right to argue that there was a great deal of overlap between mainstream medical ideas and popular attitudes in the eighteenth century.[102] (Physicians and patients had, after all, to share a certain degree of understanding.) But Culpeper's herbal and Moore's almanac continued to be read to tatters in the cottages and tenements of the poor throughout the 1800s. Many people continued to believe that there were propitious times for the administration of drugs. And as the rise of scientific medicine has gathered momentum, complaints about the 'authoritarian' and 'impersonal' nature of health care have grown louder and louder. Patients still yearn for treatment that acknowledges the metaphysical and social dimensions of illness that astrologers catered to. I am not suggesting that those concerns could be addressed by reintroducing astrology in the surgeries of general practitioners, but I am suggesting that the career of astrology in English medicine points to a loss that is still felt and expressed in various ways, such as noncompliance and resort to alternative medicines and nostrums. It is a subject that at the very least deserves thoughtful reflection – much more than I can or have given it here.[103]

Notes

1. C.S.J. Thompson, *The Quacks of Old London*, London, 1928, ch. 7. For the satiric models, see Don Cameron Allen, *The Star-Crossed Renaissance: The Quarrel About Astrology and Its Influence in England*, Durham, NC, 1941, chs 3–4; Keith Thomas, *Religion and the Decline of Magic*, London, 1971, p. 356; Ronald Paulson, *Hogarth's Graphic Works*, 3rd edn, revised, London, 1989, pp. 62–3 and pl. 89; J.C. Eade, *The Forgotten Sky: A Guide to Astrology in English Literature*, Oxford, 1984: pp. 215–16.

2. Thomas, *Religion and Magic*, chs 10–12. There were, of course, some earlier attempts to take astrology, particularly medical astrology, seriously: Carroll Camden, Jr, 'Elizabethan Astrological Medicine', *Annals of Medical History*, n.s., 2, (1930), pp. 217–26; Hugh G. Dick, 'Students of Physic and Astrology: A Survey of Astrological Medicine in the Age of Science', *Journal of the History of Medicine and Allied Sciences*, 1, (1946), pp. 300–15, 419–33. For important scholarship on astrological medicine subsequent to Thomas, see Bernard Capp, *Astrology and the Popular Press: English Almanacs 1500–1800*, London, 1979; Allan Chapman, 'Astrological Medicine', in Charles Webster (ed.), *Health, Medicine and Mortality in the Sixteenth Century*, Cambridge, 1979, pp.

275–300; Michael MacDonald, *Mystical Bedlam: Madness, Anxiety and Healing in Seventeenth-Century England*, Cambridge, 1981; Ronald C. Sawyer, 'Patients, Healers and Disease in the Southeast Midlands, 1597–1634', PhD thesis, University of Wisconsin-Madison, 1984; Patrick Curry, *Prophecy and Power: Astrology in Early Modern England*, Princeton, 1989; Michael Hunter and Annabel Gregory (eds), *An Astrological Diary of the Seventeenth Century: Samuel Jeake of Rye 1652–1699*, Oxford, 1988.

3. This crude, two-cultures model is, of course, a simplification. Both élite and plebeian culture were riven by fault-lines of education, gender, religion and social ecology. A full account of cultural change and differentiation in this period is desperately needed, but in this context the simpler model will do for us as it served for Thomas, *Religion and Magic*, ch. 22.

4. Hilary M. Carey, *Courting Disaster: Astrology at the English Court and University in the Later Middle Ages*, London, 1992, esp. pp. 23, 162.

5. For knowledge of astrology in late medieval England see T.O. Wedel, *The Medieval Attitude toward Astrology*, New Haven, 1920; J.D. North, *Chaucer's Universe*, Oxford, 1988.

6. Thomas, *Religion and Magic*, p. 288; Capp, *Astrology and the Press*, pp. 22–34; Allen *Star-Crossed Renaissance*, ch. 4.

7. Charles Goodall, *The Royal College of Physicians of London*, London, 1664, pp. 337–9; George Clark, *A History of the Royal College of Physicians*, 2 vols, Oxford, 1964, vol. 1, pp. 167–8. Assuming – and it is a big assumption – that the examination was fair, this judgement of Forman's astrological competence may have been due to the fact that there was no single, authoritative text that all astrologers followed. Indeed, it may have been this incident that prompted Forman to write the textbook setting out the method he used. It is obvious from an unbiased examination of his case notes for this period that he was an extremely competent astrological doctor. The same cannot be said with such confidence of John Lambe, who was failed for the same reason (Goodall, *Royal College*, pp. 397–401; Clark, *College of Physicians*, vol. 1, p. 259).

8. Dick, 'Students of Physic and Astrology'; Thomas, *Religion and Magic*, p. 354; Capp, *Astrology and the Press*, pp. 51–2, 205–8, 242–3, 428, Appendix I: Biographical Notes, pp. 293–340.

9. For Dee, see Frances Yates, *The Occult Philosophy in the Elizabethan Age*, London, 1979; Peter French, *John Dee: The World of an Elizabethan Magus*, London, 1972; Nicholas H. Clulee, *John Dee's Natural Philosophy: Between Science and Religion*, London, 1988.

10. Napier met Dee personally in 1604: Bodleian Library, MS Ashmole (hereinafter Ashml.) 1488, art. II, fol. 21^v; Lilly says he knew him well: William Lilly, *History of His Life and Times*, London, 1715, pp. 52–4. It is very likely that Forman was personally acquainted with Dee; he apparently possessed some of his manuscripts.

11. A.L. Rowse, *Sex and Society in Shakespeare's England*, London, 1974, is unfortunately the only full life. See also *Dictionary of National Biography*, (hereafter *DNB*); Clarke, *College of Physicians*, vol. 1, pp. 146, 167–8, 199, 214, 216.

12. Simon Forman, 'The Astrological Judgements of Diseases and Other

Questions', Ashml. 389. There are several manuscript versions of this work, all of them somewhat different. Napier's own copy was Ashml. 403; the fullest extant text was written out by his nephew, Sir Richard Napier: Ashml. 363. See also British Library (hereafter BL) MS Sloane 99.

13. The best account of Napier's practice, indeed of any contemporary medical practice, is Sawyer, 'Patients, Healers and Disease'. See also MacDonald, *Mystical Bedlam*.

14. Forman's extant practice books, covering March 1596 to November 1601 are (in chronological order) Ashml. 234, 226, 195, 219, 236, 411; Napier's run to 60 volumes and are listed in MacDonald, *Mystical Bedlam*, pp. 300–2 and Sawyer, 'Patients, Healers and Disease', pp. 610–11. Both collections are usefully calendared in William H. Black, *A Descriptive, Analytical and Critical Catalogue of the Manuscripts Bequeathed Unto the University of Oxford by Elias Ashmole*, Oxford, 1845. For a discussion of the full range of services offered by Forman, Napier and other astrologers, see Thomas, *Religion and Magic*, pp. 305–22.

15. Ashml. 240, fols 98, 101ᵛ; Ashml. 416, p. 441. The correspondence between William Bredon, an astrologer living near Napier, and both the elder and younger Richard Napier shows the strong interest that astrologers had in new astronomical findings, especially the observations of Tycho Brahe and Johannes Kepler's Rudolphine tables: Ashml. 240, fols 78, 80, 81ᵛ, 91, 96ᵛ, 97, 98, 101ᵛ. Lilly's insistence that he remained a staunch adherent of Ptolemy is wrong: Lilly, *Life and Times*, pp. 75–6.

16. Mayerne's practice notes are BL Sloane MSS 2058–76; H.R. Trevor-Roper, Lord Dacre, is engaged on a life of Mayerne, which should appear shortly.

17. George Atwell, *An Apology, Or, Defence of the Divine Art of Natural Astrologie*, London, 1660, p. 27.

18. Chapman's assertion to the contrary is simply wrong for Forman and Napier; it is probably also wrong for other élite astrological physicians. Compare Chapman, 'Astrological Medicine', p. 280 with Sawyer, 'Patients, Healers and Disease', pp. 290–3.

19. Ashml. 363, fols 2–4.

20. Sawyer, 'Patients, Healers and Disease', chs 4–5, and *passim*. Napier also used Paracelsian medicines, which he manufactured himself, in place of herbal emetics and purges, a practice sanctioned by the London *Pharmacopeia*. For a unique and all too brief contemporary description of Napier at work in the consulting room, see Atwell, *An Apology*, pp. 26–8.

21. Neither, interestingly, recorded astrological instructions for timing the administration of pharmacological remedies or even blood-letting, although they probably gave such advice, and the pattern of the substances they prescribed was determined by the wealth of the patient and to a lesser extent the nature of his or her illness, rather than by astrological considerations. MacDonald, *Mystical Bedlam*, pp. 178–98; Sawyer, 'Patients, Healers and Disease', pp. 256–68.

22. Sawyer, 'Patients, Healers and Disease', pp. 279–87; Eade, *The Forgotten Sky*; and the unjustly neglected Charles Arthur Mercier, *Astrology in Medicine*, London, 1914. Astrological textbooks were more determinis-

tic, but then they were compendia of rules, not records of actual practice.

23. Sawyer, 'Patients, Healers and Disease', chs 4–5, esp. pp. 243–56, 308–15.

24. Ashml. 363, fols 2–2ᵛ.

25. Quoted in MacDonald, *Mystical Bedlam*, p. 29 from Ashml. 1501, art. 5, fols 5–6ᵛ. See also Ashml. 1730, fols 202, 205; Ashml. 232, fol. 298.

26. See, for example, the collections of John Booker and William Lilly, listed in Black, *Catalogue of Manuscripts Bequeathed by Ashmole*, and the dozen or so anonymous astrological case books preserved in the British Library's Sloane Manuscripts and noticed in Samuel Ayscough, *A Catalogue of the Manuscripts Preserved in the British Museum*, London, 1782; Edward E.J. Scott, *Index to the Sloane Manuscripts in the British Museum*, London, 1904, which is a better guide. A useful listing of ten of the most interesting astrological and medical MSS is in Sawyer, 'Patients, Healers and Disease', p. 615. See also Lucinda McCray Beier's (1987) discussion of Dr Barker's case notes: *Sufferers and Healers: The Experience of Illness in Seventeenth-Century England*, London, pp. 120–3.

27. Peter W.G. Wright, 'A Study in the Legitimisation of Knowledge: The "Success" of Medicine and the "Failure" of Astrology', in Roy Wallis (ed.), *On the Margins of Science*, Sociological Review Monograph 27, Keele, 1979, pp. 91–2, 98. For the ideal of medical practice, which required intimate knowledge of the patient, see Harold J. Cook, 'Good Advice and Little Medicine: The Professional Authority of Early Modern English Physicians', *Journal of British Studies*, 33 (1994), pp. 1–31. Mayerne was again a partial exception to the rule. It is said that he was so fat that he would not leave his rooms, where he sat like Jabba the Hut, and was waited upon by his patients. It is a safe bet that he exacted greater tribute from them than astrologers did, though.

28. *DNB*, Case, John.

29. Thomas, *Religion and Magic*, pp. 11, 320–1; Cook, 'Good Advice and Little Medicine'. For a later discussion of pricing by a medical astrologer, see David Irish, *Levamon Infirmi: or, Cordial Counsel to the Sick and Diseased*, London, 1700, pp. 17–30.

30. Sawyer, 'Patients, Healers and Disease', pp. 293–315.

31. The classic descriptions of this world view are C.S. Lewis, *The Discarded Image*, Cambridge, 1964; E.M.W. Tillyard, *The Elizabethan World View*, 1944, repr., Harmondsworth, 1979; and Hardin Craig, *The Enchanted Glass*, London, 1960. These works, especially Tillyard's, have been much criticized of late by literary scholars who deplore their stress on the ways in which this ideology promoted a false impression of social and political stability. Those cavils are legitimate but do not diminish the significance of the scheme or its pervasive influence on both élite and popular culture.

32. Sawyer, 'Patients, Healers and Disease', pp. 308–15. Astrologers like Napier were well known for their sensitivity to problems in social relationships and were often consulted to give advice about troubled love affairs or marriages, for instance: MacDonald, *Mystical Bedlam*, ch. 4. Their insight into human affairs and the concerns of their clients is one

reason why astrology 'succeeded': Thomas, *Religion and Magic*, pp. 339–41.

33. A point not lost on the eminent Sri Lankan/American anthropologist, Stanley Jeyaraja Tambia: see his critique of Thomas in *Magic, Science, Religion, and the Scope of Rationality*, Cambridge, 1990, p. 24.

34. Capp, *Astrology and the Press*, p. 44, gives the impressive sales figures.

35. It is common nowadays for critics to complain that classic studies of ritual, such as Victor Turner, *The Drums of Affliction*, Oxford, 1968, overemphasize the extent to which healing rites are understood to invoke a fully coherent and generally held cosmology. Catherine Bell, *Ritual Theory, Ritual Practice*, New York, 1992, is a recent overview. For the limiting case, where the rituals of traditional healers remain appealing despite acculturation that has progressed so far that no one, not even the healers, can fully remember their original significance, see Murray Last, 'The Importance of Knowing and Not Knowing: Observations from Hausaland', in Steven Feierman and John Janzen (eds), *The Social Basis of Healing in Africa*, Berkeley, 1992, pp. 393–406.

36. For a broader consideration of the appeal of astrology and public tolerance for its failures, see Thomas, *Religion and Magic*, pp. 332–49.

37. *The Miscellaneous Works of Mr. John Toland*, London, 1747, p. 276. Thomas, *Religion and Magic*, pp. 9–10; Roy Porter, *Disease, Medicine and Society in England, 1550–1860*, London, 1987, pp. 14–15; Roy Porter and Dorothy Porter, *Patient's Progress: Doctors and Doctoring in Eighteenth-Century England*, Stanford, 1989, pp. 58–63. Paul Slack asks why people did not lose faith in medicine and gives similar answers to those Thomas adduces for their phlegmatic response to astrological failures: *The Impact of the Plague in Tudor and Stuart England*, London, 1985, pp. 35–6.

38. For them, see Clark, *College of Physicians*, vol. 2, index, s.v. 'empirics'. Note that some of the 'empirics' and interlopers Clark mentions elsewhere, such as Arthur Dee and John Case are not identified as astrological physicians: ibid., vol. 1, pp. 208, 216, 232; vol. 2, p. 451. See also, Matthias Evans to Richard Napier, 10 April 1621, Ashml. 223, fol. 170.

39. Lilly, *Life and Times, passim* for Evans and others; Thomas, *Religion and Magic*, p. 304.

40. MacDonald, *Mystical Bedlam*, p. 256, n. 21; Sawyer, 'Patients, Disease and Healing', pp. 272–4; John H. Raach, *A Directory of English Country Physicians, 1603–1640*, London, 1962, pp. 96–7, 111. For Bredon, see above n. 15.

41. Margaret Pelling and Charles Webster, 'Medical Practitioners', in C. Webster (ed.), *Health, Medicine and Mortality in the Sixteenth Century*, Cambridge, 1979, pp. 199, 204, 216, 234.

42. Thomas, *Religion and Magic*, pp. 302–5.

43. Many are mentioned in passing by Mordechai Feingold, *The Mathematician's Apprentice: Apprenticeship, Science, Universities, and Society in England, 1560–1640*, Cambridge, 1984, index, s.v. 'astrology'.

44. For astrological apprenticeship, see Sawyer, 'Patients, Healers and Disease', pp. 275–6; Lilly, *Life and Times*, pp. 54–60, 83–8.

45. Wright makes a good deal of this weakness as a key to the astrologers' 'failure' ultimately to thrive *vis-à-vis* 'medicine'. Although I think the argument is flawed in a number of ways, I agree with much of it and will

not explore the issues he raises in detail here (Wright, '"Failure" of Astrology').

46. This may seem obvious after Thomas's efforts, but the importance of astrological physic is still overlooked by medical historians and, on the other hand, seen as a proto-profession competing with the physicians. In this regard, Wright's suggestive article seems curiously overdetermined ('Legitimisation of Knowledge').

47. Rowse, *Sex and Society*, chs 7–10. Research by Lauren Kassell, the prelude to what will be the first proper study of Forman's practice, confirms these impressions in 'Casting Figures for Disease: The Patients of an Astrological Medical Practitioner in London, 1596–1598', MSc dissertation, University of Oxford, 1994.

48. Thomas, *Religion and Magic*, p. 319n.

49. Sawyer, 'Patients, Healers and Disease', ch. 7; MacDonald, *Mystical Bedlam*, pp. 33–71.

50. Beier, *Sufferers and Healers*, pp. 120–3.

51. Sawyer, 'Patients, Healers and Disease', chs 6–7 evaluates the pattern of illness in Napier's practice in the context of what can be learned from parish registers and other sources about the fatal and non-fatal diseases in his region.

52. See, for example, Ashml. 235, fols 186^v–193.

53. Over 20 years ago I tried to discover whether this imbalance was peculiar to the practices of astrologers. I searched the collections of the British Library and the Bodleian for every contemporary set of case notes that did not appear to be 'selected' cases and tabulated the sex ratios in them. The results were inconclusive because the numbers were too small to produce statistically meaningful ratios and because of other weaknesses in the documents. I gained the impression that wherever high cost was not a deterrent factor, women tended to seek medical treatment somewhat more frequently. I gave away my notes on this subject in about 1982. The impression is all that remains.

54. Quoted by Sawyer, 'Patients, Healers and Disease', p. 483. Sawyer's discussion of female maladies is the only study of them that has been done, pp. 482–92.

55. 'Matrix and the Pains Thereof', Ashml. 390, fols 175–85. Similar works may be found in the British Library's Sloane MSS and the Wellcome Institute for the History of Medicine's library. See, for example, 'Of the Diseases of Women', MS Sloane 421, A fols 2–25^v. For an anonymous medical practice, 1600–20, almost entirely devoted to gynaecology, see BL MS Sloane 63, fols 2–34. The standard history of these matters has little to say about actual women's illnesses and is based almost entirely on printed sources: Audrey Eccles, *Obstetrics and Gynaecology in Tudor and Stuart England*, Kent, OH, 1982.

56. Kassell, 'Casting Figures for Disease'.

57. Sawyer, 'Patients, Healers and Disease', pp. 489–92. For green sickness, see also I.S.L. Loudon, 'Chlorosis, Anaemia and Anorexia Nervosa', *British Medical Journal*, (281) (1980), pp. 1669–87; and for the 'mother' Jorden, 'Suffocation of the Mother', in MacDonald, *Witchcraft and Hysteria*; Michael Micale, *Approaching Hysteria: A Disease and Its Interpretation*, Princeton, 1995, ch. 1.

58. Sawyer, 'Patients, Healers and Disease', pp. 334–7; R.C. Sawyer

'"Strangely Handled in All Her Lyms": Witchcraft and Healing in Jacobean England', *Journal of Social History*, 22 (1989), pp. 467–9.

59. Ashml. 222, fols 196, 196; BL MS Additional 36674, fols 134–7.
60. See, for example, Anonymous Astrological Practice-Book, BL MS Sloane 3857, fol. 64 (1605), and the introduction to Michael MacDonald, *Witchcraft and Hysteria in Elizabethan London: Edward Jorden and the Mary Glover Case*, London, 1990.
61. BL MS Sloane 3822, fols 35–35ᵛ. This manuscript contains instructions for making astrological amulets, *passim*, as do several other manuscripts in the Sloane and Additional collections, compiled by Forman, Napier, Sir Richard Napier and Elias Ashmole. See also MacDonald, *Mystical Bedlam*, pp. 213–14.
62. Indeed, from a medical standpoint the history of the decline in witchcraft beliefs is the tale of the reclassification of a disparate group of unusual and alarming symptoms from the realm of the supernatural to the domain of the psychiatric. I hope to write more about this in future. Meanwhile, see MacDonald, *Mystical Bedlam*, pp. 197–8 and for a contemporary, sceptical opinion in this vein, George Castle, *The Chymical Galenist*, London, 1667.
63. Ashml. 363, fols 4ᵛ–9ᵛ.
64. For a full, contextualized discussion, see MacDonald, *Mystical Bedlam*. A second edition with a chapter of fresh reflections and *mea culpas* will be issued by the University of Michigan Press in 1996 or 1997.
65. MacDonald, *Mystical Bedlam*, ch. 4.
66. MacDonald, *Mystical Bedlam*, ch. 5. For a puritan divine's assertion that physical remedies were an essential part of treating bewitched persons, see Richard Baxter, *The Certainty of the World of Spirits*, London, 1691, pp. 173–4. Simon Forman gave a sigil to William Lilly's mistress to alleviate the 'melancholy discontent' she attributed to the 'haunting spirit' of her first husband. When she died, she was found to have a whole bagful of them under her armpit: Lilly, *Life and Times*, pp. 32–3.
67. The fullest, somewhat romanticized, discussions are [Thomas Longueville], *The Curious Case of Lady Purbeck: A Scandal of the XVIIIth Century*, London, 1909; Laura Norsworthy, *The Lady of Bleeding Heart Yard: Lady Elizabeth Hatton, 1578–1646*, London, 1935. For its political implications, see S.R. Gardiner, *History of England From the Accession of James I to the Outbreak of the Civil War, 1603–1642*, 10 vols, repr., New York, 1965, vol. 3, pp. 84–100. For its emblematic importance in modern (more or less feminist) scholarship about women and marriage, see Lawrence Stone, *The Crisis of the Aristocracy*, Oxford, 1965, p. 596; L. Stone, *The Family, Sex and Marriage in England, 1500–1800*, New York, 1977, p. 182; Antonia Fraser, *The Weaker Vessel: Women's Lot in Seventeenth-Century England*, London, 1984, pp. 12–20. I have prepared a fully documented study of this case which will form part of 'Marriage, Scandal and Female Power in the Jacobean Court' (forthcoming).
68. Norman McClure (ed.), *The Letters of John Chamberlain*, Philadelphia, 1939, vol. 2, p. 439.
69. *Calendar of State Papers, Domestic, 1623–5*, London, 1858, pp. 71, 73–4.

70. Ashml. 410, fols 81, 83.
71. For reference to Purbeck's illness and Napier's treatment and brief remarks, see MacDonald, *Mystical Bedlam*, pp. 21–2, 49, 92, 152, 192, 199.
72. The best treatment is David Lindley, *The Trials of Frances Howard*, London, 1993.
73. Ashml. 414, fol. 47.
74. *DNB*, Lambe, John; *A Briefe Description of the Notorious Life of John Lambe*, London, 1628.
75. Allen, *Star-Crossed Renaissance*; Thomas, *Religion and Magic*, ch. 12.
76. William Perkins, *The Workes of that Famous and Worthy Minister of Christ*, 3 vols, London, 1626–31, vol. 1, pp. 505–6; vol. 3, pp. 659–67; John Gaule, *Select Cases of Conscience Touching Witches and Witchcrafts*, London, 1646, pp. 25–6, 32; J. Gaule, *The Mag-Astromancer: or, the Magicall-Astrologicall-Diviner Posed, and Puzzled*, London, 1652, pp. 185–90; Thomas, *Religion and Magic*, ch. 12; Allen, *Star-Crossed Renaissance*, chs. 1–3, *passim*.
77. *Life of Lambe*, unpaginated.
78. Thomas, *Religion and Magic*, pp. 282–9; Capp, *Astrology and the Press*, pp. 204–8; Curry, *Prophecy and Power*, ch. 2.
79. Curry, *Prophecy and Power*, pp. 22–3, 30. There are popular biographies of both: Derek Parker, *Familiar to All: William Lilly and Astrology in the Seventeenth Century*, London, 1975; Olav Thulesius, *Nicholas Culpeper: English Physician and Astrologer*, London, 1992.
80. F.N.L. Poynter, 'Nicholas Culpeper and His Books', *Journal of the History of Medicine and Allied Sciences*, 17 (1962), pp. 152–67 remains the best treatment.
81. Curry, *Prophecy and Power*, ch. 2 discusses all these figures. Much useful information about astrological practice in this period may be found in the autobiographies of Lilly and Ashmole: Lilly, *Life and Times*, pp. 91–140; Elias Ashmole, *Elias Ashmole (1617–1692): His Autobiographical and Historical Notes, His Correspondence, and Other Contemporary Sources Relating to His Life*, C.H. Josten (ed.), 5 vols, Oxford, 1966, esp. vol. 2.
82. Harry Rusche, '"Merlini Anglici": Astrology and Propaganda from 1644 to 1651', *English Historical Review*, 80 (1965), pp. 322–33; H. Rusche, Prophecies and Propaganda', *English Historical Review*, 84 (1969), pp. 752–70; Thomas, *Religion and Magic*, pp. 342–3; Capp, *Astrology and the Press*, ch. 3.
83. Curry, *Prophecy and Power*, p. 27; Charles Webster, *The Great Instauration*, London, 1975, p. 200.
84. The authoritative discussion of medical reform is Webster's magisterial *Great Instauration*, ch. 4. See also Christopher Hill, *The World Turned Upside Down*, London, 1972, ch. 14; Curry, *Prophecy and Power*, pp. 23–34. Peter Elmer questions the religious motivations for reform: 'Medicine, Religion and the Puritan Revolution', in French and Wear, *Medical Revolution*, pp. 10–45.
85. In addition to reissues of Culpeper's own books, they produced new texts: Joseph Blagrave, *Blagrave's Astrological Practice of Physic*, London, 1671; Richard Saunders, *Astrological Judgment and Practice of Physick*, London, 1677; William Salmon, *Synopsis Medicinae*, London,

1671; R. Saunders, *Iatricia seu Praxis Medendi*, London, 1681, and many other works.

86. Curry, *Prophecy and Power*, pp. 80, 99.

87. Quoted in Thomas, *Religion and Magic*, p. 321.

88. Irish, *Levamon Infirmi*.

89. For a good example of the progression from attacking 'empirics' to disparaging astrology, see the digressive tirades in John Freind's much praised *The History of Physick: From the Time of Galen, to the Beginning of the Sixteenth Century*, 2 vols, London, 1725–26, vol. 1, 302–11; vol. 2, 20–1. Harold J. Cook's excellent 'The Society of Chemical Physicians, the New Philosophy, and the Restoration Court', *Bulletin of the History of Medicine*, 61 (1987), pp. 61–77 makes many pertinent observations. A balanced survey of the politics of medical practice from about 1660–1750 would be very welcome.

90. Quoted in Capp, *Astrology and the Press*, p. 281. His concise discussion of the political attitudes affecting the reputation of astrology is superb, see pp. 277–83.

91. Curry, *Prophecy and Power*, chs 2–3; Margaret Bowen, 'The Scientific Revolution in Astrology', PhD thesis, Yale University, 1974; Hunter and Gregory, *Samuel Jeake*, pp. 14–21, 73–6; Michael Hunter, *John Aubrey and the Realm of Learning* London, 1975, pp. 119–21, 144–5.

92. Henry Power, 'Some Objections to Astrology', BL MS Sloane 1356, esp. fol. 123; Michael Hunter, 'Science and Astrology in Seventeenth-Century England: An Unpublished Polemic by John Flamsteed', in Patrick Curry (ed.), *Astrology, Science and Society*, London, 1987, pp. 261–300.

93. Barbara Shapiro, *Probability and Certainty in Seventeenth-Century England*, Princeton, 1973; Michael McKeon, *The Origins of the English Novel, 1660–1740*, Baltimore, 1987, chs 1–3.

94. Quoted in Curry, *Prophecy and Power*, p. 149. Space precludes retelling the joke adequately, but Swift's fake almanac predicting Partridge's death and the subsequent pamphlets describing it dealt a heavy blow to the prestige and (it is alleged) practice of the period's most prominent medical astrologer. Curry gives an account, pp. 89–91; David Nokes, *Jonathan Swift: The Hypocrite Reversed*, Oxford, 1985, pp. 79–83 captures the jokesters' *Schadenfreude* much better. Writing with detachment, John Redwood, *Reason, Ridicule and Religion: The Age of the Enlightenment in England, 1660–1750*, London, 1976, rightly stresses the importance of ridicule in fostering scepticism.

95. Thomas, *Religion and Magic*, pp. 351–7; Curry, *Prophecy and Power*, pp. 145–52.

96. Curry, *Prophecy and Power, passim*.

97. Mary Fissel, *Patients, Power and the Poor in Eighteenth-Century Bristol*, Cambridge, 1991, p. 189, citing mainly London advertisements.

98. Capp, *Astrology and the Press*, ch. 8. Astrological lore was a staple of chapbooks in the eighteenth and early nineteenth centuries: Phyllis Marjorie Swanson, 'Popular Literature in the Eighteenth Century: The Dicey Chapbooks', PhD thesis, Northwestern University, 1985, pp. 27–8. For evidence that some people, at least, took astrological books seriously see Darcy Curwen, Untitled astrological tract, 18th cent., Cumbria Record Office, Carlisle, MS D/Cu/Acc 1964.

99. Jon Butler, *Awash in a Sea of Faith: Christianizing the American People*,

Cambridge, MA, 1990, p. 83. For astrology in the American colonies, see also David Hall, *Worlds of Wonder, Days of Judgment*, New York, 1989.

100. Francis Guybon, *An Essay Concerning the Growth of Empiricism: or, the Encouragement of Quacks*, London, 1712, p. 58. Despite his name and French, Guybon was English.

101. Curry, *Prophecy and Power*, chs 7–8; J.F.C. Harrison, *The Second Coming: Popular Millenarianism, 1780–1850*, New Brunswick, NJ, 1979, pp. 21, 40, 47–9.

102. Roy Porter, 'Laymen, Doctors and Medical Knowledge in the Eighteenth Century', in R. Porter (ed.), *Patients and Practitioners: Lay Perceptions of Medicine in Pre-industrial Society*, Cambridge, 1985, ch. 10; R. Porter, 'Lay Medical Knowledge in the Eighteenth Century: The Evidence of the *Gentleman's Magazine*', *Medical History*, 29 (1985), pp. 138–68; Porter and Porter, *Patient's Progress*, chs 11–12. See also the classic articles by Norman Jewison, 'Medical Knowledge and the Patronage System in Eighteenth Century England', *Sociology*, 8 (1974), pp. 369–85 and 'The Disappearance of the Sick Man from Medical Cosmology 1770–1870', *Sociology*, 10 (1976), pp. 225–44.

103. This may seem a peculiarly American conclusion, especially coming from an author who was educated in California. And the dissonance between doctor/patient mentalities does seem to be a hotter topic amongst medical researchers in the USA. For some recent discussion, see, for example, Margaret Gereis et al., (eds), *Through the Patient's Eyes*, San Francisco, 1993, esp. ch. 2; Robert A. Hahn, *Sickness and Healing: An Anthropological Approach*, New Haven, 1995, chs 4, 9, 10. But see also for the UK, J.B. Loudon (ed.), *Social Anthropology and Medicine*, London, 1976, pp. 1–48, 150–89.

CHAPTER FOUR

Institutional Structures and Personal Belief in the London College of Physicians

Harold J. Cook

The institutional fortunes of the College of Physicians of London have a number of similarities to the fortunes of the Church of England. Both experienced a steep decline in their public authority both during the mid-seventeenth-century civil wars and following the Glorious Revolution. The legal and political changes that most immediately caused the decline in the public power of the College had little to do with the religious outlook of its members, and were not directly caused by religion. But the similarities between the College and the Church of England suggest that the College's authority as a regulatory body was associated with a particular constitutional structure that connected the authority of learned men with the English monarchy. The very establishment of the College took place at a moment when the prestige of learned humanism was high in England and associated with good monarchical government; when such Latinate learning no longer impressed those in power, the fortunes of the College physicians, like their clerical brethren, declined precipitously. The juridical authority of the College was derived from the authority of a sacerdotal monarch, with a part of the monarch's godly duty to preserve his or her subjects extended to the College. To extend the analogy only slightly, it would seem that the Fellows of the College of Physicians were like the bishops of the Church, exercising their authority over other medical practitioners as the bishops used theirs to keep the clergy in line. In James I's famous phrase, 'no bishops, no king'. From the point of view of the medical bishops, the phrase meant that without a king or queen who supported the public authority of the learned chiefs, no power for them. Thus, while the institutional structure of the College of Physicians did not change because of the religious orientation of its members (nor did it change the Fellows' religious outlook), the deeper religious constitution, which placed paternalistic powers in the hands of learned authorities, played a fundamental part in the fortunes of the College. As a result, the College remained a conservative force in medicine, being associated first with Catholic humanism, and then with priestly Anglicanism.

From its beginnings, the College of Physicians of London had political and academic connections to the new humanists who were assuming public authority in Church and State. The humanists argued that men trained in ancient methods of analysing the *vita activa* were necessary for shaping the policies that would guide the generality of royal subjects toward the common good (the 'commonwealth'). It was the non-noble former Master of Magdalene College, Lord Chancellor and papal legate, Cardinal Wolsey, who arranged for the College's 1518 charter and for its confirmation in Parliament in 1523, because 'the making of the said Corporacion is meritorious and very good for the com[m]en Welth of this your Realme'. Physicians, the Parliament agreed, should be 'p[ro]founde, sad and discrete, groudlie lerned, and deplie studied in physyk'.[1] Rooted in civic humanist ideals as modified by the learned counsellors of the king, and modelled on the example of colleges of physicians in Italy, the London College was to be a body that would encourage the most exacting medical learning and offer expert advice to the Crown on matters of public importance.[2] As on the Continent, so in Renaissance England, medical policy became an important part of governmental thinking about the public good.[3] As a body of élite medical scholars and royal physicians, including the deservedly famous medical humanist Thomas Linacre,[4] the College offered no pretence of bringing within its folds the many ordinary medical practitioners of London: its right to forbid the practice of physic to anyone in London or within seven miles who was not a member seems at first to have been mainly meant as a rule to encourage physicians who had obtained a classical education.

When public religion became a subject of deep concern at the end of the 1520s, the College kept quiet: during the uproar over Henry VIII's divorce, the fall of Wolsey and the rise of Thomas Cromwell, the parliamentary grant of the Act of Supremacy of 1534, Cromwell's own beheading and the dispossession of the monasteries, the College obtained no further institutional grants. During this period, some of the learned clergymen who left the Church took up the practice of physic, but the College provided no home for them. This must not be ascribed, however, to any repugnance for Catholicism but to the practice of admitting to the Fellowship only those 'deeply studied in physic' (most of whom held medical doctorates, something that the ex-clergymen did not possess). In John Caius's later summary of the records of the College, nothing at all was noted as occurring between 1531 and 1541, suggesting either that the College held little or no interest for the new chief minister Cromwell, or that the physicians – like many other learned men of the time – had little enthusiasm for Cromwell's views of government, or that Caius simply suppressed any record of their relations with Henry's chief minister.[5] But about the time that Cromwell fell in 1540, the College obtained further public authority from Parliament: as people who served the public by their medical attendance, the physicians of the College became exempt from the civic duties of watch and ward, constable and other municipal obligations in London; they obtained the right to elect four censors to examine apothecary shops (together with a warden of the Grocers' Company); and they gained recognition for being able to practice all parts of medicine, including surgery (this being necessary because of the act of the same Parliament incorporating the Barber-Surgeons' Company).[6] The first record of empirics being fined for practice without the College's licence is in December 1541, when the Court of Exchequer acted twice.[7] The College also obtained its coat of arms in 1546. During the reign of Edward, however, it again showed little life.

The College records (which are particularly scanty for the first half of the century) suggest that it was reinvigorated following the accession of Mary in 1554. Mary's adviser, Cardinal Pole, was not only a learned humanist himself, he had been educated in part by the College's own Thomas Linacre. Under Mary, the College began to fine illicit practitioners again, and through the efforts of three royal physicians, George Owen, Thomas Wendy and Thomas Huys, it obtained a parliamentary Act giving it the right to commit offenders to prison.[8] It was also under Mary that the President, John Caius, reinvigorated the College's public activities: he waged war on empirics in London; he circulated a printed notice to all justices, mayors, sheriffs, bailiffs, constables and others, requiring their aid in fining and imprisoning those practising without the College's licence; he began a process of commissioning people outside London to take action against empirics; he obtained a letter from the queen requiring the College once again to inspect the London apothecary shops; he got Pole to support the College's demand that medical degrees not be awarded at Oxford and Cambridge without the students having followed a prescribed course of study; and he laid down rules for governing the internal business of the College – its ceremonial behaviour, the marks of authority of its officers, the feasts it would celebrate, and the fees it would require for entry.[9] Under learned Dr Caius, too, the College stood as a bastion of medical learning rooted in the ancient authors. While an excellent natural historian and philologist and fine anatomist, Caius objected to Vesalius's criticisms of Galen. In late October and early November of 1560, he also led a three-day disputation (it would be too much to call it an inquisition) against John Geynes, who held that Galen had been wrong on a number of counts.

An MD of Oxford in 1535, Geynes sought admission to the College, but was first forced to sign a document recanting his opinion that Galen had erred, which he finally did only after the three days of argument.[10] Physicians might be entitled to their personal views, but under Caius the College would not allow its members to publicly dissent from philologically inspired medical humanism. Moreover, when the College met as a body, the President would be addressed as 'your excellency'; he would sit on a cushion, hold a silver caduceus, and use the College seal (all presented to the College by Caius); and the other members would be organized according to their rank and date of admission to the corporation.[11]

From Mary's reign onwards, then, the sense of priestly order and dignity embodied in the College's own ceremonies, as well as in its defence of academic medical learning and its public attacks on empirics, would carry the whiff of popery to sensitive Protestant noses. If there is a pattern here (and one must be careful, since the pattern may be in the way that John Caius kept the records rather than in the actual institutional behaviour of the College), it suggests that periods when humanist notions of an ordered commonwealth dominated the concerns of the Crown were more favourable for encouraging the physicians' corporation than were the periods concerned with introducing the new religion.

The early Fellows themselves tended, like many learned humanists educated before the Reformation, to remain adherents of the older faith. John Clement, for example, left for Louvain soon after Edward VI became king in 1547 and was not included in the general pardon issued in the king's name in 1552; he only returned to England in 1554, following Mary's accession. The only known early member of the College to have harboured strong enough Protestant beliefs to be noticed was John Fryer, who was imprisoned for his Lutheranism in the mid-1520s. But he did not become a member of the College until about ten years after that, having taken his MD at Padua in the meantime. When Fryer returned to Henrician England from Italy, he had probably already moderated his views; at any rate, in the early 1560s Fryer was imprisoned for Catholicism.[12] Although Fryer was willing to go to prison for his religious views, more commonly the members of the College seem to have survived the religious storms by 'bending in the winds'. Several early Fellows served as royal physicians to Protestant and Catholic monarchs alike: both George Owen and Thomas Wendy served as royal physicians to Henry VIII and continued under the Protestant Edward and the Catholic Mary (Wendy living long enough to serve Elizabeth I as well); Thomas Huys, who replaced the Catholic Clement in 1551 as a College Elect because of his Protestant religion (religionis gratiâ), was also described as a royal physician (regius medicus) on his death in 1558 at the end of Mary's reign. Moreover, while under Mary the College elected Catholic John Caius as President in 1555, he continued to serve until 1561, even after the Protestant Elizabeth's accession in 1558. There was, therefore, no quick purge of physicians at court or in the College following changes in the religious orientation of the monarchy. Thus, the loyalties of the mid-century Fellows seem to have been to the promotion of learned physic over and above any particular religious outlook. But from what little evidence remains, it also seems that the deeply learned men of the College tended to be personally conservative, remaining more sympathetic to the old religion or diocesan Anglicanism, with their hierarchies rooted in the judgement and *gravitas* of learned men.

This pattern of intellectual and religious conservatism tending towards Catholic humanism appears to have continued through the first years of Elizabeth's reign. The College continued to act as a learned brotherhood and to prosecute empirics, but Caius stepped down from the presidency of the College in 1564 to see to his work at Gonville (and Caius) College, and was removed from his office of physician to Elizabeth in 1568 because of his Catholicism. Caius's energetic prosecution of empirics seemingly came to an end during the years 1564 to 1568, during which time the Annals recorded only admissions to offices in the College (although perhaps it is again an illusion caused by the poor quality of the record-keeping after Caius's Presidency). But perhaps, too, the new government of Elizabeth liked the College less than Mary's had. Such would seem to be the case in 1572, when Caius had to return from Cambridge to defend the College's rights to fine surgeons for applying inward remedies in a hearing in the Lord Mayor's Court, which he did successfully against an array of royal authorities. In defending the College, Caius had to argue against a host of royal advisors: the Bishop of London, Lord James Croftes of the Royal Household, the Master of the Rolls, the Master of Requests, and a number of other lords and gentlemen.[13] After Caius's death in 1573, the College records almost cease until the office of Registrar was begun in 1581. It would seem that for the first 20 years of Elizabeth's reign, her government had little use for a kind of semi-Catholic fraternity of learned physicians.

But the College's power to act against others grew during the later 1580s as the Elizabethan regime became more conservative and more assertive, and perhaps as the College became more conformist as well. The College of Physicians obtained the blessings of the Crown for reviving its juridical powers in 1588 (apparently lapsed since the early 1570s) by gaining the grant of a 'privilege' from Sir Francis Walsingham to prosecute empirics even when they had the protection of courtiers like himself.[14] During the 1590s, one group in particular that the College began to prosecute in significant number was the surgeons, who were by statute limited to practising on outward ailments only. By the end of the reign of Elizabeth and the beginning of the reign of James I, the College was vigorously acting to exclude outsiders from the practice of physic in London, and doing so with the support of the Crown and most of the royal judges.[15]

By the beginning of the seventeenth century, too, due in part to Elizabeth's policies, the College had become overwhelmingly Anglican in membership, although many members privately continued to lean toward Catholicism. The religious orientation of the Fellows was partly the result of institutional arrangements. Over the course of the sixteenth century, as religious division became a problem in England, an unofficial College policy had come into being of requiring the MD to be from Oxford or Cambridge or to be incorporated at either of the two English universities. This assured outward conformity to the Church of England, since the oath of supremacy passed under Elizabeth in 1559 required all those holding public office or taking a degree to acknowledge the monarch as Supreme Governor of the Realm in spiritual and ecclesiastical as well as temporal matters or to forfeit their office or degree. As a consequence, non-Anglican physicians could seldom obtain a fellowship in the College. With the accession of James, the fellowship was opened to those who had taken a 'British' degree (allowing James's physician John Craige to become a Fellow), but at the same time the College reinforced its association with academic medical learning by requiring all applicants to have studied at least seven years past the MA for the MD.[16]

Despite the requirement of a learned British degree, given the superior medical education available abroad, especially at Padua, a number of English students travelled to the Continent to study for their medical doctorates, bringing them into contact with Catholicism. Some of the Englishmen who travelled abroad privately converted to the Roman religion, while others became sympathetic to it. For example, Edward de Vere, the seventeenth Earl of Oxford, left in 1575 for seven years of travels (mainly in Italy), and together with friends privately professed the Catholic faith not long after his return. Coupled with the growing threat from post-Tridentine Spain, the assassination of the Prince of Orange in 1582 by a Catholic, and the discovery of several plots on Elizabeth's own life in the 1580s, Parliament passed a proclamation 'for the revocation of sundry of the Queen's Majesty's subjects remaining beyond the seas under colour of study', while sermons were preached against 'Oure Italienated Papistes'. The 1580s and early 1590s proved dangerous for English travellers in Italy, as well, given the attention they drew from the Inquisition. Nevertheless, many defied the laws and travelled in Catholic lands, especially to Italy, with the number increasing at the end of the century.[17] Among those who left England for Padua to take medical doctorates between 1590 and 1604 (when the peace treaty with Spain allowed for foreign travel) were Edward Jordan, Thomas Hearne, William Harvey, William Clement, Simeon Foxe and Thomas Winston. (During those years, too, Sir Matthew Lister also took an MD at Protestant Basle, and Thomas Lodge did the same at Catholic Avignon, while Robert Fludd also travelled for about six years on the Continent from 1598, although he returned to take his MD at Oxford in 1605.) We need not suspect any or all of them of harbouring Catholicism merely because they studied in Italy: Simeon Foxe, for instance, was the youngest son of John Fox, the Protestant martyrologist, and himself remained a conformist Puritan.[18] But given the times, these intending physicians took some risk of being viewed as Catholic sympathizers upon their return to England.

By the reign of James I, then, the College had obtained the reputation of being a body of highly educated physicians with close ties to the Crown and the right to prosecute those who practised physic without their licence; but it also had the reputation of being an institution of ceremonial ritual, of Latinate discourse, of 'monopolistic' behaviour, and of a membership that was mainly conformist but leaning towards Catholicism. The conservatism of men who devoted long years of their lives to study in authoritative texts tended to cause them to favour learned hierarchies and traditional ways. Openly religious ideologies seem to have had little place in the College. But clearly, the College officers had come to associate their own public authority with personal attachments to the monarchy, an education in medical philology and classical texts, and a spiritual discipline derived from king and bishops. As the Church and State went, so too went the College.

Under the early Stuarts, the institutional authority of the College remained linked to service to the monarchy, although the membership grew more religiously diverse, as did that of other members of the republic of learning. Under James I, and especially under Charles I, the English Crown took on ever more responsibility for trying to preserve the health of the body politic, which included directing affairs in London using the College of Physicians. As with the individual, so too with the public body: good health was assumed to come from moderation, temperance and good order. The College therefore gradually found itself involved in the various policies that evolved into Thorough and Laudianism. While its corporate privileges grew through helping the monarchy police the public, the College's reputation as a bastion of medical conservatism also grew, despite the gradual shift toward Puritanism amongst some of its members.

The first area in which the College continued to gain authority was in its right to prevent other medical practitioners in London from practising physic without the College's licence. The famous case of Dr Bonham showed that most of the royal judges were much in favour of allowing the College to exclude from London practice even a person with an MD from Cambridge. In February of 1608–09, the College won the suit it brought against Bonham in the Court of King's Bench, although much to almost everyone's surprise it lost Bonham's famous counter-suit in a split decision by the Court of Common Pleas a year later. In the second of these cases, Chief Justice Edward Coke argued against the College monopoly in words that later had repercussions for law in the early United States but that had little effect on the College's police powers (since the king and his judges continued to support the College). Why Bonham had been refused admission to the College is unclear, but it seems to have been because of his close association with the surgeons, including the king's surgeon William Clowes, at a time when the College was acting vigorously to keep them from practising physic. Although Bonham had a degree from Cambridge, where Puritanism was becoming a force by the 1590s, there is no evidence that Bonham himself was a Puritan; his associations with Clowes and the protection offered to him by the vigorously anti-Puritan Archbishop Bancroft, who wrote to the College that Bonham had 'taken his degree ... with good commendacion', suggest otherwise.[19]

In Bonham's case, Justice Walmesley argued that the king had a duty to govern the lives and healths of all his subjects, and that since it was impossible for the king to oversee all matters pertaining to the public good himself, his duties required him to make laws and to delegate his authority to agents acting on his behalf, in this case, to the College of Physicians. People committed their lives to medical practitioners, Walmesley argued, and so for the good health of all in London the College of Physicians had obtained from Henry VIII the 'power to make laws' governing physic, 'which is the office of the Parliament, for those which are so learned may be trusted with any thing'.[20] Thus, to Walmesley and the physicians, the King's duties toward the 'public good' required him to make laws and to delegate his authority to agents acting on his behalf, even if they excluded from practice those they thought unfit. For the first four decades of the seventeenth century, then, the College had the support of the king and the royal judges in prosecuting interlopers into the practice of physic. It was only at times when legal questions caused some concern, or when Parliament met, that the College lowered its prosecutorial activities.[21]

The second area in which the College and Crown worked in tandem from the middle of James's reign, was in the formation of new medical corporations, which were subordinated to the monarchically dependent College of Physicians. The Crown continued to help the College keep the London Barber-Surgeons' Company in check, as later Tudor governments had done, and it created the London Society of Apothecaries by royal fiat and subordinated it to the College of Physicians. In turn, the College began to advise the Privy Council on matters concerning the health of the metropolis, especially those concerning plague.

A de facto corporate medical policy therefore emerged under the first two Stuarts, which began through royal rewards to court favorites: Gideon DeLaune (a royal apothecary) and Theodore Turquet de Mayerne (a royal physician). Both DeLaune and Mayerne were Huguenot émigrés. As a foreigner, DeLaune had been denied admission to the London Grocer's Company (to which the apothecaries belonged), and he and other apothecaries had tried unsuccessfully to separate themselves into a new corporation in 1610. Mayerne arrived in England to stay in that same year, taking up service to James I after the assassination of his previous royal client, Henri IV. The Privy Council had already begun to take steps signalling its view that the drug trade ought to be better regulated in London, as it was in many places on the Continent; in 1618, the officers of the Crown, with the support of the College, created the Society of Apothecaries over the strong opposition of the City of London. While the City worked through the Parliaments of 1621 and 1624 to reject the new Society (and a new and stronger charter for the College which had been granted by the king), they were disbanded before they could reverse the royal corporate medical policies. Under Charles I, the medical policies favouring the creation of medical corporations in London subordinated to the College of Physicians gained further sanction and clearer authority. The charters of the Company of Barber-Surgeons and College of Physicians were adjusted to reinforce the College's domination over medical practice in the City. Under the period of Charles's personal rule, the College and Mayerne helped to draw up plans to deal with epidemics of plague, brought the new Society of Apothecaries under the College's heel, and even created a new Company of Distillers (another of Mayerne's projects).[22] Only with the meeting of the Short Parliament did the College's close relationship with the Crown begin to shift.

Mayerne's personal involvement in most of the plans developed by Crown and College from 1610 to 1640 made him a very important figure. A protestant humanist born in Geneva in 1573 – the godson of the famous theologian Theodore Beza, educated at Heidelberg and Montpellier – Mayerne had served as physician in ordinary to Henri IV. At the French court, he had refused to convert to Catholicism like his royal master (which might well have allowed him to become Henri's first physician) and he became deeply embroiled in a controversy with the Paris Faculty of Medicine, in which Mayerne and others defended their criticisms of Galen and promotion of chemical medicine. After the assassination of Henri in 1610, James I successfully sought Mayerne's services, making him his first physician and knighting him in 1624 (probably as much for his services as diplomat and spy as for his medical advice). He quickly became James's favourite physician, and retained the post of first physician under Charles. Despite his Protestantism, he also became a favourite of Charles I's Catholic French wife, Henriette Maria (probably because of his connections in France and his fluency in her language). The College could not have avoided Mayerne if it chose, and it admitted him a Fellow in 1616 in a gracious ceremony.

Given Mayerne's personal ties to Beza and his continued affiliation with humanist Calvinism, his activist policies on behalf of the health of Londoners would seem to be an excellent example of the ways in which Protestantism began to reshape the College. Ole Grell has recently argued, for example, that Beza's Protestantism gave prominence 'to the Commonwealth at the expense of the individual', that 'the medical practitioner's duty [lay] towards the Commonwealth rather than the patient'.[23] While Grell's comments were made in the context of arguing why it became acceptable for physicians to flee plague instead (as he argues Luther instructed) of staying to give advice and consolation, they would at first sight also seem to help explain Mayerne's motivations in working for a larger role for the physicians in advising the monarchical government on issues involving the health of the body politic. Nevertheless, it would be going too far to say that such views were exclusively Calvinist. As Grell points out, similar views on the Commonwealth were held by the conservative Anglican theologian Lancelot Andrews and the 'crypto-Catholic physician and poet' Thomas Lodge.[24] The English 'commonwealthmen' had their origin in a modified civic humanism that shared much with the Spaniard Vives and the neostoic Lipsius, while medical policies of the early Stuart governments and the College of Physicians continued to develop along the lines established under the Catholic Caius and Queen Mary, and under the last years of Elizabeth's anti-Puritan government.[25] While Charles I's Privy Council included a few men of a crypto-Puritan stripe, it became known mainly for being crypto-Catholic. In short, it remains difficult to believe that the policies of Crown and College under the early Stuarts were motivated by any particular religious outlook, even with the involvement of Mayerne. The civic humanism of Italy and the Low Countries, adapted to English political institutions, affected Calvinist, Anglican and Catholic alike.

It is true, however, that the religious orientation of the Fellows of the College was becoming more diverse. The growing number of Fellows with a strong Protestant orientation, even occasionally a Calvinist one, is due to the growing influence of Calvinism at some of the Cambridge colleges and the opening of Calvinist universities with excellent medical faculties in the northern Netherlands, most notably at Leiden. These developments allowed significant numbers of young men who became learned physicians to be deeply educated in Calvinist intellectual cultures, rather than simply to defect to them. While many Fellows of the College remained conservative Anglicans, and a few even remained Catholic, an increasing number became reform-minded, and a few were even strong Puritans.

The best study of the religious affiliations of the Fellows in the early seventeenth century remains William Birken's 1977 thesis. Birken notes that 'the most problematic of all areas' to identify about the biography of the early seventeenth-century Fellows 'was that of religious background', although he concludes that the College Fellows became increasingly Puritan.[26] But while Birken stresses that there were Puritans and Puritan sympathizers amongst the Fellows, he also shows the religious diversity of the members. There were Fellows of Calvinist upbringing who belonged to the two tolerated foreign churches: French Huguenots in Mayerne, Paul DeLaune (brother of Gideon), and Peter Chamberlen; and members of the Dutch church in the persons of George Ent, Baldwin Hamey, jr, Assuerus Regemorter, and John King.[27] The three Scots (John Craige, jr, Alexander Ramsey, and Sir Alexander Fraser) all served as royal physicians to Charles I, although Birken believes that Craige and Ramsey returned to Scotland upon the outbreak of the Bishops' War, suggesting that they had Presbyterian sympathies.[28] Of the Fellows from English families, those with Puritan sympathies had almost all been brought up in Cambridge. From the Puritanical Emmanuel College came Thomas Coxe, William Stanes and Lawrence Wright (as well as Paul DeLaune and Peter Chamberlen); from similarly Puritanical Christ's College came John Clarke, Jonathan Goddard, Othowell Meverall and Samuel Rand; Simeon Foxe and Edmund Wilson attended King's College; Thomas Sheafe went to Pembroke; Theodore Goulston to Peterhouse; Helkiah Crooke to St John's, Cambridge; and Edmund Trench to Sidney Sussex. Nathan Paget came from a clerical family that favoured Presbyterianism, and he was educated in Edinburgh and Leiden.[29] Sir William Paddy occasionally supported Puritans; he had been brought up in Oxford and Leiden, but was buried in the thoroughly Anglican chapel of St John's College, Oxford. Helkiah Crooke was one of the more openly agitator-Puritans and lived in the radical London parish of St Stephen's, in Coleman

Street,[30] and the College licentiate John Bastwick was famously tried for sedition before the Court of High Commission and had his ears cut off. But as far as one can tell from Birken's account and other sources, most of the Puritan Fellows of the College, like Simeon Foxe or Theodore Goulston, were moderate in their outlook rather than openly agitating for reform or publicly opposing the crypto-papist Laudianism of the 1630s. Others are hard to pin down at all. For instance, according to Anthony Wood, George Bate practised 'amongst precise and puritanical people [near Oxford], he being taken to be one of their number',[31] but he continued to practise there when Oxford was garrisoned by royalist troops in the mid-1640s; he later became one of Cromwell's physicians, and yet he wrote books after 1660 that make him seem a Presbyterian royalist.[32]

In addition to the Puritans and their fellow travellers, however, there remained a number of quite conservative Anglicans and crypto-Catholics. Sir Thomas Cadyman, who became a physician to Queen Henriette Maria, was clearly a Catholic. Francis Prujean, who had his own private chapel (like many of the recusant gentry and nobility) was 'widely suspected of Popery throughout his professional career', Birken notes, although he thinks it probable that Prujean was 'a rather typical representative of the high-church Anglicanism that was formed by Archbishop Laud' rather than a true Catholic.[33] The Italian-educated William Harvey's close association with Thomas Howard, the second Earl of Arundel, who married a Catholic and was for a time known as a member of that faith himself,[34] suggests that Harvey was another of the conservative Anglicans, if not a Catholic sympathizer. The same is also probable for Alexander Fraser, Sir Matthew Lister, Edmund Smith, Sir Maurice Williams and Thomas Winston, all of whom remained staunch royalists during the civil wars.

Given the state of the sources, then, it is impossible to formulate a statistical table on the religious orientation of the membership. All one can say with certainty is two things. First, the members held a variety of religious viewpoints, from outright Catholicism to Puritan agitation, although the bulk of the members ranged from conservative Anglicanism to Presbyterianism. None of the Fellows is so far known to have been a separatist or a radical sectary. Second, the religious views of the membership changed over time, with a younger generation of Cambridge-educated physicians gradually bringing a more pro-Calvinist perspective to the College. But in both these respects, the membership of the College remained representative of the learned members of English society, or perhaps even tended to the conservative side during the 1630s, when growing anti-Laudian sentiments amongst the clergy and others made many into Puritans.

The general intellectual conservatism of the Fellows had been incul-
cated during their long years of study and was reinforced by the requirement for admission that they possess an MD and have it incorporated at Oxford or Cambridge. Few of the professors at these two
institutions would have considered favourably the application for incor-
poration from religious enthusiasts. The College Fellows continued to
uphold the view that the best medical knowledge remained rooted in
philological scholarship and, increasingly, demonstrative sciences like
anatomy or chemistry, rather than upon the knowledge gained by personal intuition of the divine; they preferred a path to salvation marked
out by the scholar Jerome rather than the Christian fool, the religion of
Sir Thomas Browne's *Religio Medici* rather than George Fox's *Journal*.
Given this, it is easy to agree with Birken that '[t]he strongest bond
between all of [the Fellows] was the profession of medicine and the
upholding of medical standards in London', and that '[t]he College of
Physicians unfailingly reflected the political nation'.[35] While he went
too far in claiming that the College 'was staunchly Protestant in its
religion, Calvinist in its doctrine, [and] Parliamentarian in its politics',
he was correct in noting that by 1640 the College was 'mildly and
passively Puritan, ... above all an institution trying to establish its own
integrity while eschewing extremists in both religion and medicine'.[36]

Religion did come to the surface a bit more during the tumultuous
years of the civil wars and Protectorate, and following the Glorious
Revolution. But the religiously diverse, if generally conservative, membership of the College allowed it to 'bend with the prevailing winds'
during the political storms. The College quickly shifted from petitioning
the Privy Council to petitioning Parliament, for instance, when the
latter began to meet again in 1640 after an 11-year hiatus.[37] It changed
leadership, too, so that moderate Puritans like Meverall became President. Their political outlook, perhaps conditioned by their anti-Laudian
religion (although it is not certain there was a connection), caused the
new leadership to drop the College's attempts to police other medical
practitioners during most of the 1640s, which had so disturbed the City
of London, and to turn their corporation into something more like a
learned society than a closed and autocratic brotherhood. But the king's
execution in 1649 and the threat of semi-democratic republicanism
caused the College to take a much more conservative turn, as in the rest
of the nation. A kind of counter-revolution took place in 1650, when
Francis Prujean (who had been long suspected of recusancy) became
President; at the same time, the Catholic Sir Thomas Cadyman and the
conservative Anglican Edmund Smith were voted elects. Then again,
after the Major Generals had seized the reins of power in England in
1655, the College officers shifted again, with the Cromwellian Edward

Alston taking over the Presidency.[38] His group was able to use the levers
of central power to recoup much of the College's former authority to
regulate medicine in London, and he stayed on in his office during the
early years of the Restoration. Critics of the College such as Nicholas
Culpeper charged it with upholding Latinate and hence papist privilege.
Once again, however, the course of events suggests strongly that what
was crucial to the institutional authority of the College was not so
much the religious orientation of the College members as their corporation's ability to adapt to the political conditions of the moment and to
take advantage of strong central governments – whether the king's or
Cromwell's – who wanted help in bringing order to the Commonwealth.[39]

Following the Restoration, the College officers worked closely with
Lord Chancellor Clarendon to have their legal powers over London
medicine restored to the prerevolutionary status quo. But Clarendon
depended upon the Cavalier Parliament, and the College had never
found it as easy to get its way in Parliament as in the councils of the
Crown. Despite high hopes, they found themselves unable to overcome
the opposition mounted to the College in Parliament by the Society of
Apothecaries and the Barber-Surgeon's Company. The establishment
and growth of the Royal Society also caused concern, as it became a
rival learned society, seeming to support the cause of unlearned empirics,
whose knowledge of treatments and promotion of experimental medicine appeared to fit into the programme of the new philosophy. Most
importantly of all, a rival medical corporation, the Society of Chemical
Physicians, almost came into being through the support of people at
court. With the plague of 1665, and the fire of 1666 coming on top of
these intellectual and institutional challenges, the College remained a
very weak public authority until the late 1670s.

Internally, during the early Restoration the College remained diverse
but relatively conservative in religious outlook. Many of its rivals were
more intellectually aggressive and religiously extreme. But one must be
careful about stressing the religious affiliations of the parties to the
medical disputes too firmly. For instance, while some of the members of
the Society of Chemical Physicians indeed came from the radical and
Puritan side of the revolution (such as Marchamont Nedham), others
came from the royalist but Catholic camp (such as Thomas O'Dowde),
and still other ex-royalists amongst the chemists apparently happily
conformed to the Restoration church (like George Thomson).[40]

The language of the medical disputes did, however, continue to be
framed in part in religiously charged language. Nedham, the former
propagandist for Cromwell, returned from a brief exile to take up both
chemical medicine and hounding the College as a benighted, Latinate,

and Jesuitical body of old-fashioned Galenists – and Nedham's voice was joined by those of Thomson and O'Dowde. Since the College could not counter-attack using their police powers because of their juridical weakness, their only reply was to claim to be excellent chemists themselves as well as precise anatomists, following a safer, more temperate, judicious and anti-fanatical medicine. In this very hot public medical warfare of the later 1660s and early 1670s, some began to associate the new philosophy itself with threats to the fragile new order of the Restoration. Some of the Anglican intellectuals and bishops, like some in the College, began to attack the Royal Society as a threat to the textual learning from which right reason (as they defined it) flowed. One of the public defenders of the College against the new society, Henry Stubbe, made a loud case for seeing the new philosophy as a threat to Crown, Church, and College. Yet, the Royal Society itself contained a large number of physicians (as well as clerics) who considered themselves good members of the Church and State.[41]

In the roiling disputes from 1665 to 1675, great intellectual and political stakes were wagered, and the wagers were often cloaked in religious language. Indeed, the question of whether intuition and experience or study was the best route to knowledge did reflect differences of outlook between Protestant sectarians and conservative Anglicans. But given the diverse political and religious affiliations of the participants in the various disputes over medical knowledge, religious orientation seems to have been at the bottom of these arguments only some of the time rather than always. The main question at stake for the physicians was 'What kind of medical knowledge is best, and who is to be trusted with it?' In arguing this question, the members of the College themselves were divided. But the institution's leaders generally continued to hold that study at Oxford or Cambridge established the best foundations for medical learning and gave the graduate the kind of disciplined character that could be trusted.

The general association between officers of the College and the moderate to conservative Anglican establishment therefore seems to have been forged in the furnace of English political life, in which the Crown, Church, and College counted on each other to maintain a loyal good order in the kingdom. Over time, as the Restoration settlement took firm hold and Charles II's government began to depend less on income from parliamentary grants (and to meddle less in foreign wars), the College found support for taking legal actions against non-members once again, gradually beginning to regain its public authority in the mid- to late-1670s.[42]

Internally, the Restoration College had continued to have a solid core of Anglican members with a smattering of both Catholics and dissenters. Its reputation for religious conservatism brought it suspicious official inquiries during the Popish Plot scares of the late 1670s. The House of Lords sent it (and the College of Heralds and the Doctors' Commons) an official letter ordering it to expel any who did not attend church and receive the authorized sacrament or take the Oaths of Supremacy and Obedience. John Betts and Thomas Short were singled out and ordered by the officers of the College to take the oaths at the next meeting of the College; but at that meeting, too few Fellows attended to make up a quorum, and so Betts and Short escaped their dilemma.[43] At the same time, however, the College continued to include Protestant dissenters amongst its Fellows such as Edward Hulse and Richard Morton (the first of whose Leiden MD had been incorporated at Oxford in 1670 at the request of the visiting Prince of Orange, and the second of whom had been given an MD from Oxford outright at the prince's request), and Richard Lower, who lost a good deal of his court clientele when he publicly engaged in the Catholic-hunting of the plot's aftermath. Others of a non-Anglican persuasion, even those with medical doctorates, had to content themselves with a place amongst the ranks of the licentiates or Honorary Fellows (a category created in 1664 when the Puritan-sympathizer Alston was President). For instance, the distinguished but Puritan Thomas Sydenham remained a licentiate throughout his life;[44] and many other English nonconformists, such as Isaac Chauncey (the eldest son of Charles Chauncey, President of Harvard College) and Praise Watson, and foreigners – such as the Dutch Calvinist Joannes Groenevelt, the French Huguenot Philip Guide, and the Italian Catholic Henry Morelli – stood amongst the licentiates. In 1680, a large number of members of generally nonconformist outlook were added to the role of Honorary Fellows, such as Nehemiah Grew, Henry Sampson and Thomas Gibson.

The pattern of general conformity to the religio-political establishment amongst the Fellows themselves, however, was not broken until the 1680s, and then because the Crown itself openly began to favour Catholics and dissenters. From 1682 onwards, the government of the crypto-Catholic monarch Charles II began to strike back at the defenders of the *status quo*. As it revoked and rewrote the charter of the City of London and then other corporations, people loyal to the Crown were inserted into positions of leadership in institution after institution. In corporations like the College, which avoided the first round of revocations, those with close ties to the court (such as the king's surgeon John Knight) and those with a clear sense that the moment was right for restoring the College's authority over all the medical practitioners of London (such as Charles Goodall) came to the fore.

When James II ascended to the throne in 1685, his government established an even closer political and legal alliance with the College, supporting and extending its regulatory powers in a new charter, granted in 1687. The new charter not only gave the College full police powers over medicine in London, it added many new Fellows to the College, some of whom were Catholics like the king, while others were nonconformists (a group that the king was cultivating in his attempts to trim the power of the established church). Some members of both groups had earlier been made licentiates or Honorary Fellows. Among the new Catholic Fellows were Robert Gray (Honorary Fellow, 1664), Sir William Waldegrave (Honorary Fellow, 1664), Charles Conquest, John Elliott and Fernando Mendez (physician to the queen dowager Catherine of Portugal); amongst the nonconformists were Richard Griffith (Honorary Fellow, 1664), Christopher Love Morley (Honorary Fellow, 1680), and Joseph Maucleer and Thomas Botterell (both Huguenot refugees). A few of the old Fellows and Honorary Fellows were omitted, probably because they were seen as enemies of James II's government.[45] These changes under James II led to a revivified as well as larger College.[46]

But the Glorious Revolution of 1688–89 threw all into confusion. Two of the Catholic Fellows introduced by James's charter, John Elliott and Robert Gray, were caught circulating a declaration of the new 'Pretender', James Stuart. There were also important legal questions about whether the College's new charter – unlike that of other remodelled corporations – ought to continue in effect. During the political manoeuvrings in the House of Lords, the Lords asked that all the Fellows be willing to take the sacraments according to the Church of England. The College's policy on this was to report the names of the seven Catholic Fellows to the authorities, but to avoid the issue of Protestant nonconformists. The College Fellows also quickly learnt that the court of the new monarchs, and then after Mary's death that of William, would not offer them the firm political and juridical support that earlier Stuart governments had. The College was therefore forced back on to its own devices to control medicine in London, which increasingly depended upon convincing Parliament and the public that the physicians were guardians of the general interest. In this, they ultimately failed.[47]

Part of the reason for the declining authority of the College lay in its bitter internal divisions, political divisions in which religious affiliation played a role, although once again, seldom the leading part. In the last decade of the century, there were three disputes within the College which led to vehement and bitter division: the dispute about the legality of the charter of James II; the setting up of a public dispensary to counter-attack the growing power of the Society of Apothecaries; and the attempt to discipline the licentiates that led to the malpractice trial against Joannes Groenevelt and a revision of the statutes governing the members of the College. In each of these disputes, the majority of Fellows faced a more or less organized opposition from within, which can be named.

In the controversy about the charter, a bill was entered into the House of Lords to retain the new charter of James II and the membership named therein. Of the nine people named as having helped to prepare the bill,[48] all but two (Thomas Millington and John Bateman) had not been made members of the College by virtue of the new charter. As would be expected from the heterodoxy of the new members named in James's charter, the group included at least two religious dissenters (Edward Hulse and Richard Blackmore), although as far as one can tell, most were mainstream Anglicans. They also had a slightly higher tendency to have taken their degrees abroad (William Stokeham and Blackmore, Padua; Richard Griffith, Leiden or Caen; Hulse, Leiden) than at Oxford (Millington and Bateman) or Cambridge (Walter Needham). (Francis Bernard incorporated his MD from the Archbishop of Canterbury at Cambridge, and it is not certain where Richard Blackburne took his degree.) The bill of the College was, however, objected to by a petition of the 'President and the ancient Fellows of the College'. According to the petition against the 'new College' (as they called it), the members introduced by James II included some who 'are known to be Papists' as well as older members who acted to surrender the charter so that it could be remade by James's government. The 12 who signed the petition against the bill continuing the new charter were: President George Rogers, John Lawson, Humphrey Brooke, Richard Torlesse, Josiah Clerk, Richard Field, Richard Morton, Edward Browne, Edward Tyson, John Atfield, John Downes and Thomas Alvey.[49] This group included both solid Anglicans and at least one dissenter (Morton), although – as the words indicated – no Catholics. Four in the group had taken their medical doctorates at Oxford (Brooke, Torlesse, Browne, and Alvey) while another (Morton) had had his incorporated there upon the nomination of the Prince of Orange; three had their doctorates from Cambridge (Clerk, Field, Tyson); two had Padua diplomas (Rogers and Lawson); one had graduated from Caen (Atfield); and one from Leiden (Downes). All had been made Fellows of the College before James's charter – almost all during the years from 1673 to 1675 – except for Field, who had been made a Candidate in 1685 and so would have moved on to the fellowship in the ordinary way had he not been named to it by the 1687 charter. In other words, this group of objectors seems to have wanted to preserve the College as a small, medically learned, and religiously orthodox (if slightly dissenting) body;

those who wanted to preserve the membership named in James's charter wanted the College to be larger, and perhaps less authoritarian and less religiously conservative. But clearly the most important dividing line ran between new members and a group of old members who objected to the previous regime's high-handed tampering with the charter and Fellowship.[50]

When it came to the second main controversy, during the bitter controversies of the mid-1690s over whether the College should establish a public dispensary to attack the Society of Apothecaries, most of the Fellows followed the officers of the College in favouring its establishment.[51] But 13 appear several times in the College's Annals as being opposed to the dispensary: Edward Baynard, Richard Blackmore, William Gould, Francis Bernard, William Gibbons, Edward Tyson, Robert Pitt, George How, Tancred Robinson, Peter Gelsthorpe, Hugh Chamberlen, William Cole and Salisbury Cade. A subgroup of these opposed the plans of the officers so strongly that in January 1697 they petitioned for a 'visitation' of the College: Clerk, Stokeham, Bernard, Pitt, How, Blackmore and Gibbons. Tyson had become a Fellow in 1680 and had opposed the new charter; Baynard and How had been made Fellows by virtue of that charter; and the rest had become Fellows from 1692 to 1694. Several had Oxford medical doctorates (Gould, Gibbons, Cole and Cade), a couple of others Cambridge doctorates (Robinson and Chamberlen); the rest had various educational backgrounds of a high quality. Again, as far as one can tell their religious orientation ranged from pro-dissent (Baynard and Blackmore) to conservative Anglican (Tyson). Figuring out their political affiliation is at least as difficult, but they included at least two Tories (Bernard and Pitt) and two strong supporters of William's government (Baynard and Blackmore, although as dissenters they were not Whigs). What seems to have divided this group from the rest of the College was first and foremost their close associations with members of the Society of Apothecaries or Barber-Surgeon's Company, which were threatened by the new policies of the College officers. Tyson lectured to the Surgeon's Company, Bernard's brother was a surgeon, Chamberlen practised man-midwifery and surgery, and Bernard and Gibbons were closely associated with the apothecaries. In general, then, this controversy again pitted a group which wanted to restrict the practice of physic to learned physicians (the College majority) against a group of physicians who worked much more closely with others and respected their medical abilities.

Finally, when it came to fighting the attempts of the officers to discipline the members of the College, including the licentiates, more or less the same group which opposed the dispensary stood out. The Fellows who openly supported licentiate Joannes Groenevelt in his struggles against the officers of the College were Tyson, Blackmore, Bernard and Gibbons.[52] Those who signed the 'Petition of Grievances' against the new statutes in 1702 were: Tyson, How, Blackmore, Robinson, Gibbons, Gelsthorpe, Chamberlen, Cole and Cade, plus Frederick Slare (Oxford MD and Fellow of 1685), William Dawes (Leiden and Cambridge MDs, and Fellow of 1685), and Simon Welman and Richard Carr (both Cambridge MDs, and Fellows by virtue of James's charter).[53] Once again, the dividing line in the College during these disputes seems to have been the question of what kind of medical learning would be used as the foundation for regulating medicine in London (if it were to be regulated at all), rather than religion or even the institution in which a physician had received his education.

Reviewing the first two centuries of the College's life, one is left with the distinct impression that its Fellows reflected the religious views of learned English people generally. As the realm shifted from Catholicism to the Anglicanism of the Elizabethan settlement, the College shifted, too. Perhaps it shifted more slowly than other learned groups, but that can only be ascertained by a close comparison with the membership of the colleges of Oxford and Cambridge, the College of Heralds and the Inns of Court. At the moment, there is no reason to think that the College of Physicians' membership was especially slow or quick to shift from Catholicism to Anglicanism in comparison to these other groups. Additionally, while the faith of the Fellows undoubtedly had important repercussions in their private lives, the College itself as a corporate body did not represent any particular point of view. It included Fellows of diverse convictions, although as learned men they tended to believe in the power of reason and education over intuition and grace alone, making them generally conservative in outlook. In their own lives, the religious affiliations of the Fellows helped to shape their networks of friendships and patients. But from the point of view of the institution, the diversity of religion amongst the Fellows was advantageous mainly for creating the possibility of adaptability to the shifting political and legal structures on which the College depended for its very existence.

Thus, from its beginnings, reinforced during Caius's Presidency, the College was rooted in a close association between its own public authority and the monarchy's concern for supporting learned bodies who would help it govern the commonwealth. In this sense, the College's political and intellectual conservatism connected it to both Renaissance humanism and the king-and-bishop constitution of the Tudor and Stuart monarchies. As the bishops of the English medical community, the Fellows of the College generally helped the Crown to police the streets of London and to uphold the dignity and authority of the studious, who not only founded their practice on the knowledge so gained but became the kind of self-disciplined and grave men who could be 'trusted with anything', in the words of Chief Justice Walmesley.[54] Unfortunately for the College, the failure of the Stuarts to keep king and Church together undid the learned commonwealth that the humanist physicians desired. By the end of the seventeenth century, the men of wit and sensibility were taking over from the dignified men of Latin *gravitas*. In the eighteenth century, they would create their own hierarchies based on new forms of learning and social authority. But the College physicians, like their brethren the lords of the Church, were losing their juridical power over the lives of ordinary people. In this way, at least, the fate of the College had become wrapped up with the fate of the English Church and State.

Notes

1. 'An Acte Conc[er]ning Phisicons', 14 and 15 Hen.VIII.c.5, punctuation added.
2. George N. Clark, *A History of the Royal College of Physicians of London*, 2 vols, Oxford, Clarendon Press, 1964–66, vol. 1, pp. 54–66; Charles Webster, 'Thomas Linacre and the Foundation of the College of Physicians', in F. Maddison, M. Pelling and Charles Webster (eds), *Essays on the Life and Work of Thomas Linacre, c. 1460–1524*, Oxford, Clarendon Press, 1977, pp. 198–222; and Gweneth Whitteridge, 'Some Italian Precursors of the Royal College of Physicians', *Journal of the Royal College of Physicians, London*, 12 (1977), 67–80.
3. For more, see Paul Slack, 'Books of Orders: The Making of English Social Policy, 1577–1631', *Transactions of the Royal Historical Society*, S.5, 30 (1980), 1–22; P. Slack, *The Impact of Plague in Tudor and Stuart England*, London: Routledge and Kegan Paul, 1985; P. Slack, 'Dearth and Social Policy in Early Modern England', *Social History of Medicine*, 5 (1992), 1–17; H.J. Cook, 'Policing the Health of London: The College of Physicians and the Early Stuart Monarchy', *Social History of Medicine*, 2 (1989), 1–33.
4. See Clark, *History*, vol. 1, pp. 37–53; Madison, Pelling and Webster, *Essays on the Life and Work of Thomas Linacre*.
5. Annals of the Royal College of Physicians, vol. 1. The Annals really begin with Caius's election to the Presidency of the College in 1555, but he summarized the earlier records as he saw fit on fols 2b–7a. My thanks to the members of the Royal College of Physicians for permission to quote from their records.
6. Act 'Concerning Phisicians', 32 Hen.VIII.c.40.
7. Annals, vol. 1, fol. 4a. 'Empiric' is best defined as a medical practitioner who belonged to no medical corporation and who sought monetary payment for his or her services.
8. 1 Mariae, St. 2. c.9; the acknowledgement of the efforts of the three is Caius's, Annals, vol. 1, fol. 7a. The coercive power of the College was such during the years after this act that in 1570 the College discovered

that a Fellow, Dr George Walker, had accrued over 200 silver marks from empirics through extortion, threatening to bring them to the attention of the College and then illicitly selling them the authority to practise in London. He was fined 40 shillings by the Censors: Annals, vol. I, fols 31a, 31b.

9.   Annals, vol. 1, fols 7b–20a.
10. Annals, vol. 1, fols 20b–21a.
11. Clark, *History*, vol. 1, pp. 93–4; for more general information on Caius's Presidency, see vol. 1, pp. 107–24.
12. For this and other otherwise undocumented biographical information in what follows, see W.R. Munk, *The Roll of the Royal College of Physicians*, 2 vols, London, Longman, Green, Longman, and Roberts, 1861.
13. Annals, vol. 1, fol. 33b.
14. I have found no contemporary account of the privilege; it is only mentioned many years later, in February 1626/7, when Drs Ridgley and Grent were assigned to wait on Sir Theodore de Mayerne to ask him if he would try to get Lord Conway to grant the College a privilege like Walsingham had given the College in 1588, at a time when Conway was trying to get empirics released by the College: Annals, vol. 3, fol. 70a. Walsingham had been amongst those trying to get imprisoned empirics released in 1588: Annals, vol. 2, fol. 44a.
15. Harold J. Cook, '"Against Common Right and Reason": The College of Physicians Against Dr. Thomas Bonham', *American Journal of Legal History*, 29 (1985), 301–22.
16. Annals, vol.2, fol. 189a.
17. Quoted from Edward Chaney, 'Quo vadis? Travel as Education and the Impact of Italy in the Sixteenth Century', in Peter Cunningham and Colin Brock (eds), *International Currents in Educational Ideas and Practices*, Evington, History of Education Society, 1988, pp. 16–17, quotations from p. 16.
18. William J. Birken, 'The Fellows of the Royal College of Physicians of London, 1603–1643: A Social Study', PhD. dissertation, University of North Carolina, 1977, pp. 306, 328–30.
19. Quoted from the manuscript *Annals of the Royal College of Physicians*, vol. 3, 4b, in Cook, 'Against Common Right and Reason', p. 313. See this article for more on Bonham.
20. 'College of Physicians's Case', 2 Brownl. and Golds., 262, *The English Reports*, Edinburgh and London, 175 vols, 1900–1932.
21. For more, see Cook, 'Policing the Health of London', pp. 9–11. I see little evidence of Birken's 'divorce between Court and College' after about 1620, although indeed from then on the Presidents of the College tended not to be royal physicians as well: Birken, 'Fellows', 302–3. See also Clark, *History*, vol. 1, pp. 182–258.
22. For more, see Cook, 'Policing the Health of London', pp. 12–27.
23. Ole Grell, 'Conflicting Duties: Plague and the Obligations of Early Modern Physicians Towards Patients and Commonwealth in England and The Netherlands', in Andrew Wear, Johanna Geyer-Kordesch and Roger French (eds), *Doctors and Ethics: The Earlier Historical Setting of Professional Ethics*, special issue of *Clio Medica*, 1993, p.146.
24. Ibid., p. 142.
25. Fritz Caspari, *Humanism and the Social Order in Tudor England*, Chi-

cago, University of Chicago Press, 1954; A. Ferguson, *The Articulate Citizen in the English Renaissance*, Raleigh, Duke University Press, 1965; Hans Baron, *The Crisis of the Early Italian Renaissance: Civic Humanism and Republican Liberty in an Age of Classicism and Tyranny*, 2nd edn, Princeton, Princeton University Press, 1966; J.G.A. Pocock, *The Machiavellian Moment: Florentine Political Thought and the Atlantic Republican Tradition*, (Princeton, Princeton University Press, 1975; Quentin Skinner, *The Foundations of Modern Political Thought, Vol. II: The Age of Reformation*, Cambridge, Cambridge University Press, 1978; Gerhard Oestreich (ed.), *Neostoicism and the Early Modern State*, trans. Brigitta Oestreich, H.G. Koenigsberger and David McLintock, Cambridge, Cambridge University Press, 1982.

26. Birken, 'Fellows', p. 15.
27. William Birken, 'Dr. John King (1614–1681) and Dr. Assuerus Regimorter (1615–1650)', *Medical History*, 20 (1976), 276–95.
28. Birken, 'Fellows', p. 314.
29. For a chart of the educational upbringing of the Fellows, see ibid., pp. 401–6.
30. Ibid., p. 333.
31. Quoted in Munk, *Roll*, p. 211.
32. Birken, 'Fellows', pp. 308–9, 310.
33. Ibid., pp. 324, 326–7.
34. Chaney, 'Quo vadis?', p. 17.
35. Birken, 'Fellows', pp. 335, 317.
36. Ibid., pp. 335–6.
37. I disagree with Birken's thesis that the College had become an inherently Puritan and parliamentary institution by 1640: see below, note 39; Lindsay Sharp, 'The Royal College of Physicians and Interregnum Politics', *Medical History*, 19 (1975), 107–28; and Clark, *History*, vol. 1, pp. 273–4.
38. William J. Birken, 'The Puritan Connexions of Sir Edward Alston, President of the Royal College of Physicians 1655–1666,' *Medical History*, 18 (1974), 370–4.
39. See Cook, 'Policing the Health of London', pp. 27–30; and H.J. Cook, *The Decline of the Old Medical Regime in Stuart London*, Ithaca, Cornell University Press, 1986, pp. 102–32.
40. H.J. Cook, 'The Society of Chemical Physicians, The New Philosophy, and the Restoration Court', *Bulletin of the History of Medicine*, 61 (1987), 61–77.
41. Cook, *Decline*, pp. 133–82; H.J. Cook, 'The New Philosophy and Medicine in Seventeenth-Century England', in David Lindberg and Robert Westman (eds), *Reappraisals of the Scientific Revolution*, Cambridge, Cambridge University Press, 1990, pp. 397–436; H.J. Cook, 'Physicians and the New Philosophy: Henry Stubbe and the Virtuosi-Physicians', in Roger French and Andrew Wear (eds), *The Medical Revolution of the Seventeenth Century*, Cambridge, Cambridge University Press, 1989, pp. 246–71; H.J. Cook, 'The Society of Chemical Physicians, the New Philosophy, and the Restoration Court', *Bulletin of the History of Medicine*, 61 (1987), 61–77.
42. Cook, *Decline*, pp. 183–92.
43. Ibid., pp. 192–3.
44. For a view of Sydenham as a radical, see Andrew Cunningham, 'Thomas

Sydenham: Epidemics, Experiment and the "Good Old Cause"', in French and Wear (eds), *The Medical Revolution*, pp. 164–90.

45. Clark, *History*, p. 355.
46. Cook, *Decline*, pp. 202–9; Clark, *History*, vol. 1, pp. 355–62.
47. H.J. Cook, 'Living in Revolutionary Times: Medical Change Under William and Mary', in Bruce T. Moran (ed.), *Patronage and Institutions: Science, Technology and Medicine at the European Court, 1500–1750*, Woodbridge, Boydell, 1991, pp. 111–35.
48. Annals, vol. 5, fol. 104a.
49. 'Proposed Act of 1689', *House of Lords Journals*, vol. 14, p. 241.
50. See Cook, *Decline*, pp. 211–40, especially p. 239.
51. On the controversies over the dispensary, see Cook, *Decline*, pp. 222–53; H.J. Cook, 'The Rose Case Reconsidered: Physic and the Law in Augustan England', *Journal of the History of Medicine*, 45 (1990), 527–55; Albert Rosenberg, 'The London Dispensary for the Sick-poor', *Journal of the History of Medicine*, 14 (1959), 41–56.
52. On Groenevelt's case, see H.J. Cook, *Trials of an Ordinary Doctor: Joannes Groenevelt in Seventeenth-Century London*, Baltimore, Johns Hopkins University Press, 1994, pp. 1–23, 136–57.
53. Annals, vol. 7, fol. 198.
54. H.J. Cook, 'Good Advice and Little Medicine: The Professional Authority of Early Modern English Physicians', *Journal of British Studies*, 33 (1994), 1–31.

CHAPTER FIVE

Anatomist Atheist? The 'Hylozoistic' Foundations of Francis Glisson's Anatomical Research

Guido Giglioni

Cogitur intellectus anatomicum agere ...
(F. Glisson, MS Sloane 3314, fol. 101)

Francis Glisson, the physician remembered above all for his excellent description of the liver and for his theory of tissue irritability, also wrote a quickly forgotten treatise on the living nature of substance (*biusia*).[1] While mechanical philosophers were turning life into a meaningless and merely conventional entity, he tried to give a philosophical definition of life, which could mirror on a speculative plane what he was discovering in his anatomo-physiological work. From a theological point of view, Glisson's theory of *biusia* represented one of the most audacious attempts to secularize the notion of life. It goes without saying that to some contemporaries his philosophical opinions smacked of heresy. Ralph Cudworth, the first to foresee the possibility of accusations of metaphysical, religious and political subversion in Glisson's conception of life, gave the name *hylozoism* to the new atheistic threat which proclaimed the living and perceptive nature of matter.[2]

Anatomy and philosophy of life

In early modern philosophy and bio-medical thought the *organic/inorganic* dichotomy maintains its original Aristotelian meaning, which is different from what we mean now with the same words. 'Inorganic' denotes the undifferentiated state of matter; 'organic' refers to the parts of matter with an identifiable structure. According to Aristotle, the soul (and consequently life) can belong only to an organic body, that is, a body endowed with organs. In Glisson's *De Natura Substantiae Energetica* (*On the Energetic Nature of Substance*) this dichotomy undergoes a transformation: 'inorganic' means the original active (naturally perceptive and appetitive) state of prime matter; 'organic' means the 'modes' emerging from matter.

The origins of this shift can be traced back to Harvey's *De Generatione Animalium* (*On the Generation of Animals*), where blood, as self-active matter, is said not to differ from the soul and to be 'the substance whose act is the soul or the life'.[3] The aim of Harvey's endeavour is to separate the soul as an animating principle from its necessary reference to an organic body: everthing, even the elements, can be said to be animated,[4] and it is the blood that is the most animated, traditionally regarded only as a similary part of the body. This is more apparent in the fifty-seventh *Exercitatio*, where Harvey takes into account 'certain paradoxes and problems' associated with the development of the parts of the embryo. Among these, some question the traditional assumption that the organic parts alone can be alive and endowed with sensibility: the first phases of the development of the foetus witness that 'the calidum innatum and the vegetative soul of the chick are in existence before the chick itself'; embryological observations also show the paradoxical facts that 'the blood is produced, and moves to and fro, and is imbued with vital spirits, before any sanguiferous or locomotive organs are in existence'; that 'sensation and motion belong to the foetus before the brain is formed'; that 'the body is nourished and increases before the organs appropriated to digestion, viz. the stomach and abdominal viscera, are formed'.[5] There is therefore ample experimental evidence to show that an original, vital and vegetative activity precedes the rising of the soul, understood in Aristotelian terms as the act of an organic body; that a kind of perception different from brain sensation is diffused all over the body; and, finally, that a kind of living and perceptive matter (*calidum innatum* and *humidum primigenium*) is in some ways experimentally and theoretically justified. The primacy of the vegetative soul indicates that life, being the ultimate principle of organization, is such an original and immanent process as to precede (*tempore et natura*) any definite and organized structure and to allude to something divine in nature – *Deus sive natura*.[6]

In the *Prolegomena ad Rem Anatomicam* which preface *Anatomia Hepatis* (1654), Glisson is still following the traditional division of the solid bodily parts into *similary/dissimilary* and *organic/inorganic*, regarding them, in a way that is typical of Glisson's epistemological procedure, as different ways of considering one and the same thing: with respect to matter, parts are said to be similarly and dissimilary, and with respect to form, they are said to be organic and inorganic. A similary part is, according to Aristotle's definition (*Historia Animalium*, vol. I, p. 1), 'such as may be divided into lesser parts of like nature with itself';[7] an organic part, as a form, 'is fitted or made serviceable for some agent to work by'.[8] Consequently *inorganic* means the absence of form ('inorganical is as much as informis: without form'): but 'there is no part in man's body absolutely without form, neither can *informis* and *vitalis* consist together in the same solid part'.[9] Therefore no life can be given without form. Everything in the body is organic, inorganic being the same as formless.

The situation changes markedly with *De Natura Substantiae Energetica* (1672): 'We attribute the life of nature to all bodies without distinction and we deduce the difference of plants and animals from the other bodies, not from that principle, but from the organization, according to Aristotle, and from duplicated life, *insita* et *influens*, according to Neotericks.'[10] The main aim of the treatise is to demonstrate the universal life of nature. Each being is alive, emerging from primeval life (*vita primaeva sive inchoata*) in the act of modifying itself in an endless variety of forms.[11] The distinction betweeen *similary* and *organic* does not have to do with life any more. *Organic* does not discriminate what is alive from what is not. It means a mere degree in the self-developing activity of life, corresponding to plants and animals. As we have seen in Harvey, what is organic is not the counterpart of the soul any more: all bodies, even those devoid of organization, 'enjoy natural and inorganic life alone'.[12] To indicate the non-organic but living character of matter, Glisson uses the Baconian term *schematismus*:

> The division into similarly and organic parts regards above all the parts of the animals and the plants; the former of which are the matter making up the organs and the latter the organs of life. But here we are dividing rather the accidental forms pertaining to the inanimate beings; and we are investigating certain simple differences in shape, arising from the position of the particles amongst themselves, but in no way the shape formed for the use of the soul. The organic forms in their true sense enjoy twofold life, natural and *influens*: but the shaping process (*figuratio*), that we call schematism, enjoys simple life alone; or if it is observed in animated beings, it is not considered with respect to the soul or its own organization.[13]

So section 13 of chapter 29 ('*Schematismum naturae vitam monstrare*', 'That the schematism shows the life of nature') outlines a sort of 'sub-organic' anatomy, concerning the processes of 'simple figuration'. Every natural body experiences an elemental plastic force through which it receives its own due schematism – sublime natural art at work in the minutest particles of matter, constructing fibrous, striated, ramified and endless other structures. The shape is always the result of a shaping movement. It is the realization of a seminal idea, not a primary, objective quality of being; nor does it depend on an external cause or a fortuitous disposition of particles: 'nature acts from within secretly (*clanculum*) and, after attaining the idea of the species to be formed, starts working on the texture of matter in accordance with the exemplar and, if it is not hindered, reaches the specific similtude of the intended (*intentae*) thing'.[14]

The philosophical investigation of the life of nature leads Glisson to rethink his own conception of anatomy, or at least to modify significantly his original plan. From this point of view, the preface (*Epistola lectori*) to his last work *De Ventriculo et Intestinis* (1677) is very enlightening. We are given some relevant news about the origin of the treatise: that it had been almost finished 15 years before (Glisson was writing in 1676), but that it had been interrupted because 'it presupposed in many places (even though it often also demonstrated) the existence of a general natural perception, about which nothing had been written'; that, consequently, to write the 'prodrome' on the life of nature became necessary; that, finally, once having come back to the previous treatise, 'many things' are explained 'in a slightly different way and even more fully than before', 'few things' are changed, but 'a great many' are added overall. So that at last the treatise can be regarded as a 'new work'.[15] We know where to find the turning-point: the anatomy of the irritable fibres calls for the primitive and undifferentiated impetus towards shaping (*figuratio*) – namely, natural perception, acting secretly and unconsciously in every piece of matter. Natural perception is not therefore a result of the desire for novelty on Glisson's part, but is the most appropriate natural cause. 'It is more than apparent that this happens naturally and regularly, and that there is nothing miraculous (*Evidentissimum, hoc naturaliter et familiariter fieri, nihilque subesse miraculi*)'. It is true that the tract *De Partibus Continentibus* comes before and we can presume that this part of the treatise remained almost unchanged even after the inception of the new philosophical viewpoint. After all, the theory of *biusia* and natural perception concerns first the inorganic state of matter (with the consequent theological implications that drove Glisson to justify the use of natural perception in the preface) and only secondly the organs of the body. So the anatomical *administratio* can be said to be concerned more with the organic than with the similar parts, which tend to escape anatomical scrutiny. 'Therefore', Glisson declares in a rather traditional manner, 'we regard above all here the human body as an organ, a universal organ, adequately suited to all the soul's faculties'. Considered in the light of the most general bodily divisions, the human body is like a 'large machine', capable of various movements and uses. A mechanical approach is not excluded ('*corpus humanum* [...] *mechanice potissimum hic consideramus*'),[16] nor is it in contrast with the functions of the soul.

But the 'sub-organic' anatomy of the similarly parts is considered, too.[17] And the reason is now apparent. Between *Anatomia Hepatis* and *De Ventriculo* the philosophical interlude of *De Natura Substantiae*

Energetica has intervened. During the 20 years between the two strictly anatomical works Glisson had been thoroughly analysing the concept of life. Harvey's epigenesis on the one hand, and Suarez's theory of individual substance, Campanella's philosophy of nature and Bacon's concept of matter on the other, have helped in making possible an anatomy of the schematism underlying the anatomy of the organ. Glisson's philosophy is a medical philosophy, not only in the sense that it is a reflection arising from his professional activity, but also as an expression of a characteristically medical legacy. Glisson's hylozoism is much indebted to Hippocrates, Jan Baptista van Helmont and Harvey, to quote only the main sources.[18] Regarded as an energetical principle, substance is a dynamic system implying perception, appetite and movement. From this point of view, movement is an essential faculty, through which matter gives itself its own form. It is the immanent act of a natural power (*'constitutio intrinsece qualificans'*),[19] aiming at determining within definite 'limits' (*'terminus motus'*) an otherwise undetermined substratum. The limits of such original motions map the first veins of matter: thickness, thinness, heaviness, lightness, solidity, fluidity ... At a higher degree, it is the form itself that emerges, from the similary and seminal forms to the more and more elaborate organic structures involving the action of a plastic force.[20] Considered in the light of a theory of matter, *De Natura Substantiae Energetica* outlines the primitive structure of matter with its innumerable motions and forms.

Glisson's theory of substance

The basic principle of Glisson's metaphysics is the mutual convertibility of substance and activity. What subsists by itself, acts by itself. Every substance, as a substance, is the real subject of its actions, and any action witnesses to the substratum where it springs from. This is the real meaning of the scholastic axiom – *'Actiones sunt suppositorum* (actions pertain to individual substances)'* – as Glisson interprets it. We could even say that Glisson's whole metaphysics is an original rereading of this scholastic axiom.[21]

According to a statement attributed to Spinoza, scholastic philosophy started from creatures, Descartes from thought, Spinoza himself directly from God.[22] Taking this testimony as a rough description of the main streams in modern philosophy, we can consider Glisson's attempt as being included in the first category. Like scholastic philosophers, Glisson holds that metaphysics is the science of being *qua* being and that, therefore, neither God nor human thought can be the appropriate start-

ing-point. The original aspect in Glisson is that the scholastic framework conveys new contents.

Glisson's theory of substance can be seen as a *monistic* view as
regards the general nature of substance, and a *pluralistic* view as regards the number of existing substances. In this respect he follows
Aristotle's distinction between primary and secondary substances. Nevertheless the picture is complicated by the fact that Glisson distinguishes
different kinds of substances: spiritual substances (angels, demons and
rational souls) and material substances (matter).[23] They all are simple,
so that we can conclude that in the sublunar world there are a great
many individual substances displaying a common living and perceptive
nature.[24]

As far as the general nature of substance is concerned, Glisson regards substance as an undifferentiated entity that can appear to our
intellect as either *being* or *energy*. In its ultimate essence it is a principle
of movement (*nisus* or *conatus*), but as such it cannot be really represented by any human concepts. These can give us only an inadequate
image of it. What is important to note is the fact that *being* and *energy*,
'*subsistentia*' and '*natura*' arise from the same root.[25] Cudworth fully
realized that this conception of substance could be taken as a paradig-
matic instance of hylozoistic atheism.[26] Matter is inherently endowed
with life because the root of being is the original unity of *esse* and
operari. *Vita primaeva* is simply the other side of *materia prima*. Unlike
mechanical philosophies which start from the assumption that matter
and thought are really distinct attributes of being (and from this point
of view Descartes's philosophy can be considered as a paradigm),
hylozoism postulates the original interaction of the attributes and the
primordial activity of being.[27]

Distinctions are the result of a development: substance itself is a
development towards a growing distinction and individuality. Therefore
substance in the strict sense is the *individual* substance, completely
determined in its nature – the *suppositum* in scholastic terms. The *living
being*, not *life* (*vita primaeva*), is substance – or better, substance is the
process through which *life* individuates itself in a *living being*. If substances are individual living beings ('*omnia* (*prout in rerum natura
sunt) facta fuisse ab initio singularia*'),[28] the so-called principle of
individuation assumes great importance. Glisson sees the ultimate reason of individuation in a tendency towards 'confederation', meant as a
radically vital and internal act through which a nature constitutes itself
by separating from the rest.[29]

The specific act constituting each substance in its individuality ('*naturae confoederatio sibi soli*'), capable of discriminating what is one's
own from what is foreign, originates in the energetic nature of sub-

stance which is ultimately an inner 'representative' activity.[30] The foundation of natural perception as an original vital function rests on the self-representative structure of substance: substance, as deeply adherent to its perceptive faculty, is the idea through which it knows itself and its causes and effects.[31] Being a simple substance, matter, too, has a self-representative structure (*'objectiva ratio sive idea suiipsius'*), an idea that is coeval and coexisting with its being.[32]

The distinction between natural perception and sense perception parallels the distinction between inorganic and organic matter. Natural perception is the 'immediate action of substantial life'[33] and, as such, is the *inorganic* inner principle of the organization of living structures; sense perception is the result of that organization. The former is the *natura naturans*; the latter a mode and schematism of the *natura naturata*. One is pure energy prior to any kind of split between subject and object; the other is the self-duplication of life superimposing a form over another till an organ is built. One is an unconscious starting-point; the other a way toward consciousness. In order not to misunderstand the meaning of Glisson's natural perception, we should distinguish it very carefully from sensation and cognitive faculties.[34] The activity of natural perception is so deeply rooted into life as to have nothing to do with conscious perceptions at all. It is a sort of action that does not know the plan (*idea*) which it starts from and that forgets the accomplishment of the end once it has carried it out.

Mechanical philosophy and the life of nature

Universal formative motion, which every substance consists of, is an original interpretation of the peripatetic notion of *motus ad formam*. Descartes, in his battle against peripatetic science, had indeed begun by attacking this kind of vital motion.[35] And his 'devitalizing' project met with the approval of a great number of natural philosophers. Glisson's post-Cartesian attempt to give a strictly philosophical foundation to the 'life of nature' is therefore even more significant, because it is deliberately in contrast with any mechanical interpretation of life.

The radical, almost unnatural aspect or Descartes's philosophy lies in questioning any kind of natural prejudice which has forced itself upon the senses as obvious ('we began life as infants').[36] Philosophy is a backward movement which disarticulates what a lifelong experience has put together in a seemingly natural way, the search for truth being different from everyday life. Among these prejudices, one of the most characteristic is what we could call the 'animistic projection', namely to imagine that natural things can have a sort of inner life of their own,

like ours: from the fall of heavy bodies to the operations of the animals
an inner principle of movement is supposedly steadily at work. According to the Cartesian genealogy of the prejudices, not to have distinguished clearly the body from the soul led to an age-old misunderstanding of cosmology. The soul's power to act on the body is not the same as
the power one body has to act on another. Natural phenomena, which
can be explained simply in mechanical terms, have been interpreted in
the light of notions we generally make use of in knowing our body and
soul. The distinction between matter (*res extensa*) and mind (*res cogitans*)
is the real touchstone of the whole Cartesian system.[37]

Compared with Descartes's, Glisson's project, albeit just as radical,
starts from completely different premises. Descartes would have been
horrified just by reading the second part of the title of Glisson's book
on substance: 'on the life of nature and its first faculties'. To speak
about a life of nature means to disregard Descartes's dualistic approach:
there is an inner, perceptive, appetitive and motive principle in each
substance – Glisson says at the beginning of the essay – and it is caused
'by no external force, no movement and rest, no texture, schematism,
organization, proportion or nexus of parts'.[38] Descartes is directly called
into question in chapter 24, entitled significantly: 'Certain axioms commonly extolled, that are opposed to the life of nature, are examined,
rectified and brought back to their correct meaning (in order to show
the life of nature more clearly)'.[39] It is not only Descartes who denies
life to inanimate things: scholastic philosophy, recapitulated by Suarez,
had reaffirmed the difference between non-living and living things by
referring to a series of renowned 'axioms' ('*quicquid movetur ab alio
movetur*; *nihil agere in seipsum*; *idem non esse simul agens et patiens*,
... '). But much more space is given to the refutation of Descartes's
'axioms', summed up by Glisson thus: 'whatever rests, perpetually rests;
whatever moves, perpetually moves'.[40]

As Glisson well knew, the discussion of the axioms against the life of
nature involved the theological question of the relationship between
God and the created world. In Glisson's opinion, to consider the material world as inanimate, whether only partly (scholasticism) or wholly
(Descartes), means to ground natural explanations on supernatural causes
(as if God had to intervene miraculously to complete the work of the
creation, some substances being incapable of acting by themselves) and,
in Descartes's particular case, to foster strongly occasionalistic and
voluntaristic positions. In this connection Glisson's analysis concentrates particularly on sections 36 and 37 of the second part of Descartes's
Principia Philosophiae: God created matter together with movement
and rest and preserves the same proportion of movement and rest by
virtue of His ordinary concurrence ('*per solum suum concursum*

ordinarium').[41] According to Glisson, Descartes does not escape the occasionalistic pattern. God, the first cause, could have created movement as depending on matter – the second cause of material effects – but the expression 'per *solum* Dei concursum motum conservari', as Glisson stresses, betrays a view according to which the maintenance of the universe requires God's continuous, miraculous intervention. From this point of view, creatures 'are not sufficient or secondary natural principles of their own actions'.[42]

The misunderstanding of the real meaning of the principle of inertia led Glisson to reappraise all the characteristic repertory of pre-modern physics: the spontaneous capability to initiate a new movement or to end it in a state of rest,[43] the intrinsic tendencies distinguishing the natural movements of bodies,[44] the elemental vegetative operations of matter,[45] the wide range of vital actions not reducible to simple local motion.[46] As for the vegetative activity, the contrast with Descartes is at its most marked. We know that the French philosopher rejected the concept of the vegetative soul.[47] Glisson, on the contrary, highlights just this aspect: 'Because the vegetative soul is the nature of matter, the movement it produces is natural to matter itself. In fact, the soul itself is a mode of matter, and depends essentially on it, and consequently also in acting'.[48] Unlike Descartes, vegetative activity is essential to matter, being its intrinsic vital movement. In its double aspect of *prime matter* and *primeval life*, matter is an unceasingly self-organizing substratum, while the soul is an additional structure brought about by matter itself in its natural activity. The real nature of movement is to be a vital act. Following the Stagirite ('in this matter we have to agree with Aristotle'), local motion is seen by Glisson only as a kind of movement and surely cannot account for the vital phenomena. For example, it cannot account for movement accomplishing a form: this 'presupposes that matter attains a new nature, and a new idea of nature, that is, a new law whether essential or accidental of being and acting: but this new self-representing idea (*idea suiipsius*) does not seem to be brought about by local motion alone. At least the vital act, that is, the action of matter itself contributes by assuming, uniting and sustaining this new idea as its own law and nature. And this action is immanent, and does not seem to turn into local motion'.[49] The most general motion in nature is not local motion. It is the primitive vital energy pervading being prior to forms and souls. From sensitive soul through vegetative soul, to the form of every single element, the source of movement always comes before and is independent of, but productive of forms. *Motus ad formam* embraces all material substances and, even more generally, *motus antitypiae* precedes the distinction between what is spiritual and what is material.[50]

It is worth noting that the rejection of the principle of inertia, in its all-inclusive Cartesian meaning, is stated not in order to restore a world of specifically different levels of organization, but to replace that principle with a likewise all-inclusive principle: natural perception.[51] Organization is the aim of an evolution, not the result of an archetypal condition.[52] The order of the universe is the expression of the ubiquitous life of nature. To those who object that the difference between living and non-living testifies once more to God's wisdom in distributing different orders and degrees of perfection, Glisson answers that the orders of life (*vitae ordines*) can be maintained exactly by founding them on a boundless – *inorganic* and *similary* – natural life. The Creator of the universe

> assigned to the first and the most general rudiments of substances an adequate and proportionate energetic, that is, vital, nature; although he distinguished and adorned nature's superimposed degrees with increasing perfection. In this way he showed the inexhaustible treasures of his munificence, when, beginning from such a noble basis of nature, he could nevertheless raise his own work from degree to degree to such an elevated fastigium, by adding from time to time a higher and higher dignity.[53]

Glisson's theory of *biusia* is a tacit attack on the harmonious ladder of being, since the degrees of organization do not mirror an immutable scale of eternal essences.

Hylozoism, Stratonism and atheism

In his *Lexicon Philosophicum* (1613), Rudolph Göckeln listed under the entry '*vita*' the accepted meanings of the word following a threefold distinction: *physice, politice* and *theologice*. In a 'physical' sense, life is the living being itself and only in a figurative sense (*metaleptice*) indicates the soul. From a 'political' point of view, life is the same as the way of life (*ratio vivendi*). Finally, life means, 'theologically', the spiritual dimension of the human existence.[54] A rather common division. Jakob de Back, in his *Discourse* on the 'nullitie of spirits', 'sanguification' and 'heat of living things', which had by then been imbued with Harvey's 'heresy', refers to the same division when he writes: 'the soul does chiefly endeavour three things in the body, to wit, life, a better and more commodious life, and at last eternal life'.[55] But the distinction of the notion of life according to different meanings did not involve only metalepsis or other figures of speech; it hinted at a world of well-defined 'essences': material life, moral life, spiritual life. The religious suspicions against any forms of hylozoism or against the revival of conceptions which in some way implied the world soul concealed the fear that those views could represent a challenge to the hierarchically ordered structure of the universe. In particular, to regard life as one common genus meant to explode these distinctions. With his theory of *biusia*, Glisson had taken a similar step: even though material life can be considered as a substance in a different way if compared with spiritual substances, nevertheless life 'seems to be an univocal genus as regards material and immaterial life'.[56]

Hylozoism became a physico-theological question particularly from the 1670s onwards, when the religious and ideological implications associated with the emphasis on nature and life as autonomous powers came to light. The decade opened with the publication of Spinoza's *Tractatus Theologico-Politicus* (1670), where a conception of nature as an autonomous, self-productive and thoroughly immanent system was brought forth, and it closed with Henry More's *Ad V.C. Epistola Altera*, published in his Latin *Opera Omnia* (1679), where we find a significant parallel refutation of Spinoza's and Glisson's philosophical systems.[57] Through Franciscus Mercurius van Helmont the Cambridge Platonist had probably heard of the possibility that Spinozism could be interpreted as a form of vitalistic monism.[58] In Frans Cuiper's *Arcana Atheismi Revelata* (1676) he had also found confirmation of his idea that 'modern atheists' had resorted to the 'innate life of matter'.[59] Speaking of active powers and natural faculties was becoming more and more dangerous. Set against such a background, Glisson's work on the life of nature drew the attention of those who associated the emphasis on living nature with the revival of paganism or, at worst, with plain atheism. In this atmosphere Cudworth raised the alarm of the hylozoistic threat.

In his *True Intellectual System of the Universe* Cudworth shows a twofold aim, historical and theoretical. This latter was probably hidden under learning, but at all events a definite and strong theoretical ambition was at stake: the definition of the real essence of atheism (and theism). Significantly the 'historical deduction' (the analysis of the forms of atheism which occurred in history) coincides with the 'metaphysical deduction' (there are only four possible forms of atheism: atomick, hylozoick, hylopathian and cosmo-plastick). What is more, to have placed Glisson's hylozoism amongst the forms of atheism gives it a high *historical* and *philosophical* value.

Leaving aside the question of whether Glisson was upholding atheistic doctrines deliberately, his real intentions being inscrutable, a historically more accessible task would be to analyse the objective religious threat of Glisson's medical philosophy, since in this case we have two orders of facts to work on: Glisson's own writings and some reactions of his contemporaries. As for the first I have already hinted on several occasions at the risks associated with the secularization of the notion of life. Here I can only touch on two other 'heretical' aspects: the notions of prime matter and individual perceptive substance. As far as the former is concerned, it is more than apparent that Glisson regarded matter as an inherently living and perceptive substratum ('*materiam vitae radicem in se continere*').[60] The double-faced appearance of substance is represented by *prime matter* and *primeval life*: as the organic efflorescence of forms is only a progressive and temporary superposition originating from matter itself, so the living modes ('*modi vitales*'), the 'souls', are the result of the inner self-modification of life ('*originalis vita*', '*radicale vitae*'), that 'does not live on a borrowed life, but on itself'.[61] Here are just a few consequences which can be criticized from a religious point of view: the primacy of matter with respect to form,[62] the perpetuity and self-subsistency of matter,[63] the re-evaluation of the theory of the eduction of forms as a thoroughly immanent process,[64] the attribution to matter of an autonomous causal power not distinguishable from its own being,[65] the necessary and teleological self-determination of matter in its processes.[66]

As regards the notion of individual perceptive substance, Glisson's philosophy is marked by a dilemma: ontological monism or pluralism? Have we to consider substance as a whole expressing itself either as *prime matter* or as *primeval life*, or rather as an individual living principle, endowed with perception, appetite and movement? From this point of view, Cudworth and More grasped another significant aspect of Glisson's ontology, to be condemned, of course, for its unorthodox consequences. They actually found it absolutely untenable that a being characterized by substantial unity could be a composite system teeming with innumerable living and perceptive principles. We have said that Glisson's substance is a radical interpretation of the scholastic concept of 'individual' (*suppositum*). Significantly the Cambridge physician devoted many pages to the discussion of the principle of individuation and, as has been seen, the ultimate cause was traced to a vital tendency towards 'confederation'. If natural perceptive power is a *continuum*, each part of matter being capable of perception, a state of matter always corresponds to a state of perception. The counterpart of natural perception in matter is the *minimum naturale*: life is a succession of natural perceptions, matter a living tissue of *minima naturalia*.[67] The close interrelation between matter and perception is taken into account in a manuscript: 'Since all that pertains to prime matter is perpetual, the perceptive faculty itself, and the actual perception belonging to the parts of prime matter, are necessarily perpetual.'[68] Likewise prime matter and primeval life: the original perceptive faculty is unchangeable and permanent.

Both More and Cudworth criticized this aspect of Glisson's philosophy harshly. More regarded the 'primeval life of matter' as an absurdity because any minutest particle of matter must have been endowed with perfect knowledge and, what is worse, all with the same power. As a consequence, the absolute uniformity and equality of natural perceptive power would necessarily create conflicts and civil wars in the 'confederations' of *minima naturalia*. In More's opinion, Glisson's principle of individuation based on a natural tendency towards 'confederation' actually leads to a continuous state of anarchy in the natural world.[69] Even more explicitly, Cudworth had emphasized the politically and socially blameworthy aspects underlying Glisson's conception of 'the life of matter'. Since it is impossible that *'greater perfections* and *higher degrees* of being should rise and ascend out of lesser and lower'[70] without a complete overthrow of the natural order, and since 'conscious and reflexive life or animality' cannot be considered as a result of a natural perceptive power ('from the *modification* thereof alone by *organization*'), the *'Common-wealth* of *percipients'* envisaged by Glisson – nothing else but 'a heap of innumerable percipients' – was considered still more absurd than Hobbes's covenant of 'atom-subjects', each of which is, at least, endowed with consciousness and will.[71]

According to Walter Charleton, Glisson had a conciliatory nature,[72] and his writings endorse this image. *De Natura Substantiae Energetica* contains many references to Suarez, Van Helmont, Harvey and Bacon, to quote only the main sources. He also tried to reconcile the medical systems of Hippocrates (particularly his theory of the healing power of nature) and Galen (his conception of the natural faculties) with those of Neoterics.[73] If Glisson's conciliatory endeavour never gives the impression of a patchwork, it is only because the basic ideas are original.[74] Nevertheless, the richness of references helped to overshadow the original philosophical core. Was this premeditated? Again, the inscrutability of Glisson's real intentions does not allow us to give a definite answer, but in such an age when philosophers had often to present themselves in disguise, the influence of tradition was not to be underestimated. The choice to write in heavy scholastic Latin can be considered another device in order to circumscribe and screen his own readers.[75] Of course, the operation worked so well that almost nobody (except for More and Cudworth) noticed the heterodox implications of Glisson's theory of life and matter. And, finally, by a trick of history, the person who should have unmasked Glisson as a 'hylozoick atheist' helped in camouflaging him with a further mask, that of Strato. So 'Strato's ghost', portrayed by Cudworth as 'the rising sun of atheism', was taken for Spinoza, thanks also to the authoritative intervention of Bayle and Leibniz.[76]

Anatomical research and philosophical inquiry grew and interacted together in Glisson's work. The long philosophical parenthesis of the 1660s, culminating in *De Natura Substantiae Energetica*, was not a momentary digression or, at least, if it was, it was in the sense given by Glisson himself in a passage from *De Ventriculo*, where he speaks of his style of writing characterized by so frequent 'philosophical digressions':

> it happens that whether by an apparent need to clarify my thought or by the lure and sweetness of speculation, I have strayed far from the aim which I had intended at the beginning. But I hope that the kind reader will not unwillingly forgive me this: it being something that seldom occurs, except for matters of great importance and not at all of common speculation, which I would find difficult to talk about elsewhere.[77]

Notes

Acknowledgement: I would like to thank Dr Andrew Cunningham and the staff of the Wellcome Unit in Cambridge for their kind hospitality during a stay, in the summer of 1994, that proved invaluable for my knowledge of Francis Glisson's work. The University Library of Cambridge deserves special mention not only for its efficient service but also for its congenial atmosphere. I am also indebted to Paul Bowley for his kind assistance with the English.

1. *De Natura Substantiae Energetica*, London, 1672. Other published works: *De Rachitide*, in collaboration with G. Bate and A. Regemorter, London, 1650; *Anatomia Hepatis*, London, 1654; *De Ventriculo et Intestinis*, (London and Amsterdam, 1677, from which edition I shall be quoting). As for the manuscript sources kept in the British Museum, they have been only partially published: see the lecture *Doctrina de circulatione sanguinis haud immutat antiquam medendi methodum* (1662), J.M.N. Boss (ed.), *Physis*, 20 (1978), pp. 304–36; and *English Manuscripts of Francis Glisson: 1. From 'Anatomia Hepatis (The Anatomy of the Liver)'*, 1654, Andrew Cunningham (ed.), Cambridge, 1993; *English Manuscripts of Francis Glisson: 2. Lectures and other papers*, A. Cunningham (ed.) (forthcoming). For Glisson's philosophical manuscripts, which are often referred to in the present chapter, see G. Giglioni (ed.), *Latin Manuscripts of Francis Glisson (1). Philosophical Papers. Materials related to De Natura Energetica (On the Energetic Nature of Substance)*, 1672, Cambridge, 1996. On Glisson's life see N. Moore, 'Glisson, Francis', *Dictionary of National Biography*, vol. VII, pp. 1316–17; Owsei Temkin, 'Glisson, Francis', *Dictionary of Scientific Biography*, New York, 1970–1981, vol. V, pp. 425–7. On Glisson's medical work see O. Temkin, 'The Classical Roots of Glisson's Doctrine of Irritation', *Bulletin of the History of Medicine*, 38, (1964), pp. 297–328; Walter Pagel, 'Harvey and Glisson on Irritability, with a Note on Van Helmont', *Bulletin of the History of Medicine*, 41 (1967), pp. 497–514; N. Mani, 'Biomedical Thought in Glisson's Hepatology and in Wepfer's Work on Apoplexy', *A Celebration*

of Medical History, L.G. Stevenson (ed.), Baltimore and London, 1982, pp. 37–63. On Glisson's philosophy of nature see C. de Remusat, *Histoire de la Philosophie an Angleterre depuis Bacon jusqu'à Locke*, Paris, 1875, vol. II, pp. 163–8; H. Marion, *Franciscus Glissonius*, Paris, 1880; H. Marion, 'Francis Glisson', *Revue Philosophique de la France et de l'Étranger*, 14 (1882), pp. 121–55; Arrigo Pacchi, *Cartesio in Inghilterra*, Rome and Bari, 1973, pp. 150–5; John Henry, 'Medicine and Pneumatology: Henry More, Richard Baxter, and Francis Glisson's Treatise *On the Energetic Nature of Substance*', *Medical History*, 31 (1987), pp. 15–40 (with further bibliographical references); G. Giglioni, 'Il *Tractatus de natura substantiae energetica* di F. Glisson', *Annali della Facoltà di Lettere e Filosofia dell'Università di Macerata*, 24 (1991), pp. 137–79; Roger French, *William Harvey's Natural Philosophy*, Cambridge, 1994, pp. 286–309.

2. R. Cudworth, *The True Intellectual System of the Universe*, London, 1678. References to Glisson's theory of 'life of the matter' are scattered throughout the treatise; see pp. 62, 72, 105–9, 132, 145, 172–4, 666–9, 687, 728–9, 755, 758, 829–30, 838–41 (p. 839 is the only place where Glisson is almost expressly quoted: 'Which point (that all life is not a meer accident, but that there is life substantial) hath been of late with much reason and judgment insisted upon, and urged by the writer of the life of nature'), 870–1.

3. W. Harvey, *The Works*, translated from the Latin by R. Willis, London, 1847, (repr. New York and London, 1965), p. 511; W. Harvey, *Opera Omnia*, London, 1766, p. 532.

4. *Works*, pp. 508–9 (*Opera Omnia*, pp. 529–30).

5. *Works*, p. 428 (*Opera Omnia*, pp. 446–7).

6. The following remark makes us think of a pantheistic concept: 'Lastly, not only is there a soul or vital principle present in the vegetative part, but even before this there is inherent mind, foresight, and understanding' (ibid.). See also *Works*, p. 285 (*Opera Omnia*, p. 330); *Works*, p. 370 (*Opera Omnia*, p. 385): 'Nor do I think that we are greatly to dispute about the name by which this first agent is to be called or worshipped; whether it be God, Nature, or the Soul of the universe, – whatever the name employed, – all still intend by it that which is the beginning and the end of all things'.

7. *Anatomia Hepatis*, p. 14. I quote from Glisson's own English original manuscript of *Prolegomena* (Sloane 3315, fol. 182r.), translated into Latin by George Ent, and now edited by Andrew Cunningham (*English Manuscripts of Francis Glisson*, p. 41).

8. *Anatomia Hepatis*, p. 15; Sloane 3315, fol. 183r.; *English Manuscripts*, p. 43.

9. *Anatomia Hepatis*, p. 22; Sloane 3315, fol. 175r.; *English Manuscripts*, p. 57.

10. *De Natura Substantiae Energetica*, p. 226 (translations from *De Natura Substantiae Energetica* and *De Ventriculo* are mine).

11. Ibid., pp. 239–44.

12. Ibid., p. 244.

13. Ibid., pp. 425–6.

14. Ibid., p. 431.

15. *Tractatus de Ventriculo et Intestinis. Cui Praemittitur Alius, De Partibus*

Continentibus in Genere; et in Specie de Iis Abdominis, Epistola lectori (I quote from the Amsterdam edition). From this short autobiographical sketch we can also assume that an earlier version of the treatise on the stomach had been written about the first years of the 1660s (1661–62) and that Glisson moved on to devote himself to the 'nature of life' for ten years till 1672 when the treatise on the energetic nature of substance was published (see also *De Ventriculo*, p. 433). But the sketchy treatise on the stomach continued to be neglected. In fact Glisson spent almost two more years in epistemological reflections('Verum aliis, ut fit, cogitationibus, et imprimis fidis inveniendis indicantibus, quibus Ars Medica certius innitatur, admodum intentus, prioris Tractatus evulgationem aliquandiu neglexi'). His pressing old age ('anhela ingruens senecta') and his inability to support the rigours of winter ('impotentiaque hyemis frigora tolerandi') eventually persuaded the Cambridge physician to finish his work on the stomach, leaving aside the methodological speculations ('ne nova perficiendi spe deceptus, quod sub manibus erat perdam').

16. *De Ventriculo*, p. 2.
17. Ibid. See especially p. 394, where the generational process through which the dissimilary parts result from the similary ones is traced back to the plastic virtue of the *Archeus*.
18. *De Natura Substantiae Energetica*, Ad Lectorem, § 18; pp. 191–2.
19. *De Natura Substantiae Energetica*, p. 185; see also pp. 169–72.
20. Ibid., pp. 185–6.
21. Significantly the discussion of this principle can be found in a great many places: in *De Natura Substantiae Energetica* (pp. 56, 248–9), of course, but also in *De Ventriculo* (p. 363) and in the manuscripts (Sloane 3312, fols. 157, 196, 199–200, 203).
22. 'Vulgus philosophicum incipere a creaturis, Cartesium incepisse a mente, se incipere a Deo', in *Gespräch mit Tschirnhaus über Spinoza's Ethik*, in L. Stein, *Leibniz und Spinoza*, Berlin, 1890, p. 283.
23. *De Natura Substantiae Energetica*, pp. 11, 18–19, 188, 190, Ad lectorem §§ 7–8.
24. This 'crowded' ontology is another sign that distinguishes Glisson's theory of substance from post-Cartesian ones. On seventeenth-century views on substance see R.S. Woolhouse, *Descartes, Spinoza, Leibniz. The Concept of Substance in Seventeenth-century Metaphysics*, London, 1993.
25. *De Natura Substantiae Energetica*, pp. 77, 187–8. Sloane 3311, fol. 90: 'Quare basis materiae et formae una atque eadem natura substantialis est quanquam sub diverso formali conceptu'.
26. *The True Intellectual System*, p. 105.
27. I have dealt with this particular aspect in 'Panpsychism *versus* Hylozoism. An Interpretation of Some Seventeenth-Century Doctrines of Universal Animation', *Acta Comeniana*, 11 (1995), pp. 25–45.
28. *De Natura Substantiae Energetica*, p. 58.
29. Ibid., pp. 54–8. Sloane 3314, fols 43–4.
30. *De Natura Substantiae Energetica*, pp. 66, 68–69. Sloane 3314, fol. 41: 'generalis perceptio haec convenit substantiae, quo substantiae: est adeo tum corporibus tum spiritibus communis'. Sloane 3315, fol. 99: 'cum facultas percipiendi qua sic, fundatur in essentia rei primo substantiali qua viva et dein in essentia rei modificata, fit ut facultas percipiendi, a

nulla re alia dependeat, nisi a constitutione essentiali et accidentali sive qualificata'.

31. *De Natura Substantiae Energetica*, p. 194; *De Ventriculo*, Epistola lectori; Sloane 3315, fol. 98r.: 'Existimarem eam [i.e. *facultas perceptiva*] esse universam naturam entis substantialis qua vivam, ei a prima creatione inditam posse percipere, vel esse perceptivam. Nam cum essentia rei eo ipso quod est, sit perceptibilis obiective sive repraesentativa sui, cumque sibi ipsi sit intime praesens fit ut seipsam in esse suo percipiat'.

32. The following passage, drawn from *De Natura Substantiae Energetica* (p. 90), is worth quoting in full, given its importance: 'Quod materia has [*sc.* the three natural faculties: perception, appetite and movement] in sua ratione contineat, ex eo liquet, quod sit ens actu, actuque per se subsistens, nec sit per inharentiam in alio, ut modo monstravimus. Quare est objectiva ratio sive idea suiipsius. In quantum enim actu et positive est, est actu et positive cognoscibilis. Habet ergo ideam propriam sibi coaevam, qualisque est ejus entitas, talis est etiam ejus idea; nempe est actualis, positiva, et rei per se subsistentis. Non ergo cognoscitur per ideam alienam, aut per negationem alterius, ut non ens; sed in se, et per seipsam, ut intime sibi praesentem. Ipsa enim est sufficiens objectiva ratio suipsius, praesertim ubi intime unitur facultati perceptivae [...] Cum enim facultas ejus perceptiva rationi objectivae sive ideae ejusdem sit intime praesens, necessario percipit quicquid ea ratio repraesentet; actualem quippe suam entitatem quatenus per se subsistentem, eamque qua bonam et amabilem. Quare necessario quoque hanc suam entitatem appetit sive amat. Cumque ista idea repraesentet materiae subsistentiam ut naturaliter perpetuam, hac fruitur, omnique studio et industria hanc vindicat, nec ulla violentia se annihilari permittit'.

33. Ibid., Ad lectorem, §12.

34. Ibid., pp. 186–7; 209–16; Ad lectorem, §§ 10–11, 14. *De Ventriculo*, sect. II, ch. 7. Sloane 3314, fol. 23.

35. *Le Monde*, in *Oeuvres de Descartes*, C. Adam and P. Tannery (eds), Paris, 1902, quoted as AT, vol. XI, pp. 39–40; *The Philosophical Writings of Descartes*, trans. J. Cottingham, R. Stoothoff and D. Murdoch, Cambridge, 1985, vol. I, p. 94.

36. *Principia Philosophiae*, AT, vol. VIII, p. 5 (*Philosophical Writings*, vol. I, p. 193).

37. To Princess Elizabeth, 21 May 1643, AT, vol. III, p. 667 (*Philosophical Writings*, vol. III, p. 219).

38. *De Natura Substantiae Energetica*, Ad Lectorem, § 10: 'Porro, res major est, et majoris momenti, primum vitae principium cuiquam impertiri. Est enim internum principium percipiendi, appetendi, atque se movendi, ei indere. Cujus productionem nulla vis externa, nullus motus aut quies, nulla textura, schematismus, organizatio, proportio, nexusve partium, attingere queat'.

39. Ibid., p. 332: '*Axiomata quaedam vulgo decantata, quae vitae naturae repugnant, (quo clarius haec monstretur) examinantur, corriguntur, et ad sanum sensum reducuntur*'.

40. On Glisson's analysis of Descartes's concept of motion see G. Giglioni, 'Il *Tractatus de natura substantiae energetica*', pp. 146–57.

41. *Principia Philosophiae*, AT, vol. IX, p. 61 (*Philsophical Writings of Descartes*, vol. I. p. 240).

42. *De Natura Substantiae Energetica*, p. 342. That bodies are endowed with life does not belittle God's power. They are capable of perceiving since they are images of God (*causa exemplaris*) and have an autonomous substantial constitution (see Sloane 3315, fols 98v., 102, 103). Glisson's doctrine according to which to consider matter as lifeless would mean to diminish God's power is similar in many respects to Anne Conway's position as expresed in her *The Principles of the Most Ancient and Modern Philosophy*. See Sarah Hutton, *Ancient Wisdom and Modern Philosophy: Anne Conway, F.M. van Helmont and the Seventeenth-Century Dutch Interchange of Ideas*, Utrecht, 1994, pp. 6–7; S. Hutton, 'Of Physic and Philosophy: Anne Conway, F.M. van Helmont and Seventeenth-Century Medicine' in this volume.

43. *De Natura Substantiae Energetica*, p. 345: 'Non ergo repugnat legibus naturae, ut quod violenter movetur, sponte quiescat; aut quod violenter detinetur, sibi permissum se denuo moveat'.

44. Ibid., pp. 347–50.

45. Ibid., pp. 350–1.

46. Ibid., pp. 351–2.

47. *Description du Corps Humain*, AT, vol. XI, p. 250. To Plempius, 15 February 1638, AT, vol. I, p. 523 (*Philosophical Writings*, vol. III, pp. 80–1). *L'Homme*, AT, vol. XI, pp. 201–2 (*Philosophical Writings*, vol. I, p. 108).

48. *De Natura Substantiae Energetica*, p. 350.

49. Ibid., p. 352.

50. Ibid., pp. 245–6.

51. In *De ventriculo* Glisson links irritability to the refusal of the principle of inertia: 'Motiva fibrarum facultas, nisi irritabilis foret, vel perpetuo quiesceret, vel perpetuo idem ageret' (p. 168).

52. The term 'evolution' is not out of place in Glisson's case. Significantly enough, many of Cudworth's criticisms were addressed against the possibility, contained in the hylozoistic premises, of regarding what is perfect and noble as deriving from lower degrees of perfection. John Tulloch, writing in the last century, was struck by the strong similarities between hylozoism and evolutionism: 'In speaking, for example, of certain speculations which attributed the origin of life – "not only the sensitive in brutes, but also the rational in men" – to modifications of matter "by organisation alone", he [Cudworth] might be supposed characterising the theory of evolution in its latest form' (*Rational Theology and Christian Philosophy in England in the Seventeenth Century*, Edinburgh and London, 1874, vol. II, p. 264).

53. *De Natura Substantiae Energetica*, p. 221.

54. R. Goclenius, *Lexicon Philosophicum, Quo Tanquam Clave Philosophiae Fores Aperiuntur*, Frankfurt, 1613, p. 324.

55. J. De Back, *The Discourse ... In Which He Handles the Nullitie of Spirits, Sanguification, the Heat of Living Things*, London, 1653 (1st edition 1648), A Speech to the Readers.

56. *De Natura Substantiae Energetica*, Ad Lectorem, § 7.

57. *Ad V. C. Epistola Altera*, in *Opera Omnia*, London, 1679, 2 vols, vol. 1, pp. 563–614 (for the refutation of Glisson see especially pp. 604–11). See J. Henry, 'Medicine and Pneumatology', pp. 28–32. In More's opinion Glisson – 'tam diligentem naturae indagatorem' – preferred to regard

matter as an autonomously living being (that is, in More's terms, to fall into Behemenism) rather than to accept the 'shameful mistake' of the Aristotelian 'substantial forms'. (Of course, the right way to have chosen would have been Platonism) (*Enchiridion Metaphisicum, Scholia in cap. XXV. sect. I*, in *Opera Omnia*, 2 vols, vol. 1, p. 300). Other significant references to Glisson in More's work: *Philosophematum ... Examinatio, Opera Omnia* vol. II, i, pp. 340, 347. *Annotations upon the Discourse of Truth*, in [Joseph Glanvill] *Two Choise and Useful Treatises*, London, 1682, pp. 190–3, 227, 239–40. On More's interpretation of 'Behemenism' see Sarah Hutton, 'Henry More and Jacob Boehme' in *Henry More (1614–1687) Tercentenary Studies*, S. Hutton (ed.), Dordrecht, London and Boston, 1990, pp. 158–71.

58. *Ad V.C. Epistola Altera*, p. 565. See Rosalie L. Colie, *Light and Enlightenment. A Study of the Cambridge Platonists and the Dutch Arminians*, Cambridge, 1957, p. 78.

59. *Ad V.C. Epistola Altera*, p. 604. On Cuiper see R.L. Colie, *Light and Enlightenment*, pp. 74–5.

60. *De Natura Substantiae Energetica*, Ad Lectorem, § 8.

61. Ibid, Ad Lectorem, § 9. See also in particular pp. 131–63 for the relationship between prime matter and forms, and pp. 235–47 for the idea of the living modes springing from primeval life.

62. Ibid, pp. 88, 95; Sloane 3311, fol. 28v.

63. *De Natura Substantiae Energetica*, pp. 88–90.

64. Ibid., pp. 140–2.

65. Ibid., pp. 131–5.

66. Ibid., pp. 236–8.

67. Glisson's discussion of *minima naturalia* is in *De Natura Substantiae Energetica*, pp. 506–34 (at pp. 518–23 a refutation of Descartes's corpuscularism can be found). Glisson's theory of matter can by no means be considered as an atomic theory, but it is a sort of 'vital corpuscularism' (see especially pp. 512–14). On a similar vitalistic utilization of *minima naturalia* by Giordano Bruno see Hélène Védrine, 'Materie, Atome und Minima bei Giordano Bruno', in *Die Frankfurter Schriften Giordano Brunos und ihre Veraussetzungen*, V.K. Heipcke, W. Neuser and E. Wicke (eds), Weinheim, 1991, pp. 127–34 (esp. pp. 131–4).

68. Sloane 3315, fol. 105: 'De perceptione Materiae primae. Cum quicquid ad naturam Materiae primae spectet sit perpetuum, necesse est ipsa facultas perceptiva, ut et actualis perceptio quae spectant ad partes materiae primae sint perpetua'. Ibid., fol. 104v: 'Prior consideratio appellari potest facultas perceptiva originalis vel radicalis vel prima, vel facultas perceptiva materiae primae, vel etiam perceptio prima, perceptio materiae primae, perceptio immutabilis et perpetua. Est enim haec perceptio stabilis et materiae primae coaeva'. Nevertheless, the original and coeval perception and the modified and temporary perception are actually two ways of considering the same reality; see Sloane 3315, fol. 105: 'Nam materia non percipit suam primam essentiam per suam facultatem perceptivam et essentiam suam modificatam mobiliter per aliam; sed per eadem facultatem tantum ulterius modificatam utramque percipit. Quandocunque enim aut quomodocunque modificatur materia ipsa, modificatur quoque eius perceptio. Nova igitur perceptio est tantum accessoria modificatio

perceptionis primae, eidemque supervenit, et ab eadem amoveatur manente facultate originali sive prima'.

69. *Ad V.C. Epistola Altera*, pp. 609–10: 'Et sane si hoc sit, cum singula *Minima naturalia* pari sint et potentia et sapientia, omniaque totius fabricae animalis ejusque partium singularum fines atque usus, aliosque nobiliores esse et optabiliores, alios minus nobiles minusque optabiles noverint, mirum profecto est nulla inter ea oriri de ordine et primatu dissidia, nec tamen confoederare inter se velle, quam bella et lites adversus se invicem movere, adeo ut rursus necesse sit aliquid materia superius esse quod innumerae huic *Minimorum* materiae *naturalium* multitudini imperet eaque in ordinem disponat'. See also *Enchiridion Metaphysicum*, p. 301.

70. *True Intellectual System*, p. 728.

71. Ibid., pp. 839–40: 'For though voluntary agents and persons, may many of them, resign up their wills to one, and by that means, have all but as it were one artificial will, yet can they not possibly resign up their sense and understanding too, so as to have all but one artificial life, sense and understanding: much less could this be done, by senseless atoms, or particles of matter supposed, to be devoid of all consciousness or animality'. On the representation of the body as an image of the political situation see Christopher Hill, 'William Harvey and the Idea of Monarchy', *Past and Present*, 27 (1964), pp. 54–72. Roger French, *William Harvey's Natural Philosophy*, pp. 297–302 (specifically devoted to Glisson). On Hobbes's social 'atomism' see C.B. Macpherson, *The Political Theory of Possessive Individualism*, Oxford, 1962.

72. W. Charleton, *Enquiries into Human Nature*, London, 1680, p. 67: '[Dr. Glisson] who from the singular goodness of his nature took pleasure to reconcile the different opinions of the Antients'. It is interesting to note that Glisson's efforts to reconcile different positions are not simply the result of hermeneutical caution, but derive from a precise view of the historical truth: 'Veritas in multis temporis filia est' (*De Ventriculo*, p. 272). The following statement in *De Ventriculo* throws further light upon Glisson's even-tempered nature: 'Ecquis Philosophorum e tripode dictat; aut spiritu infallibilitatis in rebus naturalibus afflatur? Satis scio de meipso, me facillime errare posse. In arduis naturae, cogitationes primae fere secundis, facta pleniore inductione, cedere coguntur. Cauto est opus: ne praepropere definias, aut de aliis judices' (ibid.).

73. *De Ventriculo*, p. 389.

74. If Glisson is always ready to acknowledge his own debts to the tradition, nevertheless he is well aware of the originality of his positions too. See *De Natura Substantiae Energetica*, Epistola dedicatoria, where he lists the main results of his philosophical research: the substantial reality of the life of nature, the forms of its development and, above all, the derivation of the different kinds of soul from the life of matter: 'Verum ii pauci qui hanc naturae vitam hactenus agnoverunt, neque substantialem ejus in rebus materialibus originem declararunt, neque eandem a vita vegetabili aut animali satis discriminarunt: nedum secretioribus ejus vestigiis insistentes, quibus mediis et viis eadem a naturali ad vegetabilem et animalem provecta est, investigarunt: minime omnium, quo modo anima materialis, vegetabilis et sensitiva, e vitae materiae, gradibus essentialibus exaltata, emergunt, demonstrarunt'.

75. Cudworth adds a further reason to explain the limited success of hylozoick

atheism – its obscurity and paradoxicality: 'that life and perception or understanding, should be essential to matter as such [...] This I say, is an hypothesis so prodigiously paradoxical, and so outragiously wild, as that very few men ever could have atheistick faith enough, to swallow it down and digest it' (*The True Intellectual System*, p. 145). On the difficulties that Glisson's work had in being understood see J. Henry, 'The Matter of Souls: Medical Theory and Theology in Seventeenth-Century England', in *The Medical Revolution of the Seventeenth Century*, Roger French and Andrew Wear (eds), Cambridge, 1989, pp. 93, 110–12.

76. See P. Bayle, *An Historical and Critical Dictionary*, London, 1710, vol. III, *sub voce* 'Spinoza', p. 2782: 'All that can be concluded is, that his [of Strato] Opinion comes a great deal nearer *Spinozism*, than the System of Atoms'. [P. Bayle], *Reponse aux Questions d'un Provincial*, Rotterdam, 1704–07, vol. III, p. 1238. G.W. Leibniz *Theodicy. Essays on the Goodness of God, the Freedom of Man and the Origin of Evil*, edited with an introduction by A. Farrer, trans. E.M. Huggard, London, 1951, pp. 67, 245. On the real 'identity' of Strato see A. Pacchi, *Cartesio in Inghilterra*, pp. 150–5.

77. *De Ventriculo*, pp. 385–6.

CHAPTER SIX

The Physiology of Reading and the Anatomy of Enthusiasm

Adrian Johns

Dreams, delusions and distempers

John Rogers met God in Cambridge. Turned out of his family's Essex home in the early 1640s for consorting with Puritans, Rogers had wandered to the varsity town only to find himself reduced to eating the students' discarded quills in an attempt to stave off starvation. That was when the devil tempted him to necromancy, conjuring images of the glories of the world in Rogers's imagination. He resisted, and his resolve held fast. Whenever he felt the onset of such a *'passion'*, he told his Dublin congregation a decade or so later, 'I would fall to prayer [or] reading'. Then, at his lowest ebb, Rogers had a dream. He dreamt that he was walking, staff in hand, to his father's house. At first he could hardly see the path, and even began to question its existence; but at length he noticed footprints from others who had passed the same way before. He followed them, and as he did so the path became clearer. Before long a fine mansion appeared to his left, from which emerged a beam of light which partially blocked Rogers's path. He walked around it. But as he did so he happened to touch the beam, and the house immediately burst into flame. He was soon overtaken by an angry posse violently accusing Rogers himself of having started the conflagration. The furious mob dragged him off to prison, at which, terrified, he awoke.

Finding himself safe in his Cambridge garret, Rogers chided himself for being scared at 'a foolish *fancy*'. He fell asleep again. But immediately he sank back into the same dream, which repeated itself from beginning to end – except that this time Rogers the pilgrim found himself accompanied by an old, bearded man, who provided reassurance that God had selected him to preach His Word. This *'grave ancient man'* proceeded to interpret the whole of Rogers's dream from within the dream itself. The house represented heaven, his father, God, and his staff, God's Word. Rogers would be troubled by the various ways of men, but would follow the example (the footprints) of the saints, and would find his path becoming clearer. The magnificent house represented the '*great* ones of the world'. They were at present proud and ostentatious, and Rogers was to preach against them – the beam represented the cluster of powers and opinions he must circumvent in order to do so. The worldly powers would soon fall, but they would pursue Rogers and blame him for their catastrophe. With that, Rogers awoke again, and found that it was finally dawn.

What was he to make of this experience? Fortunately, Rogers was well qualified to know. He had been ten years old when he had his first vision, in 1637, and his life since then had been punctuated by spiritual crises. Hellfire sermons heard in his boyhood had filled him with terror, and, propelled by his fear, he had scoured the Scriptures. The young Rogers had '*read* every day', he recalled: 'I knew not what I *read*, but only thought the *bare reading* was enough.' He learnt his catechism by heart, reciting it as a talisman against the demons he knew were skulking under every bush, waiting to drag him off to Hell; he wrote down the sermons he heard, and learnt those too; he memorized morning and evening prayers, 'out of a *book*, for I knew no better yet'. All this reading threw Rogers into despair over his prospects for salvation. He was especially tormented by Matthew 5:20, which decreed that nobody could hope to enter heaven unless they exceeded the pharisees and scribes in 'righteousness'. He knew from his other reading that they had been prodigiously religious, and, confident that he could not hope to replicate their holiness, he descended into suicidal despondency. Distraught, he 'took the *Bible*', turned to the relevant pages, and 'read them over and over and over again'. It did little good: 'the more I *read* the more I *roar'd* in the *black gulf* of *despair*'. He would '*read*, and weep, and as my *usuall manner* was in the *time* of my *great despair*, fall flat (all along) with my face on the *ground*, and cry, and *call*, and sigh, and *weep*, and *call* for help'. But 'the *Lords time* was not yet come to answer', and at length Rogers gave up reading altogether, feeling tempted to conclude that 'there was no *God*' and that 'all things come by *Nature*'. He began to see demons not just under the bushes but in them, and to sit up all night in a turret in his father's orchard, wailing and drawing strange figures. Finally, just as he was about to commit suicide, he was seized and tied to a bed until his fits subsided.

From this point Rogers's condition had improved somewhat, stabilizing at an 'inward *malady*' of '*melancholy*'. And he had more dreams. In particular, he dreamt about Scripture itself – 'the *letter which killed me*' – and that the righteousness of Christ would be sufficient for his salvation. He awoke from this dream transformed. Rogers had long acknowledged that his dreams '*seised* much upon my *spirits*'. But he had regarded them as products of his own '*fancy*'. This dream was different: far from emerging out of his body, it had transformed it. 'I was so much changed that I was *amazed* at my self,' he recalled. He leapt up, exclaiming, 'Why, I am not *damned*! what's the *matter*? am I so filled with a *fancy*? ' Again his response was to turn to the Bible. He pored over its pages with new attention until, '*divine infusions ... writing* it within me', he achieved '*assurance of salvation*'. It was only now that Rogers could begin 'plainly to see *my self* (and by my self others)'. The transformation was to be completed and reinforced by his Cambridge dream – or, more precisely, the '*extraordinary token from on high* both in *dream* and *vision*'. This was 'the *call*'. The Cambridge vision – as he now called it – changed Rogers to the extent that his entire identity was transmuted: '*I am not I*', he succinctly wrote. Assured of salvation, and with his self freshly refashioned, Rogers set forth on a pilgrimage which would lead to both fifth monarchism and, eventually, medicine.[1]

At much the same time as Rogers was falling asleep to dream of God, across Cambridge another man was beginning a similar dream. This individual, like Rogers, dreamt that he was on a journey. He was staying in a house beside the road to Scotland. Perhaps it was at Grantham, which happened to be his father's town; that would make the dream directly comparable to that of Rogers. The road to Scotland served a symbolic purpose given the recent events of the Bishops' Wars. It was a bright moonlit night, and he dreamt that he left this house and wandered out into the courtyard. He was about to return, when he happened to look up into the sky. He was transfixed by what he saw. Two enormous figures had appeared in the heavens. The first, to the north, was a woman, holding a child in her lap 'with that care and tendernesse that Mothers and Nurses usually do'. To the south he then saw the second figure: an old, bearded man, lying on his side so that he was stretched out parallel to the horizon. This second 'representation', he noted (for this dreamer was a philosopher), seemed to be 'made of a very bright cloud, that had imbibed plentifully the light of the Moon'. As he 'steddily' watched the figure, it made a series of gestures with its right arm, lifting it slightly and letting it fall. Each time the old man raised his limb a little higher before releasing it. The dreamer finally turned to go back indoors. But as he did so, the figure pronounced, 'with a hollow voice much like thunder afarre off', that '*There is indeed love amongst you, but onely according to the flesh*'. Back in the house, feeling lucid and 'not at all dismaid', he recounted the vision to the occupants, and explained its significance to them – 'expounding the generall meaning of my dream in my dream', as he later remarked. He explained that the motions of the old man had been 'an Embleme of the proceedings of God when he chastises a nation', adducing 'reasons out of *Aristotles* Mechanicks', which he had just been reading, for this interpretation. What provoked this retribution, he insisted, was the people's lack of love, the spirit of Christianity.

This dream is interesting, and not only because of its superficial similarities with Rogers's: the bearded man, the central character pausing at a family home while on the road and, above all, the eery phenomenon of the dream explicating itself. This, too, was a vision. Or was it? The man who dreamt and later recounted it was Henry More, Cambridge Platonist and vehement antagonist to all varieties of visionary 'enthusiasm'. Before long, More had begun to have doubts about his own apparent vision. At length he decided that his '*Vision*' had had a terrestrial origin after all. He had been reading Ptolemy's *Geographia* the evening before and, seeing a particular figure on the engraved frontispiece, 'my fancy it seems having laid hold on his venerable beard, drew in thereby the whole scene of things that presented themselves to me in my sleep'. The 'congruity' between the supposed vision and events in Britain, at first so persuasive, was in fact 'onely casuall'.

Both More and Rogers identified their respective dreams as crucial moments of personal transformation. But they were crucial in directly contradictory ways. Rogers had moved from dismissing his dreams as artefacts of 'fancy' to respecting them as genuine visions, and simultaneously from despair at a conviction of the impossibility of his salvation to assurance that that conviction was itself mere 'fancy'. More pursued the opposite trajectory. From a belief that he had experienced a real vision, he convinced himself that his striking dream was the product of his imagination. More's 'fancy' had simply been imprinted by an image on a frontispiece. The same could happen to anybody, it seemed, and it could produce a 'vision' of convincing reality.[2]

In the years following their dreams these two figures were to become fundamental to the construction of 'enthusiasm'. As a radical minister and active fifth-monarchist, Rogers became one of the most important 'enthusiasts' of the period. As one of the foremost philosophers of his day, More made himself into perhaps the most sophisticated opponent of enthusiasm. Each played a central part in fabricating the notion of enthusiasm which has come down to us. Central to that notion is the phenomenon of the 'vision'. Enthusiasts, it was said, believed themselves to be the recipients of a revelatory inspiration by God's spirit. More and others made this claim definitive, alleging that enthusiasm was 'nothing else but a mis-conceit of being *inspired*'. And they were not altogether unwarranted in so stressing the phenomenon.[3] Rogers himself provided invaluable evidence that visions did occur within radical religious groups, and that their occurrence was regarded within those groups as of the first importance. Rogers's evidence, however, also permits the historian, who is further from the battlefront than More, to ask questions about how their participants thought visions originated, and what messages they believed them to convey.

Preaching in Dublin in the early 1650s, Rogers collected from his listeners a long series of what he called 'experiences', which he later caused to be printed. The origin of these testimonies lay in the procedure for admitting new members to his church. Before joining, he explained, every would-be congregant 'gives out some *EXPERMENTAL* Evidences of the *work* of *GRACE* upon his *SOUL* ... whereby he (or she) is *convinced*, that he is *regenerate*'. That is, everyone was expected to provide a record (often an oral record, since the person was likely to be illiterate) of a transformation such as Rogers himself had enjoyed – a transformation, that is, into a new and 'assured' self. This was summed up in a simple formula: 'Experience, we say, *proves principles*.'[4] The resulting testimonies disclose the harrowing reality of Ireland in the 1640s and early 1650s: Rogers's interlocutors had often lost entire families through incessant and merciless disease, murder and war. Yet Rogers's own Cambridge 'experience', relatively free from such ordeals, constituted his personal contribution to this effort.

The resulting accounts betray certain common features. Like Rogers himself, his subjects had often been brought up in families they described as godly. But they had at first practised merely what they called 'legal' or 'book' religion. They had then passed through a critical period, characterized as a death and rebirth, and emerged transformed, assured of their salvation. The conversions themselves generally came about by one or more of a relatively small number of possible mechanisms which, it was said, 'wrought upon' and thereby 'affected' the individual concerned. Hearing sermons, reading books and having visions were the three main mechanisms. Each was described in intimate terms. In each case success was then ascribed to God's spirit having 'wrought' within the subject: their accounts of reading Scripture, for example, often displayed a sense of helplessness before the Word. Thus one Raphael Swinfield described how he was first '*affected*' by hearing puritan preachers, becoming '*disconsolate*' and '*diseased*'. Then, he related, a 'place in *Isa*. 50.10. came into me' and '*fasten*[ed] upon me', insisting that Swinfield should trust to God. To reinforce the point, he had a dream which convinced him of his assurance. John Cooper was also converted by a dream, as were a number of others. Francis Bishop, condemned to be shot, 'turned open the *Bible*' and read a passage enjoining trust in God; when he resolved to do so, he was freed. Hugh Leeson was first 'wrought upon' by his wife, 'whom *God* made the *first Instrument* of my *good*; by her often *reading* of the *Scriptures* to me ... and by the *Spirits working* within me, with it'. Adrian Strong testified that 'by the word preached, and read out of *good Books* and the *Bible*, I was brought in to *God*'. Finally, Mary Barker was converted by all means short of visions: by '*preaching*, and *praying*, and *reading*, in *private* and *publique*'.[5]

These people, whose testimony was by all accounts either written down by themselves or taken down from their own words, claimed that visions – and inspiration in general – occurred in definite cultural and practical conditions. They stressed the experiences of reading Scripture and hearing sermons, and described in some detail their descent into 'disease' and corresponding ascent into 'assurance'. This chapter considers the character of such claims. In particular, it concentrates on a common element in their accounts which should be of particular interest, since not even the most extreme anti-enthusiast could repudiate it absolutely and still remain a Protestant. This was the stimulus of reading, and in particular of reading Scripture.

Many so-called enthusiasts found that it was reading which sparked off their inspirational experiences. Rogers, indeed, searched the Scriptures at all stages of his death and rebirth, and even dreamt about a passage from the Bible. But it was reading of a particular sort which counted. In fact, one could characterize the conversion recorded by Rogers partly as a transformation in reading practices. Another well-known religious radical, Jane Turner, likewise graduated, under the influence of reading radical works, from early 'book prayer' into a new, assured identity, characterized by an active interrogation of Scripture. 'I cannot omit to write something concerning the reading of a book,' she declared in her own account of the experience, 'by which as a means in the hand of God I received these never to be forgotten mercies.' Lent a text by an itinerant Puritan rather reminiscent of Rogers, she 'set apart a day by fasting and prayer to seek the Lord, that what was truth in it I might embrace, and that he would keep and preserve me from error', then read it. 'As I read I began to be much affected,' she remembered, 'trying' its doctrine against Scriptural passages, 'through grace I was in a great measure convinced.' So it was that Jane Turner cast herself upon Christ, thanks to a gift of God's grace manifested, she again stated, 'by reading.'[6] Other examples could be cited. Yet More's false 'vision' had also been the result of gazing at the frontispiece of a book. In that contrast lies an important issue for understanding the construction and criticism of early modern radical religion.

Christian culture in general, and English Protestant culture in particular, depended on the Word. Accounts of what constituted creditable Scripture (and what idolatrous forgery), how it should be represented and read (and by whom), and what effects it could have on the reader or hearer (and what effects it *should* have on them) – these issues lay at the heart of religious conflict.[7] Church of England Protestants of the time felt themselves under siege, and with reason. The threats posed by popery, superstition, enthusiasm and atheism appeared both all too real and all too united.[8] This chapter looks for the ways and means articulated by those trying to discriminate for themselves between enthusiasm and true religion. Central amongst those ways and means, it will contend, were arguments addressing the relation between the reading of scripture, the human frame, and the soul.

In his expert treatment of radical religious language in the Interregnum, Nigel Smith has thoroughly analysed the articulation of 'experimental faith'. For the figures Smith discusses – and Rogers is prominent among them – reading Scripture, and recording and analysing their 'experiences' as they did so, were of crucial importance. These were precisely the people whom Samuel Parker, Henry More, Meric Casaubon and others had in mind when they condemned 'enthusiasts'. As exemplified by Rogers's congregants, they spoke of being 'irradiated' by divine spirit while they scoured the pages of their Bibles. The effects of this irradiation had much in common with the self-transmutation in which alchemists reputedly attained knowledge, and indeed radicals appropriated the works of such writers as Paracelsus and Croll to articulate their own bodily and spiritual transformations. They analysed 'experience' in terms of the relation between the body and one's state of salvation or grace. That meant representing states of mind and of the body. Some radicals actually practised medicine: William Walwyn is probably the best known example, but Laurence Clarkson and Abiezer Coppe also practised physic, while Rogers himself gained medical degrees from Utrecht and Oxford. Such figures clearly thought about the body as well as the soul. Medical practitioners or not, however, radicals often described their religious beliefs and 'experiences' by reference to ideas concerning the corporeal frame and the rational and imaginative faculties. As Smith puts it, they represented themselves as 'mechanisms' affected by their exposure to Scripture. In extreme cases, they proclaimed a need for what they called 'self-annihilation': the absolute denial of the body in an attempt to become one with God.[9]

In these accounts, books did not function only as stimuli to inspiration. A common analogy was drawn between a book and the very mechanisms of the self. Radicals referred to an internal 'Book of Conscience', which was 'imprinted' by divine agency and then read by the mind. They claimed that some of them could thereby receive visions 'written by the Spirit of God upon the hearts of believers'.[10] So a vision was manifested by imprinting, or writing. But how exactly did this work? Again appropriating alchemical and Paracelsian sources, radicals referred above all to the importance of the *imagination*, or 'fancy', in representing images to the reason which could then be elaborated into knowledge. A vision, they suggested, was such an image, caused by supernatural intervention and perceived particularly vividly. Rogers gave more details. 'Uttered in *Dream, Trance, Voice,* or *Vision*', an inspiration could occur in one of two ways: it could either be mediated 'by the *senses* of the body, and so in some *visible* bodily shape', or bypass the external senses altogether, as during sleep. In the latter case subjects were 'taken up and *arrested* by the *intellectual* and *cognoscitive faculties* of their *soules*'.[11]

Visions were images in the imagination, produced supernaturally. Ironically, perhaps, such talk facilitated the conflation of sectarians with papists. Polemics against idolatry had long concentrated not only on material images, but on the idols of the mind, created by the imagination. An image of God 'feigned in the mind by imagination', the Puritan authority William Perkins had warned, 'is an idol'. Images liable to give rise to imaginings of bearded old men, in particular, were to be replaced with layouts of words which could act as their own mnemonics, that is, by printed Ramist schemes. And every Protestant was placed 'under the obligation to deal with his own imagery, to act the iconoclast on the idol-processes of his mind'.[12]

That idolatry was an internal matter raised a central question: how could one tell a true inspiration from a false one? In other words, how could one distinguish a vision from an idol of the imagination? This problem was often at the heart of anti-enthusiast polemics, which suspected either that enthusiasts' talk of inspiration was really evidence of madness or that it was deliberate imposture. The suggestion that visions appeared in the imagination was useful for such polemical purposes, too, since the imagination was well known to be unstable and capricious, the seat of 'distempers' affecting the mind. 'Without better evidence then their bare word', Joseph Sedgwick argued in 1653, 'we may modestly suspect that [enthusiasts' visions] are nothing but the distempers of a disaffected brain'.[13] He also alleged that other enthusiasts were not ill, but fraudulent, manifesting 'counterfeit inspiration'.[14] George Hickes agreed, defining enthusiasm as 'Spiritual drunkenness, or Lunacy'. It 'distemper[ed] the minds of men', he elaborated, 'with extravagant phancies'.[15] William Ramesay likewise opined that those who 'in their *Enthusiasm*' aspired to prophesy typically went mad.[16] The terminology of such attacks was deliberate: these were references to elementary, yet none the less consequential, knowledge about the human frame and the soul.

A major problem with such definitions was that they could become too broad. They threatened to outlaw much that their proponents wanted to retain as valid religiosity. Sedgwick, for instance, was prepared to acknowledge the importance (though not the necessity) of 'experience' for a minister, in much the sense in which Rogers used the word. Moreover, a notion of 'irradiation' was also important to Henry More's friend, Ralph Cudworth. Quite as much as Rogers's congregants, Cudworth went out of his way to reject the idea that religion was simply 'Book-craft'. Only when a spiritual truth was found 'within our selves' could we be said to be 'experimentally acquainted with it'.[17] 'All the Books and Writings which we converse with,' he insisted, 'can but represent Spiritual Objects to our understandings; which yet we can never see in their own true Figure, Colour and Proportion, until we have a *Divine Light* within, to irradiate and shine upon them.' Such irradiated representation could only happen in the imagination. Cudworth also defined holiness as 'nothing else but *God stamped* and *printed* upon the Soul'. Such language was strikingly similar to that of the very enthusiasts whom Cudworth, along with More, Sedgwick, Smith and Casaubon, wished to exclude. The point became a delicate one: to discriminate proper 'irradiation' from improper.[18]

Sir Thomas Browne provided one clue as to how to do this. He reckoned that grounds for discrimination lay in the mode of conveyance of candidate visions, alleging that the 'the revelations of heaven are conveied by new impressions, and the immediate illumination of the soul; whereas the deceiving spirit, by concitation of humors, produceth his conceited phantasmes'.[19] In other words, true visions partook of the immaterial soul. True inspiration could, in principle, bypass the terrene body altogether, although it did not have to do so; it always engaged at least partially with the immaterial soul. False visions, like ordinary perceptions of the outside world, relied on corporeal mediation, and therefore always arose in the body. They could never engage directly with the rational soul. Henry More likewise alleged that 'Enthusiasts for the most part are intoxicated with vapours from the lowest region of their Body', and his fellow Platonist John Smith agreed. Smith described false visions as 'seated only in the imaginative power', drawing upon Moses Maimonides to ascribe to this phenomenon the 'many enthusiastical impostors of our age'. This was no mere academic distinction: it suggested ways to discriminate in practice between true prophecy and self-idolatry. A false vision was one which could not 'rise up above this low and dark region of sense or matter'. Aristotelian reasoning straightforwardly implied that it must therefore always manifest conflict:

> from what hath been said ariseth one main characteristical distinction between the prophetical and pseudo-prophetical spirit, viz. That the prophetical spirit doth never alienate the mind, (seeing it seats itself as well in the rational as in the sensitive powers,) but always maintains a consistency and clearness of reason, strength,

and solidity of judgment, where it comes; it doth not ravish the
mind, but inform and enlighten it: but the pseudo-prophetical spirit,
if indeed, without any kind of dissimulation, it enters into any one,
because it can rise no higher than the middle region of man, which
is his fancy, there dwells as in storms and tempests, and being
αλογον τι in itself, is also conjoined with alienations and abruptions
of mind. For whensoever the phantasms come to be disordered,
and to be presented tumultuously to the soul, as it is either in a
μανια, 'fury', or in melancholy, (both which kinds of alienation are
commonly observed by physicians) or else by the energy of this
spirit of divination, the mind can pass no true judgment upon
them; but its light and influence becomes eclipsed.[20]

John Smith was not the only person to reckon that physicians were well
acquainted with the corporeal signs accompanying false inspiration.
Engagement with the very latest medical knowledge may have been rare
for both the radicals and their opponents, but reference to commonly
held beliefs about the structure of the body and a physician's role in
interpreting its signs recurred far more widely. By the end of the seventeenth-century, and probably before, such criteria constituted the main
resource for defining enthusiasm and visions.

This sort of knowledge was implicated in ideas about the proper
response to Scripture. That this was so rested on contemporary notions
of what reading itself actually was – of what happened in the mind and
the body when one confronted a written or printed page. Not just
radicals, and not just Platonists like More, found that such confrontation produced remarkable effects. Laudian polemicist and scholar Peter
Heylyn (to cite an example as far removed from both Rogers and More
as possible) found himself blinded by his reading. 'His *Brain* was like a
Laboratory', recalled his contemporaries, and had long been 'kept hot
with study' as he pored over books and papers. Hence 'his Brain, heated
with immoderate study, burnt up the Christaline humor of his Eyes'.
Others received less obvious, but still permanent, injuries. Robert Boyle
thought that he had never escaped the consequences of reading 'the
state adventures of *Amadis de Gaule*, and other fabulous stories' while
a schoolboy. These romances, Boyle recalled, 'prejudiced him, by unset-
tling his thoughts. [They] accustomed his thoughts to such a habitude
of roving, that he [had] scarce ever been their quiet master since'. The
poet Abraham Cowley, too, found that chancing upon a copy of Spenser
in his mother's parlour 'made [him] a Poet as immediately as a Child is
made an Eunuch'. Two generations later, the crypto-Jacobite virtuoso
John Byrom used laudanum to treat his sister, Ellen, for a peculiar
condition: according to his journal, 'it was their reading (for they were
reading Clarendon's history) that disturbed her'. The treatment proved
unsuccessful, and Ellen died. These are diverse incidents, traversing

place, time and social rank. Yet each illustrates a kind of impact that reading could have on an early modern human being. It could generate visions, whether divine and natural; it could determine your future character; it could blind you; and it could kill you. Strange though the series may seem, experiences like these were widely credited throughout the early modern period.[21]

That reading could have such effects was not only widely attested. It was also supported by contemporary knowledge about people and the physical world they inhabited. As Sir Thomas Browne put it, a human being was a 'great and true *Amphibium*': a soul forced to live in the alien environment of the body. It was therefore reasonable to consider all one's experiences, achievements and anxieties as simultaneously both physiological and psychological (that is, related to the soul) in character. This being so, how did contemporaries understand the effects which representations, especially printed representations, could and should have upon them? One way, widely applied, to approach such issues was to draw upon the best moral analysis of human beings then available: that in terms of the passions. John Hales, for one, reckoned that what distinguished sectarian 'schism' from 'necessary separation' (such as that of Protestantism from Catholicism) was that, though both manifested themselves in practices relating to the reading of Scripture, fundamentally the latter rested on 'weighed and necessary reasons' while the former depended on 'passion or distemper'.[22] What did such allegations mean?

A discourse of the passions

Recall Sir Thomas Browne's dictum about amphibia. To oversimplify rather drastically, physicians dealt with the body, ministers – 'spiritual physicians' – with the soul. Both, though, could and did feel themselves qualified to discourse of a branch of knowledge which, traversing the gulf separating body from soul, embraced *embodied* morality – the morality of amphibians. This was what they meant when they discoursed of the 'passions'. A large literature existed treating this subject in all its personal and social aspects – as large, probably, as that dealing with civility, and as profitable. René Descartes guessed that by its title alone his own account of the passions would sell better than any of his other works.[23]

As Bishop Edward Reynolds expressed it, introducing his own treatise on the passions, 'whereas the principall acts of mans Soule are either of Reason and Discourse, proceeding from his Understanding; or of Action and Moralitie, from his Will; both these, in the present condition of mans estate, have their dependance on the Organs and faculties of the Body'. This was the rationale underlying all discussion of the passions. With respect to the understanding, 'the whole Body is as an Eye, through which it seeth'; with respect to the will, the whole body was 'a Hand, by which it worketh'. This being so, the body, while it did not have an absolute dominion over reasoning, could exercise what Reynolds called a 'disturbing power'. Its distempers could alter the impressions perceived through the senses, and could distort habits of thinking.[24] That was why the interaction between body, reason and action was crucial to practical morality.

The word 'passion' had a specific meaning, and one which is rather alien to modern ears. Strictly speaking, passions were 'Apprehensions, resentments, or emotions of the Soul', caused by 'some motion of the spirits'. That is, they were motions of the sensitive (or sometimes the rational) soul, excited by and in response to impressions generated by the senses and other stimuli.[25] They were considered the main agencies directing human beings towards particular ends – not just unconscious or mechanical ends, like nutrition and self-preservation, but also more abstruse intellectual aims, such as the desire for knowledge or the contemplation of the self. Knowledge of the passions was therefore of fundamental importance. The philosophy of the passions, wrote Catholic priest Jean Senault, was the necessary foundation of all learning, since 'it is she that makes *Philosophers*, and which purifying their *understanding*, makes them capable of *considering* the wonders of *Nature*'. A man possessing thorough knowledge of his passions was in a good position to become 'an *honest man*, ... a good *Father* of a *family*, a wise *Politician*, and an understanding *Philosopher*'.[26]

These were large claims, and their justification was appropriately grand. For what made the passions problematic was nothing less than the post-lapsarian condition of humanity. Before the Fall, human senses had been in perfect harmony with nature, and so had 'made no false reports' to the mind. That had changed with the expulsion from Eden. Now, the senses were 'subject to a thousand illusions'. Guided by the passions generated from such illusions, the mind was almost certain to go wrong. '*False Opinions*,' according to royal physician Walter Charleton, were most often 'occasioned ... by our *Passions*'. Some correction must be provided, then, in order to achieve grace.[27]

We can characterize the issue facing such writers as a problem of knowledge. Given the essentially passionate composition of the post-lapsarian human frame, how did one distinguish true from false? Which imaginative images were accurate representations of the world, leading to a desire for beneficial objects, and which were merely 'representing as realy good, things that are so only in apparence'? We decided be-

tween the two by using our 'Understanding'. The rational soul alone
was capable of exercising this faculty (which was otherwise called
reason, right reason or the faculty of discerning). It was from this soul
that we derived 'all our *Knowledge*'.[28] The sensitive soul, though, mediated between this reasoning faculty and the body which provided its
perceptual data. It was the major seat of the passions, and a highly
unstable entity. It was subject to '*Tremblings, noddings, Eclipses, in-
equalities*, and disorderly *Commotions*' caused by the 'more violent
Passions', the most remarkable of which included both diseases and
'various impressions of sensible *Objects*'. Responding like fire to the
'fannings' of these passions, the sensitive soul would flare up (as in
anger or indignation) or fade (as in terror or grief), producing appropriate physical symptoms.[29] The rational soul could in principle intervene
– looking at impressions in the imagination as though in a mirror, it
could potentially correct their effects – but in practice one's reason was
likely to be subjugated to such phenomena.[30]

In effect, human beings contained two distinct 'faculties of *Knowing*':
the understanding, which was seated in the rational soul, and the imagination, which was seated in the sensitive. While the imagination alone
was sufficient to compound and divide sensations, thus forming ideas,
only the understanding could perform the essentially judicial processes
of constructing 'trains of notions convenient either to Speculation, or to
practice'. These 'royal prerogatives' meant that only the rational soul
was properly entitled to 'the whole *Encyclopaedia* or Zodiac of *Arts
and Sciences; Theology, Logic, Physic, Metaphysics, Mathematics, Al-
gebra, Geometry, Astronomy, Mechanics*'. All these sciences, with the
exception of theology, were properly regarded as 'the products or creatures of Mans *Mind*'. None the less, that mind still relied on the sensitive soul for the ideas with which it worked. Their relationship was
uneasy. In fact, it all too often degenerated into an '*intestin war*' on the
outcome of which rested the eternal fate of every individual human
being. If the sensitive soul won this internal civil war, then the 'divine
Politie' of the rational soul would be lost to 'triumphs of libidinous
carnality'.[31]

Since the rational soul was the seat of reason and could in principle
override the imagination, it might be thought almost certain to win this
war. In fact, writers like Walter Charleton considered this the less likely
outcome. They based this forecast on the fact that the rational soul,
although immaterial, depended fundamentally on the sensitive soul for
its information of the world. 'It is from the *Imagination* alone that she
takes all the representations of things, and the fundamental *Ideas*, upon
which she afterward builds up all her *Science*,' reported Charleton. Like
a monarch in Whitehall, the reason received 'intelligences' from the

senses in the imagination, and sent out from thence 'orders for government of the whole state of Man'. Moreover, since memory involved the repeated manifestation of images in the imagination, the mind was also dependent on the sensitive soul for this function. The corporeal character of such processes threatened to overturn the supremacy of reason itself. At the height of the internal civil war, indeed, the subject 'acted little less than like a Daemoniack possess'd with a Legion'.[32] That is he or she acted as if falsely inspired.

It was impossible to enumerate all the passions. Nevertheless, writers did frame a standard taxonomy. First, they recognized a division between *metaphysical* and *physical* passions, both of which were manifested by observable symptoms. Metaphysical passions were restricted to the rational soul, and were familiar to divines as the affections appropriate to religious contemplation. Physical passions, on the other hand, affected the sensitive soul only, and worked through material, effluvial mechanisms. As well as these two relatively simple types, though, there also existed what writers called *moral* passions. These were much more complex, since they engaged the body and the soul in concert. The first stage in generating this sort of passion occurred when the senses presented an image of a *'new* and *strange* object' to the soul, thus 'giv[ing] her hope of knowing somewhat that she knew not before'. Instantly the soul *'admire*[d]' this image. This admiration was the primary of all passions. The soul then entertained an 'appetite' to know the object better, 'which is called *Curiosity* or desire of Knowledge'. Curiosity was the second passion. On it depended all further intellectual inquiry – 'Whence it is manifest, that all natural *Philosophy*, and *Astronomy* owe themselves to this passion'. Based thus in the perceptive system of the body and in the sensitive soul, this passion was nothing less than 'the mother of knowledge'.[33]

Taxonomies of the passions then went on to recognize some six or seven simple varieties: admiration and curiosity were followed by love and hatred, desire, and joy and grief. All others were best regarded as compounds or species of these basic categories. And all had definite and distinctive physiological effects. Admiration of an object, for example, caused the animal spirits to be summoned to the imagination in the brain so that its image could be retained for prolonged contemplation. Spirits were also directed into the muscles holding the body in position and the eyes focused, so as to keep the organs in contact with the outside object. The heart and lungs were not generally affected, since knowledge was the only current objective. However, in extreme cases the withdrawal of spirits from the body could be enough to produce *'Stupor'*, and perhaps even catalepsy. A physician in Amsterdam had witnessed a dramatic example when a young Englishman repulsed by a would-be lover had been found 'congeal'd' in the same posture a day later.[34] The point was a general one: 'immoderate' passions were always harmful to the health, since they diverted the spirits from their normal duties in the body. That their physical symptoms were revelatory in normal circumstances but harmful in extreme ones was true of all the passions.

In such ways writers were able to link a wide variety of visible symptoms to the physiology of perception and imagination. Anger, for another example, resulted directly in agitation, palpitation, a burning feeling in the chest, distension of the veins, redness of the face, sparkling eyes, distortion of the mouth and grinding of teeth; in excess, it could lead to fevers, madness, apoplexy, epilepsy, convulsions, palsies, trembling and gout. All these symptoms were traced, via the passions, to processes involving the animal spirits and the circulation of the blood. They permitted early modern laypeople to become skilled interpreters of their neighbours' bodies. 'Men judg of meanings by actions,' observed Senault, 'and read in the eyes, and face, the most secret motions of the soul.' By the same token early modern laypeople also became accustomed to concealing and 'counterfeiting' their passions. Alcohol was a good way to circumvent such disguises: a drunk, John Earle said, was 'an *uncover'd man* ... the secretest parts of his soule lying in the nakedst manner visible: all his passions come out now'. Governing the passions was essential if one were not to be left vulnerable to observers able to deploy such skilled observation, and then employ what was called 'craft' to put their knowledge to evil ends. 'Craft', to be precise, was the perversion of prudence: it was knowledge of the passions dedicated to immoral ends.[35]

Passions could be generated either by sensations or by internal bodily states. The latter was certainly the case during diseases, and physicians possessed recognized remedies for such conditions. The juxtaposition, advanced by such writers as More, Sedgwick, Hickes and Smith, of enthusiastic 'visions' with the phenomena of madness and passionate 'vapours' capitalized on this. Angels, also, could manipulate images already present in the imagination in order to produce apparent visions (they could not generate new ones *de novo*). The generation of passions by external sensations was more complex. Visual perception, in particular, often seemed straightforwardly natural, as when one simply 'saw' a block of wood. But there were other cases in which some cultural conditioning must have been involved. Speaking, listening, writing and reading were such cases, in which perception must have been unconsciously abetted by conditioning. Writers discoursing of the passions did not ignore the implications of this. In such cases, they agreed, 'habits' had grown up in each individual human being. The motions of the animal spirits, and thence the imagination, in response to particular sensations had been regularized. In learning to speak, for example, the subject 'habituated' the motions of the spirits so that one only had to imagine what one wished to say, rather than specifying the individual movements of the body which made up speech. The 'habit' acquired in learning to speak, said Descartes, had 'taught us to joyn the action of the Soul, ... the tongue, and the lipps, with the signification of the words which follow out of these motions, rather than with the motions themselves'.[36] Similar habituation allowed a subject to understand without any conscious deciphering the words of others' speech, or, most pertinently for present purposes, to read them 'by the figure of their letters, when they are written'. Reading, like all perception, operated through a passion.[37]

Habituation provided a key to one of the major problems presented by the passions: that of exerting some practical 'Regulation' or 'mitigation' of them and their effects. Such action was regarded as essential for an English gentleman.[38] Habituation represented one's best hope of countering immoral, unhealthy or erroneous passions. There were two principal means by which this might be effected. First, the rational soul could imagine objects producing a contrary passion to the one experienced, thus eventually producing a habit separating the motions of the spirits from the impressions to which they would otherwise be consequent. Secondly, one could learn to delay one's response to an impression, perhaps by reciting the letters of the alphabet or the Lord's Prayer.[39] This would allow the turbulence of the spirits to recede, permitting the rational soul a more detached assessment. Either approach relied on embracing the interdependence of rational soul and animal spirits, rather than attempting to attain an unsustainable separation of reasoning from the body. In short, one could best avoid the deleterious effects of the passions by learning to exercise 'prudence'. Senault in fact proposed that the history of the arts and sciences constituted a series of 'documents' of the regulation of the imagination, urging that 'the government of Passions is of such importance, and so difficult, as the better part of sciences seem only to have been invented to regulate them'. Music had been invented to exert harmony; theatre and poetry likewise. Rhetoricians had originally acted as physicians, 'curing their auditors of all their maladies'. In short, a panoply of knowledge had been invented in the ancient world to subdue and direct the passions of the populace, and hence ensure a stable polity.[40]

There *were* ways in which the soul could be 'vindicated from the impression of the body'. The most effective of them was a sacred infusion of grace. Short of that, education and custom could mitigate the ill effects of the body. Hobbes thus made correct education essential for restraining the passions. On the other hand, John Webster argued (citing Thomas Willis) that an 'evil education' caused 'a most deep impression of the verity of the most gross and impossible things' to be 'instamped in [pupils'] fancies, hardly ever after in their whole life time to be obliterated or washt out'. This was true especially for subjects of melancholic disposition. It was a conventional enough opinion – and meshed perfectly with Boyle's diagnosis of his own reading of romances. But Webster applied it to ideas of sabbats, for example, alleging that they were 'effects of the imaginative function depraved by the fumes of the melancholick humor, as we might shew from the Writings of the most grave and learned Physicians'. Reading could serve the purpose. He even cited the case of a student who claimed that by the careful reading of sacred books he had been able to expel a devil out of his rear.[41]

The most systematic and thoroughgoing analysis of the political im- plications of such knowledge was to be found in the greatest of all discourses on the passions, Thomas Hobbes's *Leviathan*. Ward told Hobbes that his reasoning had 'never risen beyond imagination, or the first apprehension of bodies performed in the brain'.[42] He had a point, since the imagination and the passions played a central part in Hobbes's work. Since they stimulated all human actions, and no polity could ever reach such a state of perfection that they could be eradicated, the passions lay at the root of both social order and social disorder. Hobbes analysed the processes of reasoning, will and memory as dependent on them – understanding, for example, was achieved as the result of that well-known passion, the 'desire of Knowledge'.[43] And this account, as is well known, conditioned Hobbes's view of enthusiasm. Again appropri- ating the common interpretation of passions writers, Hobbes main- tained that the experience of a dream, along with false apparitions and spurious claims to prophecy, derived from the difficulty of distinguish- ing perceptions received from the outside world from imagined ones generated internally. Hobbes thus maintained that those who worshipped such non-existent spiritual beings were in effect idolaters, 'in awe of their own imaginations', and that the observable variety of such reli- gions in the world was but a simple consequence of 'the different Fancies, Judgements, and Passions'.[44] Madness, similarly, was 'nothing else, but too much appearing Passion', which could manifest itself in certain circumstances as 'inspiration'. Enthusiasts and madmen alike were liable to be 'cast out of Society' altogether, whence they existed in a state of 'perpetuall war, of every man against his neighbour'. That is, they occupied a position which was as close as Hobbes's contemporar- ies ever came to the state of nature – 'that miserable condition of Warre, which is necessarily consequent ... to the naturall Passions of men'. If unrestrained, 'singular Passions', Hobbes declared, became 'the Seditious roaring of a troubled Nation'.[45] This was why Hobbes pursued with such dedication the advocates of priestcraft and scholasticism. Their philosophy was merely 'a description of their own Passions', and therefore 'rather a Dream than a Science'. It thereby warranted claims to inspiration, whether by priests or sectaries, and led inexorably to civil war.[46]

Knowledge of the passions was widely available to the people of seventeenth- and eighteenth-century England, especially in the realm of medicine. The role of the imagination, in particular, became well known. 'There are many instances to be met with in physicians books', Robert Boyle noted, 'to shew, that imagination is able ... to alter the imagining person's body.' The effects of representing in the imagination images seen in print were also well known. Natural magic books and books of secrets suggested that would-be parents concerned to produce handsome children should place in their bedchambers 'images of *Cupid Adonis*, and *Ganymedes*, ... that they may alwayes have them in their eyes'. In the early seventeenth century, among the cases Richard Napier treated which centred on the imagination and the passions were many resulting from excessive reading, many of them concerning women whose brains had, like Heylyn's, overheated from the effort. They complained of insomnia, breathlessness, trembling, upset stomachs, vertigo, headaches, ringing ears, 'rising' sensations, swooning and general weakness.[47] Napier bombarded these women with the full battery of physical remedies available to an early modern physician: emetics, laxatives, bleeding, vomits, and the drugs recommended by Paracelsian writers, including opiates. Thomas Willis, too, found himself treating a man who had 'studied excessively and out of season', as a result of which his 'phantasy' denied him all serious reading and contemplation.

Analysis in terms of the passions had made enthusiasm an issue of knowledge about the body as well as the soul. In fact, questions of enthusiasm and inspiration became implicated in a series of researches into the body, begun in the 1650s and continued into the Restoration. The best way to convince an enthusiast or atheist, proclaimed William Dawes at the end of this period of experimentation, was to persuade him to anatomize himself: 'Let him consider his own wondrous make/ And, for a time, himself to pieces take.'[48] It is time to take this advice to heart, and examine the anatomy of visions.

Vision and visions

Talk of visions and inspiration implicated a complex set of ideas surrounding the passions. They, in turn, rested on widely available notions about perception and the body, and the relation of both to the soul. Seventeenth-century people were able to discuss the effects of reading Scripture or seeing images in terms of this material. The question raised by all this is, then, a fundamental one. It has in fact already been raised by Patrick Collinson. What was it in early modern England, Collinson asks, to 'see'? He insists that this 'is where an account of protestant culture ought to begin'.[49] In what follows it should become clear that Collinson, as so often, is right.

Seventeenth-century English Protestants had answers to Collinson's central question. They employed their answers in order to understand how seeing Scripture through the mechanisms of vision could give rise to visions. They described how it was that one perceived letters on a page; they analysed what it was that passed through the air and into the eye, and how it had an effect when it got there. They used these analyses to discriminate between true and false religiosity. As it were, antagonists to enthusiasm explained away visions by vision.

Their answers rested on a body of knowledge about optics and dioptrics which had been constructed over decades of looking at letters through eyes. Johannes Kepler, for example, following the anatomical researches of physician Felix Platter, had found that if one removed the crystalline humour from a specimen eye and looked through it at letters on a page, they could be seen clearly, enlarged by its magnifying power. This encouraged Kepler to place the faculty of vision in the retina, and to conceive the crystalline humour as a lens, the function of which was to focus rays of light from an observed object on to the retinal surface, there to 'paint' or 'imprint' its reversed image. For Kepler, the physiology of the eye thus became a matter for dioptrics. More specifically, he represented the eye as the natural equivalent of a *camera obscura*. This well-known device consisted of a darkened chamber with a pinhole in one wall. Light admitted through this hole from an object outside the chamber would form an inverted image of that object on the opposite wall. Kepler himself knew its properties well – when Sir Henry Wotton visited him on a mission from Francis Bacon, he found the Imperial Mathematician proudly displaying a painting which he had constructed using just such a camera. Kepler would sit inside its darkened chamber, tracing the image formed on a canvas stretched across the back wall, and rotating the whole apparatus when he wished to project a new segment of the outside landscape. In effect, Kepler the painter was sitting inside a model of the human eye.

The *camera obscura* analogy became the standard model for vision, common to writers who otherwise disagreed radically on the nature of light and its physics. Jesuit astronomer Christopher Scheiner was one who both constructed a model of the eye which could project images on to its 'retina' in precisely this way, and also saw the phenomenon 'most clearly' in a real human eye extracted from a cadaver.[50] Descartes agreed, saying that the identity could be demonstrated by 'taking the eye of a newly dead person', replacing the membranes at the back with a translucent material such as eggshell, and placing the reconstituted eye in the aperture hole of a *camera*. The attentive observer would then see, 'not perhaps without wonder and pleasure', a 'picture' of an outside object projected on to the eggshell in perfect perspective. At the end of the century Locke and Newton were still accepting the *camera obscura* as an accurate representation of the eye.[51]

But none of these authorities thought that the *camera obscura* was a complete account of visual *perception*. Kepler himself had realized that the 'picture' painted on the retina only became vision after it had passed 'through the continuity of the spirits' to the brain. Inside the brain there was then 'something, whatever it may be, which is called the common sense', on to which the image was 'impressed'.[52] Descartes presented the most influential account of this process, in the context of a general account of perception, as the transmission of a 'figure' through the nervous system and on to the common sense. According to this account, light was a pressure in the plenum of 'very subtle and very fluid matter' permeating the space between an object and the individual. This pressure generated an impression on the retina, which was instantly transmitted through the optic nerve to the common sense. In fact, Descartes declared, the body could be compared to the quill which he himself was using to write this very passage: no material substance passed from one end of the quill to the other, yet the movement of the feather in the air was determined by, and simultaneous with, the tracing of letters on the page. In the same way, the imagination was imprinted at the same instant as the organs, and in a way determined by the structure of the human body.[53]

Whenever the mind perceived an object, then, it was really considering an image mediated through the body. But that image could also have been produced by the imagination. Descartes insisted that the term 'idea' must therefore be applied to any such 'impressions', whether imaginative or perceptual. Either could give rise to physical actions.[54] *Camera obscura* models of vision therefore could not be as simple as their proponents had perhaps hoped: the involvement of the body and of the imagination meant that, far from having been rendered regular and even mathematical, a visual percept could be corrupted or counterfeited by the imagination, affections or prevailing exterior conditions. Qualifications to *camera obscura* models accordingly became necessary, and indeed routine. Della Porta, to whom the popularization of the *camera obscura* itself could plausibly be attributed, had noted that observers needed to be conditioned in order for the *camera* to work. One could not simply set it up and gaze at its images:

> you must stay a while, for the Images will not be seen presently: because a strong similitude doth sometimes make a great sensation with the sence, and brings in such an affection, that not onely when the senses do act, are they in the organs, and do trouble them, but when they have done acting, they will stay long in them: which may easily be perceived. For when men walk in the Sun, if they come into the dark, that affection continues, that we can see nothing, or very scantly; because the affection made by the light, is still in our eyes; and when that is gone by degrees, we see clearly in dark places.[55]

Descartes, too, observed that his anatomical demonstration worked only as long as the eye kept its 'natural' shape – 'for if you squeeze it just a little more or less than you ought, the picture becomes less distinct'.[56] Just what constituted proper 'squeezing' he left unclear. Later in the century, Isaac Newton warned that vision could be corrupted if the eye were either coloured, too 'plump', or not plump enough. Only in the proper circumstances, and only if the phenomena 'are not produced or altered by the power of imagination, or by striking or pressing the Eyes', could knowledge of colours be considered a Newtonian mathematical science. This he verified in a foolhardy series of self-experiments on his eye and his imagination. Vision now became part of a number of such experiments performed by Boyle and other virtuosi. A related case was that of William Briggs, whose theory of vision was designed to account for the construction by the imagination of one image out of the perceptual input from two eyes. It was demonstrated before the Royal Society, using sheep's eyes. As early as 1663, Wren had suggested that an artificial eye would be a good device for the Royal Society to exhibit to Charles II should the king deign to visit; such an eye was apparently made, but the king never came to see it.[57]

Acceptance of a *camera obscura* model therefore meant that to account for the construction of knowledge from perceptions one needed some appreciation of the 'affections' internal to the human constitution. The physical structure of the brain and nervous system played an essential part in the reception and manipulation of ideas. The most authoritative account of the physiology and neurology of vision and the passions came from Oxford, and the Sedleian Professor of Natural Philosophy, Thomas Willis. Willis undertook a series of dissections of the brain, news of which Henry Oldenburg spread across Europe. This work was to be of central importance to representations of reading.[58]

A convinced Anglican, Willis was engaged in what he called 'Psycheology', or the 'Discourse of the Soul'. He began from a belief in an at least twofold division of the soul, into a rational component, which was immaterial, immortal and intellectual, and a sensitive one, which was corporeal and mortal. The former could not be subjected to physiological study, but the latter could. As Willis conceived of it, this 'sensitive soul' played a wide range of roles. It was not confined to any particular organ, but 'Co-extended to the whole Body'. It conducted all the physical processes of perception and movement, acting through the vehicle of 'animal spirits' sublimed from the blood and channelled through the nervous system. These were the same spirits which transmitted perceptions to the common sense. They were like internal 'Rays of Light', Willis declared: 'For as light figures the Impressions of all visible things, and the Air of all audible things; so the Animal Spirits, receive the impressed Images of those, and also of Odors, and tangible Qualities.' Imagination and perception could thus be indistinguishable because they depended on this same vehicle.[59]

Willis wished to reveal anatomically the channels in which the spirits flowed, and thereby to identify physical features associated specifically with the functions of memory, imagination and the appetites. This required 'a new way of opening ye Brains'. Rather than producing horizontal sections through the head, Willis uncovered the brain layer by concentric layer, thereby revealing 'the order of Nature'.[60] The first structure encountered in this method, of course, was the skull. As a shield, the skull acted to 'restrain and keep within the Brain the Effluvia's of the animal Spirits, lest they should too thickly evaporate'. Indeed, so fine were they that certain intense passions could cause the spirits to escape from the head altogether. They then formed 'a sort of aetherial man' in the air. This liberated effluvial figure might be seen by others, and called a ghost. Spectres were one phenomenon amongst a cluster caused not by action at a distance, but by passion at a distance.[61]

Within the skull, Willis revealed to spectators the internal structures and channels in the *dura mater* and *pia mater*, and then in the brain itself. His audience could see the complex of vessels and folds guiding the circulation of animal spirits.[62] They could also perceive the vessels in which blood flowing into the brain was distilled to provide those spirits as a 'Chymical Elixir'. They could therefore trace the pathways of the imagination. A 'free and open space' above the callous body, at the base of the brain, was particularly important here. This was the common sensory. Here the animal spirits gathered and circulated, to be called upon to 'exercise the acts of the animal Faculties'. Their circulation made perception possible.[63]

Willis accepted the *camera obscura* theory of the eye. On seeing an object, an 'Optick Species' generated by the *camera* was transmitted, he held, through the optic nerves and into the brain. There a variety of things might happen. It might simply be reflected from the callous body back through the nervous system, yielding the sort of reflex action maintained even in sleep. But if it disturbed the spirits circulating in the common sense, then it gave rise to a passion. It could then pass further into the cortex, when 'it impresse[d] on it the image or character of the sensible Object'. This generated a memory.[64]

A passion produced in this way generated physical symptoms, since a 'fountain' of animal spirits flowed continuously from the head to the body, where it would 'irradiate' all its parts. 'As often as a violent passion … is conceived in the Brain', Willis remarked, its 'impression' would 'disturb' these spirits, and thence induce 'mutations in the Organs'. This was why someone subject to a fit of rage experienced radical changes in body temprature, heart rate, stomach functions, and so forth. Perception was thus part of a single continuing process. Seeing an object (and imagining one) could not be separated from the circulation of the blood and the state of the nervous system. The same system also underwrote the ability of seventeenth-century people to 'read' each other, decoding their passions by interpreting bodily signs.[65]

Physicians did not often get the chance to anatomize a real, flesh-and-blood enthusiast, let alone an atheist. One occasion on which they did arose in early 1657. The unfortunate subject was an ex-Leveller named Miles Sindercombe, who had been cashiered from the army by General Monck. Fired by political radicalism and atheistic zeal, not to mention underhand support from exiled royalists and Spanish papists, Sindercombe had gathered around him a band of desperate assassins and embarked on a reckless plot to murder Oliver Cromwell. The conspirators had rented a room in Hammersmith verging on the route regularly taken by the Protector's coach on its way to Hampton Court, and installed there an 'engine' of such ferocious ingenuity that it would, had it been used, have 'torn away Coach and person in it'. Failing in their primary mission, they had then attempted to burn down the palace of Whitehall, before finally being arrested. They were found to be carrying an array of advanced weapons technology which amazed their captors: 'scrued Pistols', for example, 'which upon triall, appear notable Instruments to do execution at a distance', and which could fire at the rate of 10–12 at a time 'a strange sort of long Bullets, in the nature of slugs'. Sindercombe had been given to carrying such weapons around 'in a Violl-Case', like some anachronistic Al Capone. His accomplice turned Protector's evidence, and, as the unease generated by the case provoked the first suggestions that Cromwell be offered the crown, Sindercombe himself was sentenced to death. Once interned in the Tower, he proved singularly unreceptive to the ministers who visited him. He maintained that the redemption bought by Christ's crucifixion would be universal in any case, and he told them that 'when man dieth the soule sleepeth with the Body'. Both were characteristic atheist tenets. The latter in particular was the 'wretched opinion of that sort of men whom wee (in English) call Soul-sleepers', explained *Mercurius Politicus* – an utterly unChristian doctrine, and one which purportedly conditioned its proponents to attempt 'any Treason, Sedition, or Assassination'.

In the event, Sindercombe cheated the London crowd of its spectacle. He died mysteriously the evening before his projected execution, leaving a note explaining that he 'would not have all the open shame of the world executed upon my Body'. This created a delicate problem for the authorities. In fact, Sindercombe's plot had seemed so extraordinary that there were already murmurs to the effect that it was largely fictitious: that Sindercombe was the dupe of a cunning and Machiavellian project to elevate the Protector into a monarch. His death, which cheated the crowd not only of the execution but also of the victim's all-important last speech on the scaffold, had to be shown not to have been murder. In the event, three separate groups of anatomists had to be employed before the required outcome could be found. The first discovered nothing; the second found injuries commensurate with a severe external injury to the head – hardly the right answer – and only with the third was a conclusion of suicide rendered possible. When, attended by witnesses including the physician Sir Richard Napier and the Anatomy Professor of Gresham College, Dr Ferne, the Wardens of the Surgeons' Company opened the head, they found Sindercombe's brain 'inflamed, red, and distended with Blood'. Around it they also observed 'much Extravasall, grumous, and clotted Blood, which they judged to be the effect of some very violent and preternaturall cause'. What was left of Sindercombe was convicted of self-murder, ritually paraded through the streets, and buried with a stake through his heart the end of which was left protruding from the ground as an emblem of terror.[66]

The wits then went to work. The day of Sindercombe's proclaimed suicide was a good one, Marchamont Nedham decided, for an 'Operation' of a different sort. Nedham envisaged an invasive analysis of the body politic to match that carried out on Sindercombe's own body: a radical surgical procedure aiming not just to understand, but to heal the diseases of the Commonwealth. The body politic, he explained, had been 'sorely afflicted with an infectious Itch of scribling political discourses'. This had been caused by 'a Salt humour first bottel'd in the Braine pan, and often breaking out at the fingers ends'. The magistrate had therefore decided to resort to desperate remedies, ordering the scribblers to 'the Hospital of the *Incurabili*', there 'to have their Sculls opened and searched with a long Sword'. On the appointed day, a 'celebrious meeting' took place at the hospital of 'Operators of all sorts and sizes': *'Surgeons, Apothecaries, Methodical Doctors, Quacks, Mountebanks, Leeches, Simplers, cunning Women, Midwives, Nurses, Chymists, Trepanners, Sow-guelders, and Druggers*, with all other the Appendants of the profound Mysterie.' Nothing must be left untried that might 'restore the wits of the Commonwealth'. Alas, its condition proved incurable. The next day, however – that is, the day of Sindercombe's actual autopsy – 'a jolly Crew of the Inhabitants of the Island of *Oceana*' arrived in town, in search of the reported treatment and headed by Harrington himself. In future weeks and months Nedham's *Mercurius Politicus* reported more and more such diseased figures turning up in search of a cure for their bodies politic: Hobbes, Thomas White, John Hall, even *Mercurius Politicus* himself. It provided an excellent excuse for Nedham to satirize all the alternative polities on offer in those fractious days. The anatomy of an atheist had been made the occasion for a comprehensive anatomy of politics.[67]

Enthusiasm, credit and the physiology of reading

Willis's work, technical though it was, proved influential. Gentlemen were exhorted to read it as a central part of their education. Charleton exploited Willis's findings in his treatments of the passions. The well-known anti-enthusiast Samuel Parker began to construct arguments based on neurology, while Robert Sharrock preached on the callous body. Henry More increasingly placed the passions at the centre of his analysis of enthusiasm, alleging that enthusiasm was a 'distemper': a physiological condition needing to be cured rather than exorcized or idolized. It was simply the consequence of an excess of 'ecstatical passion' coupled with an 'illusion of the imagination'.[68] While his own proferred physiology did not coincide with Willis's, which he regarded as materialist, More agreed with the Sedleian Professor that in practice reasoning could never be separated from corporeal perceptions, and must therefore always be prey to 'Phantasmes'. 'Thoughts', he believed, 'offer or force themselves upon the mind, ... according to the nature or strength of the complexion of our Bodies'. In some individuals, and in certain circumstances, imagined pictures were as strong as those sensed. An enthusiast's sensitive soul was well on the way to winning the microcosmic civil war: the *'Imaginative* facultie has the preheminence above the *Rationall'*.

Moreover, since enthusiasts effectively surrendered their reason to their passions, far from being emancipated by their 'visions', as they themselves claimed, they were in fact delivering themselves up to merely mechanical reflexes. Such a person became 'perfectly *Cartesius* his *Machina*'. More and Cudworth coined the term '*Neurospasts*' to describe such individuals: they were effectively 'Puppets' of the sensitive soul. However, More confessed that he himself had 'a natural touch of Enthusiasm in my complexion'. He had written and published Platonic poems which had seemed to 'affect *divine Visions*'. Was he then, as his magician opponent Thomas Vaughan claimed, 'sick of that Disease I would pretend to cure others of'? To establish the difference between his own experiences and the professed inspirations of the enthusiast, he recounted the dream he claimed to have had at the outbreak of the Civil War, and added a description of another dream, even closer to a '*Vision* or *Enthusiasm*', which had likewise arisen from his reading of Aristotle's *Mechanicks*. A description he had read there of a lever-based machine for timber-moving had raised such a 'Temper and frame of spirit' in him, he declared, that 'I should be prone to suspect something more then naturall in what preceded it, did I not consider that sometimes there may be of it self such a Terrour and Disposition of body, that may either suggest or imitate what is most holy or divine'.[69.]

Such an awareness of the power of reading to create visions through the mechanisms of the body was far from unique to More. Who could wonder that St Chrysostom had dreamt of St Paul, Sir Thomas Browne asked, since he read Paul's Epistles 'dayly'? These were 'butt animal visions'. In his own attack on enthusiasm, Meric Casaubon also concentrated on what he called 'the strange, but natural effects' produced by words. Metaphors, for example, worked by the 'representation of shapes and images' to the imagination – that is, they worked '*by a kind of Enthusiasme*'. Casaubon himself could testify that when he read a passage from a classical poet, 'I do not only phancy to my self, that I see those things that they describe; but also find in my self (as I phansy) the very same content and pleasure, that I should, if my eyes beheld them in some whether coloured, or carved representation of some excellent Artist'. The error of the enthusiast lay in attributing to such experiences the status of certain, even divine, truth. Such an error was at its most dangerous, needless to say, when what was being read was Scripture itself.[70]

Both Casaubon and More thus used accepted accounts of the effects of reading texts and images – accounts based in their knowledge of the passions – in order to characterize and attack enthusiasm. Enthusiasts were those who did not habituate their reading and their passions properly. Knowledge, civility and the history of reading intersected here, as More and Casaubon put their ideas of the nature and effects of reading to work in the most controversial of circumstances. And this had practical implications.

Casaubon agreed that enthusiasts were suffering from a medical condition: they should go to a 'Physician of the body'. But he did not want such a strategy to be too widely applied. In particular, Casaubon did not wish to deny the reality of demons. Those who had done so, he noted, had attempted to attribute *all* spirits, not just inspired ones, to 'a depraved fancy, or imagination'. They had pointed out 'how easily it may represent to it self Devils, and Spirits', which 'may make great impressions in the brain, and offer themselves in sleep, or when the brain is sick'. Casaubon insisted that demons did exist. They operated precisely by casting 'false *species*' into the imagination. In this he agreed with Willis, Glanvill and More. But he now found himself facing an epistemological problem. Like Browne, he believed that those doubting the existence of spirits were 'Atheists'. Yet such 'atheists' relied on almost exactly the same arguments from imagination and the passions which he himself employed to crush enthusiasts. The atheist relegated every spirit phenomenon to the imagination. But, demanded Casaubon, 'What hath he left to us, that we can call *truth*, if this be but phancy?'[71] This question – the question of what could still be trusted as truth, if experience was entirely subjected to the imagination – was fundamental.

It was especially fundamental when related to reading. Someone reading the Bible was using the eyes provided by God to 'satisfie himself and others' in matters of 'trust and consequence'. It was this that made the correct habituation of reading so important. But enthusiasts' reading practices were dangerous. Casaubon illustrated this by the example of the ancient bishop, Synesius. Synesius used to begin reading a text, then close his eyes and extrapolate from what he had read a passage so harmonious with the work that nobody listening could tell that he was no longer reading. 'It is likely that he often practised it by himself, before he adventured to do it before others,' Casaubon admitted, and the applauding audience probably did not know any more of the work being read than what they had just heard. None the less, 'what he so supplied by his extemporary wit, did sometimes prove to be the very same that he found afterwards in the book'. And that 'may very properly be referred to some kind of *enthusiasme*'.[72] This display of reading, indeed, captured the fundamentals of enthusiasm: deceit, prodigy and display.

Enthusiasts credited books too readily, thus falling foul of the sort of strong impressions which had caused More's dream (and Rogers's). By contrast, in Casaubon's world books were *not* necessarily trustworthy. Every writer was prone to believe, and even to produce, 'lyes, or frauds', if convinced that the end justified doing so, and the realm of print reflected as much. 'What a world of lyes and counterfeit books' had 'the conceit of *piae fraudes*' produced. And 'how many have been gulled and deceived by them, who doth not know, or hath not heard?' Reading must therefore be not a passive imprinting on the mind – the writing of a supposedly divine spirit – but active and critical *labour*. There was no labour more noble and advantageous than that devoted to spotting and revealing false books.

Moreover, this labour took enormous skill in obscure languages, customs and fashions. That was why Casaubon questioned the faith placed by some of his contemporaries in experimental philosophy. Shapin has convincingly analysed experimentalism in terms of the strategies of credit pursued by its practitioners. They were centrally concerned with problems of testimony and experience. This chapter ends with the credit of dreams and the credit of books interlaced with that of people. For Casaubon believed that those who (he claimed) advocated reducing all knowledge to that produced through 'natural experiments' ran the risk of losing the skill needed to ward off enthusiastic reading habits. There would then be no way to discriminate between 'Oracles' and 'abominable forgeries', and to ward off the imaginative effects of the latter. Unlike More, then, when Casaubon exploited his own experiences to expose enthusiasm he recalled, not a dream derived *from* a book, but a direct, industrious confrontation *with* a book. He described his own encounter with a work on Etruscan antiquities. Casaubon had come across this book in a shop in London. Its engravings had been so impressive that he all but lost control of his body: 'the first sight of the book did so ravish me,' he affirmed, 'that I scarce knew where I was, or what I did.' Had he left things at that, the result might have been similar to the experiences of More and Rogers. Instead, buying the volume, Casaubon began to read it as he embarked on a boat for Gravesend. Before long he had realized his mistake. 'The truth is, when once the heat or violence of my expectation (which did almost transport me) was once over,' he recalled, 'I began to wonder at my self.' In truth, every line of the work was fraudulent. But the point was that many other readers did credit it, to the extent, apparently, of going to Italy to see the monuments it purported to represent. That indicated how 'prone' people were, not only to 'entertain an imposture', but to resist its overthrow thereafter. 'What wonder then,' Casaubon asked, 'if *Christianism* was so soon turned into *Mahometism*', when so little skill existed 'to discover the impostures of pretended *Enthusiasts*?' The implication of his own experience when confronting the Etruscan forgery was, then, both clear and immense. 'Had these *Antiquities* been received generally, as a true piece,' Casaubon warned, 'half the world would have been Conjurers, and *Enthusiasts* by this time.'[73]

Notes

1. J. Rogers, [Hebrew] *Ohel or Beth-shemesh*, London, 1653, pp. 419–38. Rogers would gain MDS in Oxford and Utrecht.

2. [H. More], *Enthusiasmus Triumphatus, or, A Discourse of the Nature, Causes, Kinds, and Cure, of Enthusiasme*, Cambridge, 1656, pp. 309–12.

3. [More], *Enthusiasmus Triumphatus*, pp. 1–2; M. Casaubon, *A Treatise Concerning Enthusiasme*, London, 1655, pp. 3, 17.

4. Rogers, *Ohel*, pp. 354–5, 362, ("Expermental": *sic*).

5. Rogers, *Ohel*, pp. 396–8, 398–9, '390'–402, 407, 409, 411–12, '2' (new pagination), '9'–'10', 413–14. Margaret Aston describes the articulation of death and resurrection as a motif in iconoclasm: M. Aston, *England's Iconoclasts. I: Laws Against Images*, Oxford, 1988, p. 460.

6. J. Turner, *Choice Experiences of the Kind Dealings of God Before, In and After Conversions*, London, 1653, pp. 11–13, 49–58, 64. For Turner's insistence on searching the Scriptures and trying doctrine by the Bible, see also ibid., pp. 82–3, 86, 198.

7. This is adumbrated in R.W.F. Kroll, *The Material Word: Literate Culture in the Restoration and Early Eighteenth Century*, Baltimore, 1991.

8. E.g. G. Hickes, *The Spirit of Enthusiasm Exorcised*, London, 1680, sig. A2ᵛ, pp. 37–9; R. Baxter, *A Holy Commonwealth*, W. Lamont (ed.), Cambridge, 1994, p. 31; [W. Ramesay], *The Gentlemans Companion*, London, 1672, pp. 19, 21.

9. N. Smith, *Perfection Proclaimed: Language and Literature in English Radical Religion, 1640–1660*, Oxford, 1989, pp. 5, 11, 13–17; N. Smith, 'The Charge of Atheism and the Language of Radical Speculation, 1640–1660,' in M. Hunter and D. Wootton (eds), *Atheism from the Reformation to the Enlightenment*, Oxford, 1992, pp. 131–58, esp. pp. 157–8. Some radicals even displayed themselves as contracting 'divinely instituted madness': N. Smith, *Perfection Proclaimed*, pp. 26–9, 32–5, 38–9, 50, 56, 57n.117. For other examples see Turner, *Choice Experiences*, pp. 36–8; J. Henry, 'The Matter of Souls: Medical Theory and Theology in Seventeenth-Century England,' in R. French and A. Wear (eds), *The Medical Revolution of the Seventeenth Century*, Cambridge, 1989, pp. 87–113, esp. pp. 89, 95.

10. Smith, *Perfection Proclaimed*, pp. 73–8. For an example of the analogy of printing in the heart, see Rogers, *Ohel*, pp. 375–6.

11. Rogers, *Ohel*, pp. 449–50.

12. Aston, *England's Iconoclasts*, pp. 452–66, esp. p. 460 (italics added). For details of the production, origin and use of images in frontispieces and broadsheets, see T. Watt, *Cheap Print and Popular Piety, 1550–1640*, Cambridge, 1991, esp. pp. 131–216, 217–53.

13. J. Sedgwick, *A Sermon, Preached at St. Marie's in the University of Cambridge May 1st, 1653. Or, An Essay to the Discovery of the Spirit of Enthusiasme*, London, 1653, pp. 5–6.

14. Sedgwick, *Sermon*, pp. 1, 31.

15. Hickes, *Spirit of Enthusiasm*, p. 2.

16. [Ramsesay], *Gentlemans Companion*, pp. 40–1.

17. Sedgwick, Επισκοτθ Διδακλικοζ. *Learning's Necessity to an Able Minister*, London and Cambridge, 1653: bound and paginated with Sedgwick,

Sermon, p. 51; R. Cudworth, *A Discourse Concerning the True Notion of the Lord's Supper*, 3rd edn, London, 1676, pp. 39–41.

18. Cudworth, *Discourse*, pp. 52, 55. Hickes was an exception, since he repudiated the need for any sort of inspiration at all: Hickes, *Spirit of Enthusiasm*, pp. 34–5.

19. T. Browne, *Pseudodoxia Epidemica*, 2nd edn, London, 1650, p. 30.

20. H.G. Williams (ed.), *Select Discourses by John Smith*, 4th edn, Cambridge, 1859, pp. 194–6, 200–1; Henry, 'The Matter of Souls', pp. 92–5, 98–100; H. Schwartz, *Knaves, Fools, Madmen, and that Subtile Effluvium: A Study of the Opposition to the French Prophets in England, 1706–1710*, Gainesville, FA, 1978, pp. 31–70, esp. pp. 50–1.

21. J. Barnard, *Theologo-Historicus: Or, the True Life of the Most Reverend Divine, and Excellent Historian Peter Heylyn*, London, 1683, pp. 258–64; G. Vernon, *The Life of the Learned and Reverend Dr. Peter Heylyn*, London, 1682, pp. 6–7; *The Works of Mr. Abraham Cowley*, 8th edn, London, 1684, pp. 143–4; R. Parkinson (ed.), *The Private Journal and Literary Remains of John Byrom*, 2 vols in 4, Manchester, 1854–57, vol. I, pp. 46–8. Other examples are provided in C. Condren, 'Casuistry to Newcastle: "The Prince": in the World of the Book', in N. Phillipson and Q. Skinner (eds), *Political Discourse in Early Modern Britain*, Cambridge, 1993, pp. 164–86.

22. C.A. Patrides (ed.), *Sir Thomas Browne: The Major Works*, Harmondsworth, 1977, pp. 103–4, 129; *The Works of the Ever Memorable Mr. John Hales of Eaton*, 3 vols, Glasgow, 1765, vol. I, p. 116.

23. R. Descartes, *The Passions of the Soule in three Books*, London, 1650, sig. B3^v. For the notion of ministers as 'spiritual physicians' see, for example, M. Heyd, 'The Reaction to Enthusiasiam in the Seventeenth Century: Towards an Integrative Approach', *Journal of Modern History*, 53 (1981), 258–80, esp. 277–8.

24. E. Reynolds, *A Treatise of the Passions and Faculties of the Soule of Man*, London, 1640, pp. 3–5.

25. Descartes, *Passions*, p. 23.

26. J.F. Senault, *The Use of Passions*, trans. Henry, Earl of Monmouth, London, 1649, sig. C^v; Kroll, *The Material Word*, pp. 219–23.

27. [W. Charleton], *Natural History of the Passions*, London, 1674, sig. [A3^r]; Senault, *Use of Passions*, sigs. C2^r–C4^r, pp. 61, 105.

28. [Charleton], *Natural History of the Passions*, sigs [A3^v]–[A4^r], pp. 2–3.

29. [Charleton], *Natural History of the Passions*, sigs [A4^v] ff, sigs bb4^v–[bb5^r] (where Charleton cites Bacon, Hammond, Gassendi and Willis in support of his opinion of the soul), pp. 9–10, 22–5.

30. [Charleton], *Natural History of the Passions*, pp. 30–2; Descartes, *Passions*, pp. 7–14, 20.

31. [Charleton], *Natural History of the Passions*, sig. [A4^v]ff, pp. 48–50, 54–9.

32. [Charleton], *Natural History of the Passions*, pp. 62–4, 86–7; Descartes, *Passions*, pp. 25–9, 33–5; T. Willis, *Two Discourses Concerning the Soul of Brutes, Which Is That of the Vital and Sensitive of Man*, trans. S. Pordage, London, 1683, p. 43.

33. [Charleton], *Natural History of the Passions*, pp. 75–89, 164. See also the similar genealogies in Descartes, *Passions*, pp. 47–55, and [Ramesay], *Gentlemans Companion*, pp. 139–82.

34. [Charleton], *Natural History of the Passions*, pp. 89–91.
35. [Charleton], *Natural History of the Passions*, pp. 113–14, 159ff; Descartes, *Passions*, pp. 88–90; Senault, *Use of Passions*, pp. 159–62; [J. Earle], *Micro-Cosmographie, or, A Peece of the World Discovered* (5th ed) London, 1629, s.v. 'A Drunkard'; [W. Charleton], *A Brief Discourse Concerning the Different Wits of Men*, London, 1669, pp. 31–2, following Thomas Hobbes, *Leviathan*, ed. C.B. Macpherson, Harmondsworth, 1985; this edition reprints the original text of 1651, pp. 137–9. See also pp. 40–6 for citation of Willis on the site of the soul and the mechanisms of perception. For the practices of prudence see S. Shapin, *A Social History of Truth: Civility and Science in Seventeenth-Century England*, Chicago, 1994.
36. H. Lawrence, *An History of Angells*, London, 1649.
37. '[Les] parties du corps ... ne sentent tous, à proprement parler, que par une passion': Descartes, 'Règles pour la Direction de l'Esprit', in F. Alquié (ed.), *Oeuvres Philosophiques*, 3 vols, Paris, 1963–73, vol. I, pp. 67–204, esp. p. 136; Descartes, *Passions of the Soule*, pp. 43–4.
38. [Ramesay], *Gentlemans Companion*, pp. 183–214, esp. p. 183.
39. Descartes, *Passions*, pp. 36–7, 171; [Charleton], *Natural History of the Passions*, pp. 182–5; [Ramesay], *Gentlemans Companion*, pp. 184–5.
40. Senault, *Use of Passions*, pp. 105, 165–73. For Hobbes on the possibility of 'imprinting' passions on the mind of an audience, see *Leviathan*, pp. 142, 177.
41. Reynolds, *Treatise*, pp. 8–10; Hobbes, *Leviathan*, pp. 717–18; J. Webster, *The Displaying of Supposed Witchcraft*, London, 1677, pp. 32–4, 313, 321–2, 343–5.
42. [S. Ward], *A Philosophicall Essay Towards an Eviction of the Being and Attributes of God*, Oxford, 1652, sig. A3ᵛ–[A4ʳ]. For *Leviathan* and the passions see also N. Smith, *Literature and Revolution in England, 1640–1660*, New Haven, 1994, pp. 159–62.
43. Hobbes, *Leviathan*, pp. 85–90, 93, 100, 108–9, 118–34, 139, 147–8, 160–1, 297–8.
44. Hobbes, *Leviathan*, pp. 91–3, 168, 172.
45. Hobbes, *Leviathan*, pp. 134–42, 209, 214–16, 223, 266, 272, 317.
46. Hobbes, *Leviathan*, pp. 150, 241, 686.
47. R.G. Frank, 'Thomas Willis and his Circle: Brain and Mind in Seventeenth-Century Medicine', in G.S. Rousseau (ed.), *The Languages of Psyche: Mind and Body in Enlightenment Thought*, Berkeley, 1990, pp. 107–46, esp. p. 141; T. Willis, *The Remaining Medical Works of that Famous and Renowned Physician Dr. Thomas Willis*, trans. S. Pordage, London, 1681, p. 134; Robert Boyle, *The Works of the Honourable Robert Boyle*, ed. T. Birch, 5 vols, London, 1705–66, vol. II, pp. 174–6; R. James, *A Medicinal Dictionary*, 3 vols, London, 1743–45, s.v. 'IMAGINATIO'; Browne, *Pseudodoxia Epidemica*, p. 277; J.B. Porta, *Natural Magick*, London, 1658, pp. 53–4; M. MacDonald, *Mystical Bedlam: Madness, Anxiety, and Healing in Seventeenth-Century England*, Cambridge, 1981, pp. 174, 181–3, 185–6, 288 n.59. For women's experiences of illness and remedies see also L.M. Beier, *Sufferers and Healers: The Experience of Illness in Seventeenth-Century England*, London, 1987, ch. 8. For the construction of passions and sensibility in the eighteenth century, see also

G.J. Barker-Benfield, *The Culture of Sensibility: Sex and Society in Eighteenth-Century Britain*, Chicago, 1992, pp. 1–36.

48. [W. Dawes], *An Anatomy of Atheism*, London, 1694, pp. 5, 21–2.

49. P. Collinson, *The Birthpangs of Protestant England: Religious and Cultural Change in the Sixteenth and Seventeenth Centuries*, Basingstoke, 1988, p. 122. An interesting examination of the physiology of viewing for a slightly earlier period is D. Summers, *The Judgment of Sense: Renaissance Naturalism and the Rise of Aesthetics*, Cambridge, 1987.

50. J. Kepler, *Ad Vitellionem Paralipomena*, Frankfurt, 1604, pp. 176–7; S.M. Straker, 'Kepler's Optics: A Study in the Development of Seventeenth-Century Natural Philosophy' PhD thesis, University of Indiana, 1970, pp. 425, 450–60; A.C. Crombie, 'Expectation, Modelling and Assent in the History of Optics – II: Kepler and Descartes', *Studies in History and Philosophy of Science*, XXII (1991), 89–115; Porta, *Natural Magick*, pp. 363–5; C. Scheiner, *Rosa Ursina*, 1626–30, vol. II, pp. 23, 110–12 (cited in Crombie, 'Expectation', 106).

51. J. Cottingham, R. Stoothoff and D. Murdoch, trans. and eds, *The Philosophical Writings of Descartes*, 3 vols, Cambridge, 1985–91, vol. I, p. 166; I. Newton, *Opticks*, London, 1704, pp. 9–11; J. Locke, *An Essay Concerning Human Understanding*, London, 1689. Compare S. Alpers, *The Art of Describing: Dutch Art in the Seventeenth Century*, Chicago, 1983, pp. 50–1.

52. J. Kepler, *Dioptrice*, 1611, pp. 372–3 (cited in Crombie, 'Expectation', p. 103).

53. R. Descartes, 'Rules for the Direction of the Mind', in Cottingham, Stoothoff, Murdoch (eds), *Philosophical Writings*, vol. I, pp. 39–42, 152–6.

54. Cottingham, Stoothoff, Murdoch (eds), *Philosophical Writings*, vol. I, pp. 42, 105–6.

55. Porta, *Natural Magick*, p. 363.

56. Cottingham, Stoothoff, Murdoch (eds), *Philosophical Writings*, vol. I, p. 167.

57. Newton, *Opticks*, pp. 9–11; R.S. Westfall, *Never at Rest: A Biography of Isaac Newton*, Cambridge, 1980, pp. 93–5; S.J. Schaffer, 'Self Evidence', *Critical Inquiry*, 18 (1992), 327–62; S.J. Schaffer, 'The body of natural philosophers in Restoration England', in C.J. Lawrence and S. Shapin (eds), *Bodies of Knowledge*, Chicago, 1997; W. Briggs, *Ophthalmo-Graphia*, Cambridge, 1676, pp. 73–4; W. Briggs, *Nova Visionis Theoria*, London, 1685; T. Birch, *The History of the Royal Society of London*, 4 vols, London, 1756–7, vol. I, pp. 288–91, 391; vol. IV, pp. 136, 137, 203.

58. T. Willis, 'The Anatomy of the Brain' and 'The Description of the Nerves', in *Remaining Medical Works*, pp. 55–136, 137–92. For the circumstances surrounding this work see K. Dewhurst, *Thomas Willis's Oxford Lectures*, Oxford, 1980, pp. 37–49, 52ff; Robert G. Frank, 'Thomas Willis', in *Dictionary of Scientific Biography*, ed. C.C. Gillespie, 16 vols, New York, 1970–80, vol. 14, pp. 404–9; W.F. Bynum, 'The Anatomical Method, Natural Theology, and the Functions of the Brain', *Isis*, LXIV (1973), 444–68, and R.G. Frank, *Harvey and the Oxford Physiologists: A Study of Scientific Ideas*, Berkeley, 1980; Birch, *History of the Royal Society*, vol. I, pp. 416, 421–2, 436, 444; A.R. Hall and M.B. Hall (eds), *The Correspondence of Henry Oldenburg*, 13 vols, Madison and London,

1965–86, vol. II, pp. 141–5, 300–9, 631–3; G.S. Rousseau, 'Nerves, Spirits and Fibres: Towards Defining the Origins of Sensibility', *Studies in the Eighteenth Century*, III (1976), 137–57; G.S. Rousseau, 'Science and the Discovery of the Imagination in Enlightened England', *Eighteenth-Century Studies*, III (1969), 108–35; J. Mullan, 'Hypochondria and Hysteria: Sensibility and the Physicians', *The Eighteenth Century: Theory and Interpretation*, XXV (1984), 141–74; C. Lawrence, 'The Nervous System and Society in the Scottish Enlightenment', in B. Barnes and S. Shapin (eds), *Natural Order: Historical Studies of Scientific Culture*, Beverly Hills, 1979, pp. 19–40.

59. Willis, *Two Discourses*, sigs. [A3]ᵛ–[A4]ᵛ, pp. 5, 23–4, 38ff.

60. Willis, *Remaining Medical Works*, pp. 55–62, 91, 95–7; Willis, *Two Discourses*, pp. 23–5, 33, 75–86; H. Isler, *Thomas Willis, 1621–1675*, New York: Hafner, 1968, p. 25.

61. Willis, *Remaining Medical Works*, pp. 56, 77–8; Dewhurst, *Willis's Oxford Lectures*, pp. 125–6; Isler, *Willis*, p. 159.

62. Willis, *Remaining Medical Works*, pp. 57–62, 81.

63. Willis, *Remaining Medical Works*, pp. 79–80, 82–3, 87–8, 91–3. See also Dewhurst, *Willis's Oxford Lectures*, pp. 65–7, 93, 138–45.

64. Willis, *Two Discourses*, pp. 33, 35–6, 77–8; Willis, *Remaining Medical Works*, pp. 63–4, 96, 139–40; Dewhurst, *Willis's Oxford Lectures*, pp. 54–6.

65. Willis, *Remaining Medical Works*, pp. 80, 84–5, 89, 95–6, 101–4, 108–17, 134–6, 140–3; Dewhurst, *Willis's Oxford Lectures*, pp. 145–50; T. Willis, *De Anima Brutorum quae hominis vitalis ac sensitiva est, exercitationes duae*, Oxford, 1672, pp. 154–65; Willis, *Two Discourses*, pp. 55–60; Dewhurst, *Willis's Oxford Lectures*, p. 100; Frank, 'Thomas Willis', p. 134.

66. *Mercurius Politicus*, 345 (22 January 1657), 7541–3; 347 (5 February 1657), 7561–2, 7575–6; 348 (12 February 1657), 7587–92; 349 (19 February 1657), 7604–8; M. Hunter, 'Science and Heterodoxy: An Early Modern Problem Reconsidered', in D.C. Lindberg and R.S. Westman (eds), *Reappraisals of the Scientific Revolution*, Cambridge, 1990, pp. 437–60, esp. pp. 440–3; Henry, 'The Matter of Souls', p. 96. Sindercombe's explanation reminds us that the ritual of execution inscribed the nature of the crime on the body of its victim: see P. Hammond, 'The King's Two Bodies: Representations of Charles II', in J. Black and J. Gregory (eds), *Culture, Politics and Society in Britain, 1660–1800*, Manchester, 1991, pp. 13–48, esp. p. 38. For Sindercombe, see also: D. Underdown, *Royalist Conspiracy in England 1649–1660*, New Haven, 1960, pp. 192–4; A. Marshall, *Intelligence and Espionage in the Reign of Charles II, 1660–1685*, Cambridge, 1994, pp. 285–7, 290; M. MacDonald and T.R. Murphy, *Sleepless Souls: Suicide in Early Modern England*, Oxford, 1990, pp. 48, 104, 226.

67. *Mercurius Politicus* 352 (12 March 1657), 7641–4; 353 (19 March 1657), 7657–9; 354 (26 March 1657), 7673–5.

68. [Ramesay], *Gentlemans Companion*, pp. 127–9; Frank, *Harvey and the Oxford Physiologists*, pp. 182–3; H. More, 'The Immortality of the Soul', in H. More, *A Collection of Several Philosophical Writings of Dr. Henry More*, 4th edn, London, 1712, sig. [L14]ᵛ, Casaubon, *Treatise*, pp. 28–9, 211; [More], *Enthusiasmus Triumphatus*, sigs [A5]ᵛ–[A6]ᵛ, 2–20; M.

Casaubon, *Of Credulity and Incredulity, in things Natural, Civil, and Divine*, London, 1668, pp. 29–30. For More's appropriation of Descartes in the fight against enthusiasm see A. Gabbey, '*Philosophia Cartesiana Triumphata*: Henry More (1646–1671)', in T.M. Lennon, J.M. Nicholas and J.W. Davis (eds), *Problems of Cartesianism*, Kingston, 1982, pp. 171–250.

69. T. Tryon, *A Treatise of Dreams and Visions*, 2nd edn, London, 1695, pp. 9, 20, 44, 48–51, 203–4. [More], *Enthusiasmus Triumphatus*, pp. 2–5, 27 40–1, 43–6, 50–1, 294–5, 309, 312–6; More, *Collection of Several Philosophical Writings*, pp. x, 132–3; R. Cudworth, *A Discourse Concerning the True Notion of the Lord's Supper*, 3rd edn, London, 1676, p. 64; N. Ingelo, *Bentivoglio and Urania, in Six Books*, 4th edn, London, 1682, p. 91. Compare [J. Trenchard], *The Natural History of Superstition*, London, 1709, pp. 12–14. See also A. Gabbey, 'Cudworth, More, and the Mechanical Analogy', in R. Kroll, R. Ashcraft and P. Zagorin (eds), *Philosophy, Science and Religion in England 1640–1700*, Cambridge, 1992, pp. 109–27. For conflicts between More and Willis see Henry, 'The Matter of Souls'.

70. Patrides (ed.), *Sir Thomas Browne*, p. 476. Casaubon, *Treatise*, pp. 135ff, 150–1, 170ff, 175–6, 182–4.

71. Casaubon, *Of Credulity and Incredulity*, pp. 29–30, 38, 44; Reynolds, *Treatise*, p. 27; Thomas Willis, 'An Essay of the Pathology of the Brain and Nervous Stock', in *Dr. Willis's Practice of Physick*, London, 1684, separately paginated, 43–4; Patrides (ed.), *Sir Thomas Browne*, p. 98. For insistence on the reality of witchcraft, compare J. Glanvill, *Saducismus Triumphatus*, 2nd edn, London, 1682, pp. 25–6.

72. Casaubon, *Treatise*, pp. 160–1. For the use of books to create atheism, and the attribution of miracles to the imagination, see M. Hunter, '"Aikenhead the Atheist": The Context and Consequences of Articulate Irreligion in the Late Seventeenth Century', in Hunter and Wootton (eds), *Atheism*, pp. 221–54.

73. Casaubon, *Treatise*, p. 160; Casaubon, *Of Credulity and Incredulity*, pp. 294–300; Steven Shapin, *A Social History of Truth: Civility and Science in Seventeenth-Century England*, Chicago, 1994, *passim*. The work in question was C. Inghiramius, *Ethruscarum Antiquitatum Fragmenta*, Frankfurt, 1637; it was exposed in L. Allatius, *Animadversiones in Antiquitatem Etruscarum Fragmenta*, Paris, 1640; 2nd edn, Rome, 1642. Casaubon also identified as an important example Annius of Viterbo, who has recently been studied by Grafton as a key figure in the history of both forgery and criticism: 'Traditions of Invention and Inventions of Tradition in Renaissance Italy', in A. Grafton, *Defenders of the Text: The Traditions of Scholarship in an Age of Science, 1450–1800* (Cambridge, MA, 1991), pp. 76–103. Compare Sedgwick, *Sermon*, for stress on the need for 'industry' in reading Scripture. For a slightly later example, compare also [Trenchard], *Natural History of Superstition*, pp. 8–9, 28, on the effects of the 'Forgeries of the Papists, and the Frauds and Follies of some who call themselves Protestants'. Such falsities could not have enjoyed so great a success, Trenchard felt, 'unless something in our Constitutions made us easily to be susceptible of wrong Impressions'. So he felt that 'it is incumbent upon us, first of all to examine into the frame and constitution of our own Bodies'. Trenchard described from this how

'a poor Enthusiast with his Brains intoxicated with reading the Revelations' could seem to make 'a lucky discovery that the last Day is at hand'.

CHAPTER SEVEN

Piety, Physic and Prodigious Abstinence

Simon Schaffer

Wherefore have we fasted, say they, and Thou seest not? Wherefore have we afflicted our soul, and Thou takest no knowledge? Behold, ye fast for strife and debate: ye shall not fast as ye do this day, to make your voice to be heard on high.

(*Isaiah* 57: 3–4)

The miraculous chameleon

Dr Thomas Browne's *Pseudodoxia epidemica*, produced in several versions between 1646 and 1672, was a remarkable confrontation between erudite Christian humanism and vulgar beliefs. It was directed not to 'the people whom Bookes doe not redresse and are this way incapable of reduction, but unto the knowing and leading part of Learning'. A good example of the Norwich physician's method was his criticism of the general opinion that 'the Chameleon liveth onely upon ayre'. The chameleon's anatomy visibly possessed the appartus for nutrition and 'the wisedome of God' dictated that no part should be useless, so the fact was improbable. Indeed it was impossible, since though air could sustain flame it could not feed living matter. The opinion had gained ground merely because the chameleon so often held its mouth open and was certainly 'a very abstemious animal'. Then at the end of this essay on the chameleon Browne suddenly turned his attention to episodes of remarkable human fasts. He conceded at once that the humours of some might let them survive without food: 'wee read of many who have lived long time without aliment, and beside deceites and impostures there may be veritable Relations of some, who without a miracle, and by peculiarity of temper, have far outfasted Elias'. The key term here was 'miracle'. For in his careful account of the natural causes which sustained life and allowed abstinence, Browne was equally concerned to preserve a space for the divinely sustained fast. 'That may be miraculously effected in one, which is naturally causable in another'.[1] His aim was to correct error and ground judgement in the knowledge of natural causes, not solely to scotch false belief but also to secure the genuine possibility of miraculous wonders.

The comparison between the chameleon and the human abstinent was a rather delicate matter. When physicians offered plausible accounts of such phenomena, they were in danger of explaining away truly divine acts. Browne's sources included Laurent Joubert, a Montpellier physician who in the 1560s produced a lengthy treatise defending medicine against popular errors, and the Paduan natural philosopher Fortunio Liceti, author of a 1612 essay on survival without food. They followed Aristotle's argument that since living beings depended on their inner heat, those with less heat, such as old men and young women, would need less nutriment. Joubert also referred to Pliny for evidence that the chameleon, too, was full of cold humours, survived without food, and could even live off the air. But Joubert, whose work was targeted against surgeons and midwives, was well aware that malicious readers and those who were 'ignorant of natural philosophy and medicine' might fear lest the long fasts of Christ, Moses or Elijah 'would no longer be taken as miracles if through some natural cause fasts can be endured for several months or years'. The learned physician responded that his stories only applied to those who wasted away during long periods of abstinence. The truly miraculous abstinent combined fasting with perfect health: 'we believe that Christ had a very temperate and pure body'. 'Exempted from the weakness of the flesh for a time', he explained, 'their condition was thus other than that of humankind'. Late Renaissance texts were well stocked with accounts of abstinents not obviously exempt from the human condition. Some, such as a young German woman, Eva Fleugen, who claimed in the early 1630s to have lived for three decades off the smell of a rose, were judged merely fraudulent, and were used by Browne in his *Religio Medici* (1642) as examples of 'the spirit of delusion'. In better attested cases, such as that of a 14-year-old girl in Poitou whose fast in 1599 drew the attention of the eminent royal physician François Citois, there was considerable debate about the balance to be struck between medical causation and the work of the spirit.[2] To live off airs or odours, to waste away voluntarily and spectacularly, were widely recognized marks of sanctity. In cultures where the deportment of the body and judgement of its capacies were crucial marks of grace and social rank, these stories carried considerable philosophical, medical and theological messages. In what follows, I examine one case of a young woman's wonderful abstinence much discussed in Restoration England, in order to show how the relation between testimony, natural knowledge, deceit and the miraculous was negotiated by learned physicians and their community. Chameleons might not be miraculous, but miracles, like chameleons, were highly coloured by the setting in which they appeared.

Bodies, spirits and vulgar errors

'A MIRACLE is a work of God, (besides his operation by the way of Nature, ordained in the Creation) done for the making manifest to his elect, the mission of an extraordinary Minister for their salvation'. In mid-seventeenth century England, there was no single agreed way of dealing with such work. It was possible that the age of miracles was past, it was scarcely easy to determine which phenomena lay within 'nature's way', nor were there sure means of telling 'manifest missions' from cheats and errors. In his *Leviathan* (1651), where this definition is to be found, Thomas Hobbes characteristically set out to assign the problem of miracles to the judgement of trust, and therefore to the power of the Commonwealth.

> In these times, I do not know one man, that ever saw any such wondrous work, ... that a man endued but with a mediocrity of reason, would think supernaturall: and the question is no more, whether what wee see done, be a Miracle ... but in plain terms, whether the report be true or a lye. In which question we are [to make] the Publique Reason, that is, the reason of Gods Supreme Lieutenant, Judge.[3]

There has been considerable interest in the role of miracles in the fortunes of secular and divine authority. The Oxford divine and some-time Secretary of the Royal Society, John Wilkins, reckoned that the miraculous 'often serves for the Receptable of lazy Ignorance which any industrious spirit would be asham'd of', while in his Restoration defence of the society, Thomas Sprat condemned 'this wild amuzing mens minds, with Prodigies and conceits of Providences'. It was 'one of the most considerable causes of those spiritual distractions, of which our Country has long bin the Theater'. During the seventeenth century, inexplicable but significant signs became increasingly associated with secular wonders, their apparently supernatural quality blamed on Satan and ultimately attributed to nature. Causal stories about such events depended on accounts of those who could rightly judge, or be duped by, strange phenomena. Thus, five years before Hobbes, Browne argued in *Pseudodoxia epidemica* that the Devil 'made the ignorant sort beleeve that naturall effects immediatly and commonly proceed from supernaturall powers ... which being of themselves, the effects of naturall and created causes ... are alwayes looked on by the ignorant spectators as supernaturall spectacles'.[4]

The distribution of trust in miracle stories helped map the distribution of spirits and bodies. Hobbes argued that the vulgar wrongly reckoned that bodies were whatever could be touched or seen. So they attributed corporeality to 'Idols of the brain, which represent bodies to us where they are not, as in a Looking-glasse', and spirituality to air, wind, or breath. 'Such is the ignorance and aptitude to error of all men, but especially of them that have not much knowledge of naturall causes, and of the nature and interests of men; as by innumerable and easie tricks to be abused'. And the abusers, Hobbes continued, were the divines and their allies who exploited ignorance for their own purposes, 'as men fright Birds from the Corn with an empty doublet, a hat and a crooked stick'. Ignorant and dangerous superstition flowed from the wrong map of body and spirit. Browne agreed that this map was crucial, but the pious physician took an opposite line on its meaning. The 'grossenesse' of vulgar 'comprehensions' meant that 'things invisible ... have been degraded from their proper forms, and God himselfe dishonoured into manuall expressions'. So for Browne vulgar incapacity meant the idolatrous materialization of true spiritual religion. 'Being erroneous in their single numbers', Browne expostulated against the incorrigible plebs, 'once hudled together they will be errour itselfe'.[5]

The new philosophy privileged particulars over nature's ordinary course, so it was obsessed by problems of imposture and of the doctrine to be learnt from spectacular signs. These signs were tried by a range of authorities. In 1634 William Harvey had led a team of five physicians and ten midwives during the investigation of the body of the Lancashire witch Margaret Johnson. Three decades later his admirer Browne testified during a witch trial at Bury St Edmund's that the young female victims were indeed bewitched, that 'the devil in such cases did work upon the bodies of men and women upon a natural foundation', and that in this case, motions of the womb were 'only heightened to a great excess by the subtlety of the devil'. Though the presiding judge, Matthew Hale, proposed testing the blindfolded victims by having them touched by substitutes for the two accused women, convincing many that the possessed were frauds, the accused were nevertheless convicted and executed. Physicians were often used in such cases to decide whether symptoms were natural, involving the sacred disease, melancholy or motion of the womb.[6]

As D.P. Walker points out in his brilliant study of the case of John Darrel, gaoled by the Anglican regime for allegedly fraudulent acts of exorcism, such medico-juridical decisions about the scope of 'nature' were politically charged. Darrel, a Cambridge Puritan, defined spiritual events as 'a hard and unusual work surpassing all faculty of created nature, done by the divine power to that end that it may move the beholders with admiration and confirm their faith'. His enemy, an Arminian cleric Samuel Harsnett, was much concerned to damn both Puritan enthusiasm and papist ritual, and riposted that Christ's original gift of spiritual power to his apostles had granted them the capacity to drink poison with impunity. He suggested to Darrel that if he were genuine he should give an 'experimentall demonstration' of the same thing. Ritual trials and body techniques were bound up with the authority and meaning of spiritual wonders. Denying genuine witchcraft, Harsnett explained how a woman could learn to seem possessed, with 'a little helpe of the Mother, Epilepsie or Cramp', to 'role her eies, wrie her mouth, gnash her teeth, startle with her body, hold her armes and hands stiffe, make anticke faces, grin, mow and mop like an Ape, tumble like a Hedgehogge, and can mutter out two or three words of gibridg'. James I's new canon law banned fasting and prayer against possession, and by the later seventeenth century established churchmen increasingly withdrew from these rituals of spiritual action. Though a firm believer in spirits and sure that the age of miracles was not past, Browne nevertheless saw in contemporary rituals the threats of papism. 'That may have some truth in it that is reported by the Jesuites of their Miracles in the Indies, I could wish it were true, or had other testimony than their owne Pennes', he wrote in *Religio Medici*. 'They may easily beleeve those Miracles abroad who daily conceive a greater at home, the transmutation of those visible elements into the body and blood of our Saviour'. While the miraculous was minimized and naturalized by those hostile to papism and enthusiasm, divines and naturalists still had to explain the true role of spirit and its workings in the visible world.[7]

At a range of extremely sensitive moments, such as eucharist, childbirth and deathbed, defining spirit's powers was an urgent and nice matter. Mistakes could be appalling. In 1668 the Somerset cleric Joseph Glanvill explained in his widely read essay on witchcraft and possession that 'the Sin against the Holy Ghost' was just 'a malicious imputation of the Miracles wrought by the Spirit of God in our Saviour to Satanical Confederacy and the power of Apostate Spirits'. This was why the Royal Society should compile a history of 'the World of Spirits', because 'we know not any thing of the world we live in but by experiment and the Phaenomena, and there is the same way of speculating immaterial nature by extraordinary Events and Apparitions'. The fear of such a sinful error also affected Henry More's response to faith healing and Robert Boyle's attitudes to the investigation of the agency of spirit in alchemy.[8] Reporting 'Events and Apparitions' was never innocent but polemical, because of their widespread use in political and religious debate. Sixteenth-century texts such as Foxe's *Book of Martyrs* (1554) and the *Mirror for Magistrates* (1563) had carried stories of special providences meted out to unjust rulers and virtuous martyrs. Their precedent spawned numerous lists of marvels. During the Civil Wars, and notably at the Restoration, rival compilations of prodigies were distributed to make manifest the divine mission of a wide range of parties. In the 1660s these best-selling collections were subject to hostile scrutiny by the licensers of the press.[9]

The issue of trust was acute. Vendors commonly urged that 'the truth of the substance of the relations ... is credibly certified by several persons, though some would obscure the works of the Lord'. Some collectors, such as the pre-eminent Presbyterian Richard Baxter, tried to mobilize a country-wide network of reliable ministers to gather and verify reports of remarkable prodigies. According to Charles II's ultra-royalist biographer, a brief but dramatic thunderstorm, which inter-rupted his coronation in 1661 was 'taken by the most Judicious and discerning part of Mankind for a very auspicious and promising Omen, notwithstanding the mad Remnant of the Rebellion'. The difference between madness and discernment was politically charged.[10] In 1663 'some Hobbians' were allegedly convinced of spirits by visiting a haunted house in Wiltshire, the householder Mr Mompesson was taken to meet the king, Glanvill printed versions of the events, but at the end of the decade Baxter told his close if 'sometimes much overvaluing friend' Glanvill that sceptics 'at Court and the Innes of Court' held that Mompesson 'hath confessed that it was all his own jugling, done onely that he might be taken notice of'. Both Boyle and Mompesson strenu-ously denied such imputations. Glanvill and his ilk used the fragile authority of the Royal Society because 'the relations of your Tryals may be received as undoubted Records of certain events, and as securely be depended on, as the Propositions of Euclide'. This was wildly over-optimistic. Judgement of the credibility of wondrous accounts and the precise definition of the scope of matter and of spirit posed important social, moral and philosophical problems.[11]

Such problems touched on the rights of priests and physicians in their relations with each other and with the laity. Though the Reformation might be interpreted by some as the moment when the healing power of the Church was withdrawn, and established canons rule against priestly agency even in cases of possession, much debate continued about the apparent infringement of medical rights by churchmen, whether the clergy should tend their flocks' bodies and, ultimately, on the body's role in apparently spiritual affairs.[12] Sometimes the insistence on the bodily, and thus potentially medical, source of apparently spiritual phe-nomena was designed to discredit them. This was Harsnett's strategy in 1599, his allies explained that the afflicted 'imagine themselves to be vexed of some hurtful spirits' because their minds were 'troubled by means of noisome fumes', and such materialist accounts were used in Hobbesian ridicule of spirit stories. In 1649, at the establishment of the Commonwealth, Henry More explained the hypocrisy of the self-styled 'godly' party by 'childish humours, and melancholick impressions upon their disturbed spiritts'. But in the later 1660s, writing just after the plague, More's ally Glanvill offered a humoral account of possession exactly to raise its spiritual status. Familiars infused 'some poisonous ferment' and 'vile vapour into the body of the witch'. This let the witch's 'infected imagination, heightned by melancholy and this worse cause', produce 'the separation of the soul from the body' and so directly affect the vulnerable, especially children, 'because their spirits and imaginations being weak and passive are not able to resist the fatal invasion'. 'Men of bold mindes who have plenty of vigorous spirits', Glanvill reassured his readers, 'are secure from the contagion, as in pestilential Airs clean bodies are not so liable to infection as are other tempers'. With this timely interpretation of possession as pestilence, Glanvill did not intend to let physicians monopolize its management nor to secularize its meanings. Indeed, in 1668 he followed up his essay on witches with a defence of the new philosophy widely read as a direct assault on the College of Physicians. Thus Glanvill's sketch of a complex continuum between bodily and spiritual agents was designed to show that spirits could become apparent as witnessable phenomena under the careful interpretation of pious divines and experimenters. Such a design was inevitably troubled, because these phenomena so often specifically involved those subjects held by genteel convention to be distinctly unreliable – poor, infirm, young and female.[13]

The relation between these definitions of the scope of body and spirit and of the rights of physicians, priests and naturalists is well illustrated in some of the best publicized wonders of the 1660s. Such stories show how trust in individual accounts of strange phenomena was connected with the authority attributed to rival subjects, interpreters and healers. Such a case was that of Martha Taylor, a young Derbyshire woman whose spectacular fast and spiritual conversation between late 1667 and mid-1669 attracted the attention of a remarkable range of gentry, divines, physicians, philosophers and pilgrims. Never slow to exploit public appetite for such marvels, metropolitan printers issued a range of reports of her deeds and sufferings. These reports allow an examination of the ways in which Restoration culture established the meaning of singular spiritual and bodily phenomena. Taylor's 'prodigious abstinence' reveals an important connection between gradations of social hierarchy and of attitudes to the presence of spirit in this case. Populist pamphleteers and the devout who attended her routinely saw her as angelic, speaking through God's spirit. A Presbyterian minister practising physic in distant Worcestershire, who never saw her in person, used recent medical chemistry to explain how vital matter could sustain such a long fast without the need for a miracle. A Tory physician from South Yorkshire visited Taylor, subjected her body to the most strenuous examination, and reckoned her a fraud, while Hobbes himself saw no difference between her experiences and his own mundane illnesses. The route of this story therefore ends in London with the Royal Society, but it starts in the Derbyshire village of Over Haddon. Divine agency was more apparent there in Taylor's own village than in more distant and socially elevated circles, and as attention switched from her state of grace to the intimate details of her body, so judgement shifted from plebeian faith to clerical prudence and the judicial violence of the state. This range of judgements formed an important part of the construction of terms such as 'miracle' at a moment of intense religious and political crisis.[14]

Martha Taylor, 'Wonder of Wonders'

Martha Taylor was born in early 1652 into the family of an Over Haddon lead-miner. She was baptized at nearby Bakewell, a centre of dissent in northern Derbyshire. Close to the Manners estates at Haddon Hall and the Cavendish lands around Chatsworth, the lead-mining communities of the high Peak and its surrounding hills were often judged barbarous. 'The very Breeding of that Country has been noted for something more than Rustick', wrote one reporter on Taylor's career, 'the Religion of very many there is but few degrees beyond ignorance'. For 'ignorance' read recalcitrance. In the year of Taylor's birth, the lead-miners organized a major campaign against the tithes of ore claimed by local clergy to pay for prayers for successful digging, while the priests' spokesmen responded that their own rights were warranted because lead 'grew and renewed in the veins'. In his later description of the region, Daniel Defoe singled out these lead-miners for graphic and atypical moralizing, detailing their almost troglodyte existence, his unwonted charity on their behalf, and that 'the uncouth spectacle' of a miner, 'who looked like an inhabitant of the dark regions below' and gave him 'room to reflect how much we had to acknowledge to our Maker, that we were not appointed to get our bread thus'. Devout pamphleteers made much of the contrast between the district's 'very thick and homespun' language, and endemic poverty and irreligion, and Martha Taylor's 'courtesie, her candour, and comely carriage', which 'quite overacted her original as to place and persons'. Her language 'was of a finer unaffected make'. Sceptics and critics, on the other hand, used anecdotes of vulgar cunning precisely to deprive her story of credibility. They made her part of her community to undermine her status, while her own community treated her as a transcendent and thus spiritual being.[15]

The details of Taylor's history seemed widely agreed. When she was 11 years old a neighbouring corn miller struck her so violently on her back that she began to suffer fevers and lameness, permanently taking to her bed in May 1662. Then in November 1667 she began to experience extraordinary bleeding and vomiting, wept 'tears of blood', and by the following month 'the very approach of Meat or Drink was a great trouble to her, the very sight or smell of either, though at a remove, would beget her sorrow; yea, the very thoughts of either would make her sick'. By the time public reports began being distributed, in autumn 1668, she had barely taken more than a few drops of water or honey, or, as one report had it, 'for six weeks in the summer [of 1668] she did not take a drop of liquid, but pursued the life of an angel, being revived by the smell of flowers'.[16] Just as her diet was rather carefully detailed – plum juice at Christmas 1668, syrup in February 1669, claret in the following April – so her body was subject to exceptional scrutiny and her family's small cottage increasingly packed with wardens and visitors. Taylor's experiences did not happen in an obviously withdrawn and private space and, intriguingly, the possibility of deceit was contemplated from the very beginning. During 1668 local gentry nominated about 20 girls to watch her bedside in turn 'to see how she lived, that they might be the better satisfied in the truth'. Thirteen came from her own village – Martha's entire generation there, it has been estimated. Later in the year, more eminent neighbours took a hand, when the Earl of Devonshire, hare-hunting from Chatsworth, came to Over Haddon, visited the celebrated abstinent, and promptly assigned a watch of over a dozen women to attend her in pairs, day and night, during an entire week. Eventually the Earl's tutor, Thomas Hobbes, came too. Ultimately as many as 60 women seem to have been involved in the guard, 'for several weeks at differing seasons'. Reporters seeking to establish the veracity of the fast never failed to stress these witnesses, and the Earl's scrutiny was important enough to appear on the title page of some accounts; others simply failed to mention them. By January 1669, Taylor's deeds were being reported directly to the Government: 'she lies in bed talking much, although worn to a skeleton'.[17]

The spirit which emerged from Martha Taylor was at least as important as the matter she did not consume. This 'Wonder of all Wonders' attracted hosts of visitors keen not merely to watch but to converse with an apparently spiritual mystery, and often to testify to their experience. This part of Derbyshire was not only wild, it was famously full of natural wonders – deep holes, wells, caves and hills which from the mid-seventeenth century were organized as a tourist trail, sung by Hobbes in Latin verse, lauded by Charles Cotton, and soon satirized by Defoe who judged that 'the greatest of all wonders of the Peak' was the remarkable power exercised by the local courts over the 'turbulent, quarrelsome' lead-miners.[18] Taylor's career was easily absorbed into this vocabulary of wonders, citations from Hobbes's poem on the Peak appeared as epigraphs for her own story, and she was subject to much more than 'the inspection and circumspection of physitians, chirurgeons and midwives'. They included 'the curious from many parts as also ... the Religious of all perswasions', her deeds becoming fit matter for local enthusiasts' spiritual autobiographies. Among these was Leonard Wheatcroft, veteran of the New Model Army, then tailor and parish clerk at Ashover, some ten miles distant, who recorded in a history of his 'Life and Pilgrimage' that in January 1669 he 'had much discorse of God, & Jesus Christ, of hir selfe and of hir distemper' with Martha Taylor.[19] John Gratton, 'servant of Christ', lived two miles west of Over Haddon at Monyash, where he kept a journal recording his spiritual quest during the 1660s. Temporarily discouraged by the reflection that Interregnum clergy had insisted that the age of miracles had ceased, and 'that it was presumption for any Man to look for the spirit of God to be given him now as formerly', he encountered the radical millenarian followers of John Reeve and Lodowick Muggleton, spent some time with the local Baptist community, and in 1669 he visited Taylor where he reported meeting many different sectaries. Gratton, the 'Apostle of the Peak', was soon to see the light as a Quaker, and was equally swiftly convinced that the Presbyterian deniers of miracles, expelled from their livints after 1662, were in any case 'physicians of no value'. His testimony, posthumously issued by one of London's leading Quaker publishers, confirms the significance of the Over Haddon marvel as a temporary but important centre of religious ferment, enthusiasm and debate.[20]

There was a connection between the young women who sat with Taylor and the spiritual meanings so many found in her words and deeds. In such cottages it was common to set the bed in the parlour, and there, before the fire, Taylor was surrounded by an interestingly transformed version of the typical scenes of transition, of birth and death. As Adrian Wilson points out, the seventeenth-century lying-in chamber, a place of female collectivity, was a profoundly consecrated space, the gossips present there as witnesses and members of a wider community. Local women treated their presence there as a vital duty and right. In accounts of their spiritual conversions, too, pious women often stressed their place in the domestic setting, where enthusiast men such as Grattan wrote of removal from home and a more wandering existence. One of her visitors was the Derby surgeon Percival Willughby, an ambitious authority on midwifery and kinsman by marriage of Over Haddon's largest landowner, though the only record of his experience there is that he 'almost fell into a swoon' on seeing Taylor's physical condition. The presence at Over Haddon of eminent physicians and the gentry was not uncommon in idealized deathbed scenes, and may have served rather to emphasize the liminal, and thus sacred, status of the saintly abstinent whose good death was a public scene of struggle for salvation. 'Nothing she can be likened to but to the picture of death all her body over', as though she was practically pursuing the *ars moriendi*.[21] The principal pamphlets therefore sought to represent her as a peculiarly holy figure, hovering between life and death, stressing the virtues of conduct and conversation which could safely be accounted part of a relatively stand-ard vocabulary of pious morality. 'The ultimate manifestation of the prophet as a passive and entirely purified receptable of divine energy', writes the historian Phyllis Mack, 'was the maiden who preached prone, holding forth from a sickbed'. The publicists often appealed to this divine energy to steer their readers away from the equal – and present – dangers of sectarian enthusiasm and sceptical atheism.[22]

These reports included the pseudonymous *Mirabile pecci*, published in spring 1669 by the Presbyterian stationer Thomas Parkhurst, and two pamphlets composed during winter 1668–69 by Thomas Robins, variously described as a Derby ballad-maker or divine, 'a well wisher to the gospel of Jesus Christ'. They followed the common style of won-drous reports issued in London in the form of letters from the prov-inces: 'I should be worse than an Infidel if I should set out any such a miraculous thing as this if it were a Fabel'.[23] These stories made much of Taylor's capacity, though unlettered, to converse expertly with the clergy on matters of scripture and the faith. Even Hobbes, otherwise dubious of Taylor's deeds, wondered 'how her Piety without Instruction should bee so eloquent, as 'tis reported'. The image of Christ and the doctors was used to suggest her holiness by stressing her unwonted transcendence of the conventional female exclusion from the sphere of debate. 'She is very ready in the Scripture, is able to discourse with any of the Clergy, and yet very small Learning, when it pleased the Lord to strike her into this condition, and yet now as ready as if she had gone seven years to the School.' It was much remarked that she had lately learnt to read, and 'hath attained some Knowledge in Sacred Mysteries, but nothing of Enthusiasm that she pretends to'.[24] The point was to strike a balance between the insistence that here was a spiritual wonder and that this was no matter for dangerous sectarianism, 'between the two dangerous extreams of unadvis'd credulity and sensless credulity'. Robins turned her sufferings into a sermon: 'she is fed with Angels food and the power of Heaven is with her and the Angel of the Lord is her door keeper and without doubt there is a place provided amongst those blessed Angels where she shall receive life everlasting world without end'. The publicists' strategy was thus to surround Taylor with the apparatus of hagiography. *Mirabile pecci* cited previous well-confirmed cases, including Citois's famous report of the Poitou girl. The pamphlet listed Taylor's more salient religious sayings and insisted that 'she seems to be made up of Prayer'. Her emaciated body was the evacuated receptacle of a rarified and purified spirit.[25]

Taylor's sanctity established, it thus became possible to use 'the Almighty power of a wonder-working God' against those too 'ready to hiss everything off the stage of the world which doth not fall within their own cognizance or experience'. Enthusiasts and sceptics were both to be equally damned as diabolical tempters hovering round her bed, devilish 'instruments, heretical ones, who did their utmost to proselite her to their Whimsies and Conceits', and those 'who employed themselves to vilifie her and cry her up for a Cheat'.[26] No cheat or sectary, and certainly an agent of divine grace, Taylor's person was distinctly wondrous, yet not quite miraculous. Dedicated to a noblewoman noted for her skill 'in the puzling Architecture of the Humane Body, as your judicious, prosperous and charitable Applications do sufficiently demonstrate', the pamphlet released by Parkhurst gave a standard list of patristic and classical precedents of remarkable abstinence. It mentioned the marvels of perpetually burning lamps as analogues for the survival of natural objects without fuel, and stated in good Reformed manner that the age of miracles was probably past. 'The seeming Miracles of these latter Ages of the World' were not supernatural but due to nature 'mightily improved, supported or success't by the holy Skill and art of Sacred Providence'. The important conclusion was that such events 'may deservedly be called wonders, though they have not been advanced so high as to be undoubted miracles'. To sustain this complex and prudent lesson, it was necessary that the scope and contents of providentially guided nature be established, in just the same way as the reliability of the natives of Over Haddon.[27]

Asceticism and the odours of sanctity

The construction of Martha Taylor's wonderful abstinence and modest piety as the signs of a truly providential and spiritual event drew on some traditional resources, notably conventional hagiography, put to use at a very specific conjuncture, the crisis of Restoration dissent. As Caroline Walker Bynum has argued, late medieval Christendom developed an especially somatic female spirituality, 'so much so that the emergence of certain bizarre miracles characteristic of women may actually mark a turning point in the history of the body in the West'.

She attributes these events to the identification of the female with the flesh, but also to the increasing sensibility that grace would be achieved and marked through bodily transformation. Asceticism in general, and wondrous fasts in particular, were especially common in these stories. Such fasts might often mean little more than departure from normal diet, and a rich vocabulary emerged for representing the saintly woman's withdrawal from food, denial of the flesh and, like Martha Taylor, the gradual enclosure of her body against all intrusion or extrusion.[28] Taylor, virginal and abstinent, was following a well-understood pattern when she produced no sweat and took no meat. She was reported as saying that 'I look upon my preservation without the use of creatures to be the manifestation of Infinite Power for the benefit and advantage of them that fear God'. These processes of self-containment became, after the Reformation, increasingly vital weapons in the hands of male interpreters who would use the lives of female religious for their own propagandistic purposes. In Restoration England it was often judged hard to balance the ways of female virtue and of authorship. Taylor was scarcely allowed to represent herself, but was represented by a host of spokesmen.[29]

In the representation of the saint, nutrition was a key term. Augustinian texts were especially devoted to the imagery of spiritual, as opposed to secular, food. Divinity and consumption were peculiarly close in a religion whose central rite was a sacramental meal. Mathurine Riverain, an Angevin girl who went for four years from 1580 without food, began her fast after taking the host on Easter Day. It was crucial in these narratives that asceticism be successfully seen as a deliberate choice. One medieval saint, whose abstinence was rumoured to be due to a blocked bowel, not a state of grace, deliberately and quickly ate large amounts of food 'so that all would know he could eat if he chose to'. As this anecdote suggests, canonization and miraculous work were the result of complex and increasingly regulated negotiations between local communities and church authorities, with their apparatus of petitions from the faithful, surveys of the saint's life, and juridical decisions on the legitimacy of wondrous cures and other events. Miracles had to be edifying and linked to the saintly person, reinforcing true doctrine and clearly drawn from God, and, in particular, should stand up to official enquiry. Concerns with local interest and cunning were endemic in the process through which miracles were authorized and canonization established. The possibility of explaining an apparent wonder through natural means was very closely linked with the omnipresent need to deal with local aspirations, politics and cultures.[30] Canonization thus involved an intriguing series of displacements. In life, the abstinent saint was often deliberately cut off from her immediate surroundings and as frequently lay between this world and the next. After death, her body would literally be translated from home to a ceremonial interment. Christian missions in the New World, where an unfamiliar terrain was scarcely capable of providing familiar signs of divinity, including bread and wine, often faced the puzzles of sustenance and sanctity. In the process of saintly authentification the contingencies of local and communal belief were to be institutionalized within the pantheon of the universal church.[31]

But the holy body leaked. Across the strong boundaries which divided the saint from her mundane world moved a range of aromas, scents and fluids which were widely seen as the specific mediators of true holiness. The great Anglican poet George Herbert, author in 1632 of an important handbook for country parsons, used these images in lauding Christ as an 'Odour', an 'oriental fragrancy', 'this broth of smells, that feeds and fats my mind'. Saints' bodies were notoriously aromatic, a symbol of their resistance to the corruption of death, and equally a means through which they were nourished. The odour of sanctity was apparent most in moments of ecstasy, and when the saint's corpse was translated to burial. One celebrated English abstinent of the mid-1650s exclaimed to her bedside companions that 'the scent of dead souls was still in my nostrils'. In close association with such aromas were the oils and unguents used in the great ceremonies of the Church and State, during the Mass, at the moment of supreme unction, and at the coronation of the monarch.[32] Thomas Browne made gentle fun of such beliefs when he included 'a transcendent Perfume' of divine significance in his fanciful collection of unobtainable rarities, the *Musaeum clausum*, and his discussion of the chameleon in *Pseudodoxia epidemica* contemplated the link between aerial food and holy abstinence. Though the Church authorities might increasingly reject such odours as signs of sanctity, these oils and fragrances were popularly seen as means for linking the two worlds spiritual and corporeal, for effecting a connection which transgressed, and sometimes effaced, natural boundaries. If virtue was accompanied by good smells, then evil must stink. Sweet smells kept the plague at bay. In mid-seventeenth-century England, the natural philosophical distinction between matter and spirit was often just as porous as these boundaries around the persons of the holy and the afflicted. Thus Glanvill could easily propose a model of witchcraft based on pestilential effluvia, and Martha Taylor could be 'revived by the smell of flowers'. Such fluids were useful means of representing the virtues of abstinence and chastity and making it clear how the immured body could become holy, then survive 'without the use of creatures'.[33]

Asceticism and contested prodigies

Taylor's deeds and sufferings were understood as conventional episodes in the history of saintly ascetism, but the Restoration crisis of enthusiasm and dissent gave the events at Over Haddon their peculiar significance. Baxter explained the predicament of the later 1660s, when what he called 'the malice and unreasonable implacable violence' of high Anglican persecution forced his fellow moderates into silence and their flocks into the arms of extreme enthusiasts: 'the common people (though pious) are so apt to be led by outward palpable appearances, that they forgot both former principles and sad effects and practices'. Baxter, who had once been offered a bishopric by Clarendon, now reckoned that the Anglican persecutors were 'sect-makers', and that while the Presbyterians who tried to survive Restoration discipline might be seen by 'the people as lukewarm temporisers', the radical sects were encouraged by 'driving the poor people ... into these alienations and extremes'. He judged Quakers as all but identical to Ranters. During 1668–69, in particular, there was much public concern with the activities of nonconformists, including both the moderate Presbyterians and the apparently more visible and enthusiast Quakers and sectarians. In March 1668 the king issued a proclamation against conventicles, and the Commons soon passed a new bill to ban dissenters' meetings. Wilkins and Baxter debated comprehension of the more moderate nonconformists. During the year the government heard reports of active nonconformist gatherings and of public disorder associated with their activities. Stiff provisions were taken against the dissenting press. In July 1669, a few months after he had distributed pamphlets on Martha Taylor, the printer Thomas Parkhurst, one of Baxter's publishers, was prosecuted by the Government for selling texts against the persecution of moderate nonconformists. The principal publicists of Taylor's fast, including Parkhurst and Thomas Robins, were closely linked to the cause of moderate Presbyterianism, and many were publicly opposed to the Quakers. Their aim was to direct her story in favour of reformed religion and against extreme spiritual illumination.[34]

Baxter spoke for many divines and physicians who saw enthusiasm as a form of disease: 'Certain experience telleth us, that most in our age that have pretended to prophecy or inspirations ... have been melancholy, crack-brained persons near to madness, who have proved deluded in the end'. And he was not alone, either, in linking this weakness with the dangers of sectarianism: 'No person more fit for a Quaker, a Papist or any sectary to work upon, than a troubled mind'. An overestimate of the miraculous, combined with a large and vulnerable populace, was seen as a recipe for disaster. Sprat, for example, echoed a

Restoration commonplace when he complained that 'the enthusiast goes neer to bring down the price of the True and Primitive Miracles, by such a vast, and such a negligent augmenting of their power'.[35] The Friends were notorious for their public witness and were singled out for ferocious persecution because of their refusal to conform or worship privately. Their living signs and enacted parables, whether going naked in public or, especially, engaging in spectacular public fasts, maintained the interregnum culture of personified wonders. Because potentially freed from sin, Quaker men and women possessed regenerate bodies. Since Christ had been able to fast for 40 days, Quakers could do so too. Margaret Fell published on the virtues of such fasts in 1655, and whole families of Friends took up the practice. Their leader James Nayler, notorious for his restaging of Christ's entry into Jerusalem at Bristol in 1656, engaged in public fasts 'as a signe to people who lie given over to fulfil the lusts of the flesh'. In the same year, the Quaker James Parnell died after fasting for ten days in Colchester gaol, and many travelled there expecting to witness his resurrection. In 1661, Charles Bayly fasted for almost three weeks to demonstrate to sceptics that the practice was not necessarily fatal. The significance of such demonstrations of the strength of regenerate bodies was bolstered by Quaker cultivation of faith healing. George Fox himself recorded almost 150 such cures, including touching for the King's Evil. Resurrection and wondrous healing were taken as evidence of spiritual power.[36] Despite their leaders' increasing delimitation of such powers, apparently miraculous cures and public fasts continued well after the Restoration and were sustained during the persecution of the later 1660s. The prevalence of anti-Galenic and chemical medicine within the Quaker networks underscored their faith in the unity of the spiritual and physical body and the possibility of dramatizing and then redeeming the sufferings of the flesh. In his discussion of sectarian prodigies of the mid-seventeenth century, Keith Thomas juxtaposes the experiences of James Nayler and Martha Taylor. The Quaker John Gratton may not have been the only pilgrim at Over Haddon during 1668–69 who saw there another sign of remarkable workings of the inner light, and thus of confirmation of the faith delivered to the Saints.[37]

Prodigious abstinence was a sensitive theme in Restoration England. There were fewer reports of 'black fasts', in which abstinents forswore sustenance so as to act malevolently against a specific victim, but public fasts, involving abstinence, chastity, prayer, and avoidance of work and sleep, remained a well-understood practice amongst the dissenters, subject to strict communal codes. The Fast Sermons of the Commonwealth were occasions for homilies on spiritual reformation and political rhetoric. It was said the Cambridge divine Ralph Cudworth gained such parliamentary preferment from his 1647 sermon that 'he hath gott more at a fast then others can gett at a feast'. Such public fasts were carefully controlled by the restored Church.[38] Precedents for Taylor's deeds included several episodes of spectacular fasts which had not been linked to Quaker enthusiasm but, instead, had been taken as providential signs to be interpreted within the capacity of divinely heightened nature. *Mirabile pecci*, for example, appealed to the cases of Protestant martyrs under Marian persecution who had gone long without food. The very titles of the Taylor pamphlets, such as *Wonders of Wonders*, were also used to describe these episodes, some including apparent resurrection from death, others of strenuous abstinence, all used to teach moral lessons. In 1647, a young Londoner, Sarah Wight, fasted for 53 days, was described as 'an empty nothing creature' only sustained by 'the spirit of grace'. She was visited by Baxter's doctor Thomas Coxe and by the reformist physicians Benjamin Worsley and Gerard Boate, associates of the Boyle clan both soon to be appointed medical officers to the Parliamentary Army in Ireland. Wight's publicist, the Baptist Henry Jessey, a leading faith healer and independent preacher, used her remarkably widely known deeds to attack the claims of Quakers and Ranters alike. Jessey also made sure to build up Wight's credit: 'the reason of naming many, was that some more incredulous might sooner believe and reap benefit'. During the 1650s, several such well-attested cases of spectacular fasts and resuscitations were reported, occasionally used against the Quakers themselves.[39]

During a two weeks' fast in 1652 a young Yorkshire woman, Martha Hatfield, was visited by followers of the local Quaker preacher Richard Farnsworth and was much praised for her resistance to their blandishments. 'Jesus Christ will be my physician', exclaimed Hatfield. The local Congregational minister James Fisher, who spread news of her deeds, reported that she had been resuscitated by his prayers. He concluded that 'God's presence is with his Ministers', not with the disciples of the free spirit such as Farnsworth. The following year Farnsworth attacked the future chronicler of Martha Taylor's fast, Thomas Robins, as 'England's blind guide' because of his stalwart Calvinism. In 1655 Farnsworth became embroiled in a similarly fierce debate with Baxter at Worcester, and initiated a competitive fast with East Anglian sectarians over a space of two weeks, 'neither party taking any sustenance but a little spring water, nor looking in a book during the time' they preached. Fasting and cognate wonders, such as resurrection, were signs of extraordinary regeneration and sites of contest between the sects.[40]

At just this moment, in 1655, Baxter's colleagues began to contemplate collecting records of such wondrous events from reliable fellow ministers, since 'many pious persons are too credulous'. The project was revived in 1657 with an ambitious nation-wide 'Design for registring of Illustrious Providences' to be gathered by county secretaries and co-ordinated at their metropolitan headquarters at Syon House. The calamities of the Restoration made contests over interpretation of these events even more urgent. In late 1660 Jessey, the veteran spokesman of the visionary Sarah Wight, and publisher of a prophetic *Scripture-Calendar* (1649) throughout the Commonwealth, compiled a catalogue of portents and prodigies directed against the restored regime. Jessey listed the sufferings of the godly alongside extraordinary signs in heaven and on earth. His project, deeply suspect not only to the Government but to many dissenters, was continued in a series of volumes, *Mirabilis Annus* (1661–), which reported a host of such events as the sudden speechlessness and death of a Worcester woman who had drunk the king's health. The aim was to show that 'the Lord's immediate preaching to us from heaven' had made up for the expulsion of godly ministers. Jessey and his collaborators were gaoled, his publishers were temporarily silenced, and Baxter judged that these 'many volumes' of wonders, 'with the mixture of so many falsehoods and mistaken circumstances ... turned them to the advantage of the Devil and ungodliness, and made the very mention of Prodigies to become a scorn'. The recipe was to manage, discipline and distribute the reports of spiritual wonders lest their effect be debased or else the faith in providential guidance be abused.[41]

Presbyterian piety and medical chemistry

The most eloquent public attempt to exploit Martha Taylor's abstinence against these twin dangers of radical enthusiasm and arrant atheism was produced in early 1669 by Baxter's ally John Reynolds, a Worcestershire minister turned physician. His was no parochial story of a Derbyshire wonder, indeed he never saw Taylor in person. 'A just Reverence to Reformed Theologues asserting a total Cessation of Miracles' prevented Reynolds seeking 'a supernatural Asylum' in this case, yet 'a prejudicate Opinion of human Bodies in this animal State' meant that Taylor's experience could not be explained by 'Physical Causes clubbing together'. His ornate *Discourse upon Prodigious Abstinence*, designed to reconcile this puzzle, was released by Baxter's publisher Nevill Simmons, a Kidderminster bookseller. Reynolds's career was typical of the Presbyterian fate. After reading divinity at Oxford in the early 1650s, he was a minister at Wolverhampton in the later part of that decade, joined Baxter's Worcestershire Association and was ejected from his living at the Restoration. In 1663 he was presented for holding conventicles and in the midst of the renewed persecution of 1669 had a public fight with a Wolverhampton apothecary, Richard Bracegirdle, in which Reynolds's stout defence of dissent and the Good Old Cause was so violent that it was used as a pretext by the bishops to have his patron Baxter briefly gaoled. These events followed Reynolds's retirement to his native town of King's Norton, where, like some other expelled Presbyterians, he took to practising medicine. His income came 'from noble and rich Patients, that made use of him as a Physician'.[42]

Reynolds was connected with the eminent Shropshire anatomist Walter Needham and read widely in contemporary authorities, especially the Oxford professor Thomas Willis, whom he called 'the great reformer of Physick'. An Oxford student just when Willis was working on medical chemistry and promoting the view of the physician as a manager of ferments, Reynolds 'laboured to advance the antique Glory of the Heart' with his own experiments on blood chemistry. He discussed with Needham the distinction of blood and seed to help resolve puzzles in the doctrine of the resurrection of the individual body. For such a godly practitioner, the link between medicine and priestcraft was not merely one of a temporary switch in employment rendered convenient by adversity. In the 1640s Baxter, who read widely in learned medicine, offered his parishioners free medical care, but since he could not bear the risk of miscarriage recruited a 'godly diligent physician' in his stead. Priestcraft and physic seemed complementary. Baxter insisted that 'it is the Ministers office to oversee each members [sic] of the flock ... as Physicians care for mens health and lives', while at the end of the 1660s Reynolds welcomed Baxter's attempt to reconcile the dissenters as the extension of 'your *manum medicam* to the cure of the Churches wounds'.[43]

These views were shared by the King's Norton curate, the fierce Presbyterian Thomas Hall, also expelled in 1662. Like his fellow collegiate Hall, who had penned a notorious defence of gown-learning and orthodox physic against the sectarian John Webster in 1654, Reynolds was a pugnacious opponent of the Quakers and other enthusiasts. In 1662 Reynolds quizzed two Worcestershire Friends on key points of doctrine and policy, including the need for ordination, churches, sermons and orthodox baptism, the virtuous sufferings of the Presbyterians, reckoned no less than those the Quakers so loudly trumpeted and, above all, the supremacy of the Scriptures. The Quakers' spokesman, Thomas Taylor, answered that 'the body of thy Divinity' was made up of 'deceit, of Philosophy, Traditions of Man, Rudiments of the World and false sciences. You are both in the Fighting and Persecuting nature, as all idolaters are'. But then 'how shall we know', Reynolds responded, 'whether the Spirit that speaks in us be the Spirit of God, or an evil

spirit, but by trying them by the Scriptures?' Baxter also insisted that
'we must not try the Scriptures by our most spiritual apprehensions, but
our apprehensions by the Scriptures', which he judged 'only a trying of
the Spirit by the Spirit; that is, the Spirit's operations in ourselves and
his revelations to any pretenders now, by the Spirit's operations in the
apostles'. And Hall had eloquently denied the possibility of any immediate illumination: 'the spirit of God works by meanes ... Who ever
expects helpe from God must not sit still and dreame the spirit will help
him'. In the same fashion Reynolds insisted that preaching the Lord's
Word from the pulpit, convincing the congregation's 'Consciences, Melt-
ing the Hearts, Humbling the Spirits, and turning them from Darkness
to Light', was the only sure way of sustaining the true faith against the
seductions of false light and the terrors of persecution.[44]

Reynolds's *Discourse* on Martha Taylor was part of this campaign to
discipline inspiration by textual authority and thus to trace a path
between 'that uncharitableness which presumes to write *falshood* upon
all humane testimonies' and 'those in the contrary extream that believe
a century of such reports with a faith almost as miraculous as these
miracles themselves'. His very term 'prodigious abstinence' was a seventeenth-century coinage designed to balance the claims of nature and the
divine. He continued the careful project on special providences discussed by Baxter, and sought to avoid the extremes of enthusiasts'
dubious wonder-mongering. 'Some persons as scant in their reading as
they are in their travels, are ready to deem everything strange to be a
monster, and every monster a miracle.'[45] Reynolds, like other pamphleteers, began by listing the large number of reliable stories of remarkable
abstinents garnered from scripture, the Fathers and more recent medical
authorities such as Daniel Sennert. His appeal to 'the learned world'
had two targets. Against what he called 'miracle-mongers' he pointed
out that, if truly miraculous, those who fasted should intervene in
doctrinal debate or successfully prophesy, 'but not a Cry of these from
most of our abstinents'. In Taylor's case, for which he cited just one
report received from an eyewitness, 'there's no cause from any anteced-
ent sanctity to ascribe this mirandous production to miraculous causes'.
Christ and His apostles had fasted but not wasted away. As many prior
authorities confirmed, their deeds were real miracles. Here Reynolds
was close to Baxter, who debated whether miracles were now necessary
to convince the faithful and sought to distinguish between evidence of
spirits and false or exaggerated wonders. Reynolds was especially keen
to deny that anything angelic was happening to this 'Ethnick' at Over
Haddon. Taylor was obviously not getting visible food, otherwise her
companions would have seen it, and 'if it were invisible, then altogether
incongruous to our Bodies, and therefore miraculous', an obvious im-

possibility.[46] The guards' presence helped Reynolds attack his other enemy, the sceptics. 'Abstinents have been watcht by the most wakefull eyes and jealous ears to detect their fraud, if guilty of any'. Scholarship, prudence, but above all contemporary medical doctrine confirmed the plausibility of her story. Her modesty and willingness to be visited 'may serve to occlude, not only the Mouths that are so Unevangelical, as to cry her up for a Miracle, but those also, that are so Unphilosophical, as to cry her down for the Cheat of a Faction'.[47]

To show that Taylor's abstinence was neither supernatural nor physical, Reynolds used resources from the principal texts of Restoration medical chemistry. Unlike populist pamphleteers or devout pilgrims he was not interested in what Taylor said or foresaw, but solely in her tightly enclosed body. He described her atrophy, her restraint and, above all, her domestic and physical insulation. 'These persons are ... environed with a thick Wall, whose very Crevises, and much more Gates, and publick Outlets, are ... close shut up and barricadoed.' Using Willis's 1659 theory of ferments, its 1665 defence by Richard Lower and Needham's anatomy of the foetus published in 1667, Reynolds depicted Taylor's body as a physically closed but spiritually porous laboratory whose system of fermentation was entirely mastered by medical authority. Taylor scarcely sweated or defecated, so there was no loss to be made up by food, nor was there any danger from a build-up of excrement, since, as Needham had shown, the foetus absorbed nutriment without excretion. Reynolds used his discussion of how fermentation was maintained without chyle to list the fashionable ferments much in vogue in London and Oxford. Blood was capable of an innate fermentation and so, according to Willis, was the brain. Reynolds's own trials on mixing acid with the blood of one of his patients confirmed that the spleen could help blood ferment. In his 1641 defence of the circulation, the eminent London physician Georg Ent had argued that both atmospheric air and the seminal principle contained nitrous virtues, so Reynolds concluded that both simple respiration and 'the seminal humours in these Virgins may, by a long abode in their vessels, ... thereby supply the blood with a more than ordinary ferment'. Indeed, Taylor's age 'confirms the probability of a ferment in the seminals'.[48]

Reynolds's chief puzzle was to define the role of this virginal abstinent's heart. His essay appeared just at the same time as Lower's long-awaited and much publicized *Tractatus de corde* (1669), which summarized recent debates with Needham and others to show that the blood was entirely responsible for all activity and life and deny the heart any innate heat. Here, therefore, Reynolds had to treat his authorities with care. He cautiously denied any innate ferment or fire in the heart, agreed with Needham that it was simply a muscle, but set out the range of means through which cardiac activity did generate fermentation. According to Reynolds, the heart functioned as a cistern, loom and furnace, as an alembic or filter 'to raise and exalt the vital spirits'. The point was to establish the spiritual agents at work inside any abstinent's body. Just as 'Nature hath furnished several Parts with an attractive Power, the Blood with fermentation, and several vessels with a Kind of vermicular Motion of their own', so nourishment could be recouped through chemically active agents. 'When higher Causes shall disjoin what Nature usually conjoineth, and exalt one Principle and depress another, then very astonishing Results appear upon the stage of human Bodies.' Reynolds reworked the traditional link between sanctity and aromatics in newfangled chemical terms. 'It is notorious that Scents do hugely affect the Brain', and 'the most philosophical doctor' Willis himself had argued that scents could affect the nitro-sulphureous particles in the nerves, so, asked Reynolds, 'why may not these Abstinents be relieved by such inriched Fumes also?'[49]

Reynolds's careful essay used Reformed theology and recent medical chemistry to balance humble piety and erudite judgement. 'The long Finger of powerful Providence', Reynolds insisted, 'is undoubtedly to be observed in the Production of these wonderful Effects; though these be not advanced to the Zenith of Divine Miracles, wrought by the immediate Hand of Omnipotency'. Taylor would not fall into the hands of enthusiasts nor be ridiculed by sceptics. He cited the common doctrine of providence proffered by Willis and his colleagues, especially their view that the Deity directed the motions of spirits in the animal economy. But he also stressed the medical chemists' account of vital matter, inherently active and imbued with seminal powers. This was just what Reynolds and Baxter both needed to reinforce their views of real spirits and of the igneous ferments in the blood. Baxter's views on the blood were rather close to those of these medical chemists. Reynolds and Needham specifically discussed how their account of the blood's activity could be used to defend the resurrection of the body. After reading and learning to admire Francis Glisson's 1672 treatise on active matter, Baxter controversially wrote that 'in your Blood' such an active and fiery substance 'is the prime part of that called the Spirits ... And if the Soul carry away any Vehicle with it, it's like to be some of this'. For Reynolds, in the same way, the intermediate place of such vital matter between the divine and earthly worlds helped define the intermediate place of Martha Taylor's body between the dangerously miraculous and the brutally mundane.[50]

The abstinent anatomized

When Reynolds had completed his essay in February 1669, he cast it in the form of a letter to Needham and sent it to London as a 'humble offering to the Royal Society', of which Needham had recently been proposed anatomy curator. While in the wake of Glanvill's publicity during 1669, storm clouds gathered over the Society, the College of Physicians and the London apothecaries, soon to burst in violent pamphlet wars, the Society remained important as a public broker of such tales, and some attempt was made to direct the form of intelligence received from the provinces. Though never discussed at the Society, the *Discourse* took its place alongside a series of comparable provincial reports to the Society, some penned by those dissenters who had turned to medicine and natural philosophy after 1660.[51] The Society proved peculiarly receptive to accounts of remarkable abstinence. They had already heard from Hobbes, whose highly sceptical account of Martha Taylor reached the Society's treasurer at the end of 1668 via a Yorkshire justice of the peace and keen naturalist, John Brooke. In January 1669 it was one of their fellows, Joseph Williamson, who as manager of the Government's communication network received reports about the Derbyshire marvel.[52] Now, in summer 1669, a further story was received from the nonconformist physician Nathaniel Fairfax, a Suffolk curate ejected in 1662 who then acquired a medical licenciate, an extensive East Anglian practice, and a ready audience at the Royal Society. Like his contact Thomas Browne, Fairfax set out to correct vulgar errors and use spirit stories against atheists. Three months after Reynolds's report, Fairfax wrote to Henry Oldenburg, the Society's secretary, with another 'relacion of an attempt of self starving'. In March of that year Jane Naunton, a young gentlewoman staying in Fairfax's house, began to fear that her income would no longer allow her to maintain the status of a lady, contemplated suicide and tried to starve herself to death. Fairfax recorded the details of her diet, her weakened spirits, and his eventually successful attempts to wean her back to sustenance. 'She is now taking dyet with as much warynes, as she had foresaken it with rashnes, being at present as great an instance of a trifling resolver, as she was before of an adventurous faster.' Unlike Reynolds's letter, and like that of Hobbes, this was a thoroughly secular story, its moral found in the woman's proud concern with her social status and her addiction to 'Romances, with the life & soul whereoff she was as practically spiritted as a good Christian is with that of the Bible'. With other reports Fairfax sent Oldenburg on remarkable anatomies of young women, including hermaphroditism, or the story received later in summer 1669 from a

Plymouth physician about 'a maid's breasts excessively swelled in one night', the experience of Jane Nauton reinforced the Society's convention of gathering remarkable medical narratives from which no significant spiritual lesson would be expected or offered.[53]

Barely a week after Fairfax's letter on self-starving was read, the Society received the most detailed clinical report on the more celebrated events at Over Haddon. This, the final public account of Martha Taylor, was written from south Yorkshire by Nathaniel Johnston, a Cambridge MD of impeccably high Anglican credentials, an indefatigable antiquarian and naturalist of his native county. Johnston's letter was written in Latin, as befitted a report from one scholar to another, and his metropolitan correspondent was the Oxford-trained physician Timothy Clarke, protagonist of the Society's interests in blood transfusion, energetic coordinator of its medical correspondence and a ferocious enemy of vulgar empirics. Johnston reached Derbyshire prepared with his reading in past accounts of abstinents notably that of the French authority Citois, and with his mind already set on the possibility that the whole story was a fraud fomented by dangerous sectaries. He began by listing Taylor's diet. His letter was cast as a highly dramatic narrative of unveiling and detection, written not as a pious meditation on a local saint, nor a learned discourse in contemporary medical doctrine, but a direct and circumstantial report of a remarkably destructive encounter. In two hours' questioning of Martha Taylor, he noticed 'how lively was her face, how bright her eyes, how full her lips and also her cheeks'. Taylor told the Yorkshireman that her spirits were uplifted, while he guessed that her occasional coughing fits were merely for show. Taylor's pulse 'was in every way like that of healthy people', and when 'she told me that her intestines had fallen out and her bladder removed from its place, without being overheard by those watching I said that the bladder could not come out without there being an ulcer in the womb'. Here, Johnston reckoned, were good grounds for real suspicion.[54]

Taylor evidently resisted Johnston's questions, so he returned the next day to examine her manually, leaving her family outside. 'But the light was so low and the opening so narrow that I could not make out either the colour or shape, nor feel anything; yet though I scarcely touched her, she was overcome by an intense pain, and as far as I could judge I only gently touched the raised lips of her vulva.' Johnston's questions became more intense, Taylor insisted that he could see quite well enough already, refused to allow him to examine her mouth, but conceded that she was bandaged regularly with poultices of milk, cream, whey or ale. At this point, Taylor's mother burst in, and, according to Johnston, 'complained with a snarl that her daughter was in no way a hypocrite, since she had fully satisfied the whole region, indeed all of England'.

This was the climax of the interrogation. Martha's mother, elsewhere described as of rather high birth and 'cautious about her words and actions', exclaimed to Johnston that 'she often felt that her stricken girl was wasting her strength in talking too much by publicizing her miracles in God's honour'. Johnston tried to bribe the woman into letting him examine her daughter's uterus, but 'the cunning woman' answered that 'my daughter well knows how wretchedly I am affected by her suffering, and so she has not shown it to me and I don't want to see it'. When she mentioned the pity Percival Willughby had felt when he'd seen the tumour, Johnston simply noted that this showed that the Derby physician had surely been careless in his examination. He gave over his inquisition, offering to help cure the girl 'so that I might try whether she really wanted to be healed', then went off to interview a local woman who had been tending Martha Taylor. She confirmed that there was a tumour on the young woman's uterus, but its size scarcely matched the stories he'd heard from the sufferer herself.[55]

These severe conclusions were rather similar to those of Hobbes, whose views on what Johnston called 'the great Leviathan of Government' and the role of the law he later hesitantly endorsed. Like Hobbes, too, Johnston judged vulgar use of portents and prodigies a key cause of sedition. Hobbes's letter of the previous year to the Yorkshire justice John Brooke may have been seen by his fellow-Yorkshireman Johnston, who shared many of Brooke's interests in natural history, antiquities and a 'rich and well stored Cabinet of Art & Nature'. 'To know the certainty', as Hobbes put it, would require a detailed investigation of Taylor, but no law 'authoriseth a Justice of the Peace or other subject to restrain a sick person, so farr as were needfull for a discovery of this Nature'. As he had already argued in *Leviathan*, the question of miracles should be judged by the state church. Hobbes did point out, however, that it would be very easy to administer food secretly and 'the shrunken Intestine may easily bee kept clean'.[56] Johnston fully confirmed these suspicions. 'The most ingenious spectators' had been deceived by Taylor's family, while she secretly took in food and drink and relieved herself into 'some attached bladder'. The cure for this scandal lay with the executive powers of law. 'While the girl is alive it is not certain, I judge, that the virtuosi will be able to bring the controversy to an end, and after her death (unless she comes under the anatomist's knife) the controversy will grow.' Johnston reminded Clarke, recently made physician-in-ordinary to the king, of the monarch's grant of a new charter to the Royal Society, which seemed to promise them fresh powers. Charles II should be persuaded to appoint investigators, preferably a commission made up of a physician, a justice of the peace, and other 'reliable witnesses'. 'Knowing the certainty' here was a crucial political matter. 'In this case', Johnston insisted, 'when not only the vulgar but also wise men vacillate, and others, who are given over to religion, persist in their opinion of a miracle, it seems necessary that the certainty of the thing be known, so that an opportunity for everyone to doubt can be forestalled'.[57]

So Dr Johnston's prescription was simple. The false saint should be tried by the learned, examined by the State and, if possible, anatomized. 'So fierce are men, for the most part, in dispute, where either their learning or power is debated, that they never think of the laws, but as soon as they are offended, they cry out, *crucifige*.' Thus Hobbes, who prepared this analysis of the relation between power and dispute in summer 1668, after being told by the government that none of his works could be published in English and arranging for their release in a Latin edition at Amsterdam. Much concerned with the threats of persecution and the control of public belief, he visited Over Haddon barely three months later. At the end of his remarks on the legal rights of inquiry into Taylor's case, Hobbes added his own judgement of the matter. He recalled that 20 years earlier, when ill and in exile in Paris, he had kept to his bed for six weeks without eating. '6 Months would not have made it a Miracle. Nor do I much wonder that a young Woman of clear memory hourely expecting death, should be more devout, then at other times. 'Twas my own case.'[58] This was an apt epitaph on the whole story. A range of commentators turned Taylor's case into their own. Their concerns, their experience, and even their own bodies, were used to judge hers. Devout Derbyshire villagers saw her as a divine presence fed by angels. London stationers used her deeds to market their pamphlets. Presbyterian ministers, fearful lest the case be used to undermine true spirit or foment enthusiasm, used medical chemistry to explain her vitality. At the Royal Society, her case was juxtaposed with other provincial reports of remarkable female bodies. High Anglican physicians treated her case as an opportunity for juridical and medical inquest designed to establish certainty against subversive dispute. Taylor's voice and her person were translated and appropriated. Even her fate remained obscure. Hobbes guessed that she would soon die, other records suggest that she may have survived until the 1680s. The prodigious abstinent was avidly devoured by her culture, which used her to establish trustworthy versions of the proper capacities of bodies, spirits and marvels. 'We are what we all abhorre', wrote Thomas Browne in his discussion of the mystery of the resurrection, 'devourers not onely of men, but of ourselves, and that not in an allegory, but a positive truth'.[59]

Notes

Acknowledgement: thanks to Roger Chartier, Andrew Cunningham, David Harley, Adrian Johns, Adrian Wilson and Michael Wintroub for their generous help.

1. Thomas Browne, *Pseudodoxia epidemica*, ed. Robin Robbins, 2 vols, Oxford, Clarendon, 1981, vol. 1 pp. 3, 242–51. 'Elias' is Elijah, who fasted for 40 days and nights: see 1 Kings 19.

2. For Browne's sources see *Pseudodoxia epidemica*, vol. 2, pp. 646, 864; there is a 1661 discussion of the chameleon in Thomas Birch, *History of the Royal Society*, 4 vols, London, Millar, 1756–57, vol. 1, pp. 47, 52. For Aristotle's doctrine see Everett Mendelsohn, *Heat and Life*, Cambridge, MA, Harvard University Press, 1964, pp. 11–14. For Joubert and Citois see Gérard Rudolph, 'Histoire mémorable d'une fille d'Anjou, laquelle a été quatre ans sans user d'aucune nourriture, que de peu d'eau commune: anoréxie mentale (?) au 16e siècle', *Comptes rendus, 93e Congrès national des sociétés savantes, 1968: section des sciences*, Paris, 1971, vol. 2, pp. 17–29 and Caroline Walker Bynum, *Holy Feast and Holy Fast*, Berkeley, University of California Press, 1987, p. 211. Natalie Zemon Davies, *Society and Culture in Early Modern France*, Cambridge, Polity Press, 1987, pp. 224, 258–62. For Fleugen see Thomas Browne, 'Religio Medici', in C.A. Patrides (ed.) *Major Works*, Harmondsworth, Penguin, 1977, p. 98, n.186, and Walter Vandereycken and Ron van Deth, *From Fasting Saints to Anorexic Girls: The History of Self-Starvation*, London, Athlone, 1994, pp. 62–4.

3. Thomas Hobbes, *Leviathan*, London, Andrew Crooke, 1651, pp. 235, 237. For the cessation of miracles as an anti-Catholic view see P.H. Kocher, *Science and Religion in Elizabethan England*, San Marino, Huntington, 1953, pp. 104–7.

4. John Wilkins, *Discourse Concerning a New Planet*, London, 1640, p. 248; Thomas Sprat, *History of the Royal Society*, London, J. Martyn and J. Allestry, 1667, p. 362; Browne, *Pseudodoxia epidemica*, vol. 1, p. 67. See R.S. Westfall, *Science and Religion in Seventeenth Century England*, New Haven, Yale University Press, 1958, pp. 96–100; R.M. Burns, *The Great Debate on Miracles*, Lewisburg, Bucknell University Press, 1981; Peter Dear, 'Miracles, Experiments, and the Ordinary Course of Nature', *Isis*, **81**, (1990), 663–83; Lorraine Daston, 'Marvellous Facts and Miraculous Evidence in Early Modern Europe', *Critical Inquiry*, **18** (1991), 93–124.

5. Hobbes, *Leviathan*, pp. 207–8, 236, 373; Browne, *Pseudodoxia epidemica*, vol. 1, pp. 16–17.

6. Thomas Howell, *Collection of State Trials*, London, Hansard, 1810, vol. 6, p. 697. See Garfield Tourney, 'The Physician and Witchcraft in Restoration England', *Medical History*, **16** (1972), 143–55; Barbara Shapiro, *Probablity and Certainty in Seventeenth-Century England*, Princeton, Princeton University Press, 1983, p. 207; Michael Macdonald, *Mystical Bedlam*, Cambridge, Cambridge University Press, 1981, pp. 174–5, 198–9. For Harvey see C. l'Estrange Ewen, *Witchcraft and Demonianism*, London, Heath, Cranton, 1933, pp. 248–50.

7. D.P. Walker, *Unclean Spirits*, London, Scolar, 1981, pp. 66–71; Keith

Thomas, *Religion and the Decline of Magic*, Harmondsworth, Penguin, 1972, pp. 576–9. For the later fate of the miraculous, see Eamonn Duffy, 'Valentine Greatrakes, the Irish Stroker. Miracle, Science and Orthodoxy in Restoration England', *Studies in Church History*, 17 (1981), 251–73, esp. pp. 253–7 and David Harley, 'Mental Illness, Magical Medicine and the Devil in Northern England 1650–1700', in Andrew Wear and Roger French (eds), *The Medical Revolution of the Seventeenth Century*, Cambridge, Cambridge University Press, 1989, pp. 114–44. For Jesuits see Browne, 'Religio Medici', p. 95.

8. Joseph Glanvill, *A Blow at Modern Sadducism*, London, E.C. for James Collins, 1668, pp. 69, 95. For Boyle, see Michael Hunter, 'Alchemy, Magic and Moralism in the Thought of Robert Boyle', *British Journal for the History of Science*, 23 (1990), 387–410.

9. Thomas, *Religion and the Decline of Magic*, pp. 109–10.

10. Jerome Friedman, *Miracles and the Pulp Press During the English Revolution*, London, UCL Press, 1993, p. 251; William Lamont, *Richard Baxter and the Millenium*, London, Croom Helm, 1979, p. 33; Gerard Reedy, 'Mystical Politics: the Imagery of Charles II's Coronation', in P.J. Korshin (ed.), *Studies in Change and Revolution*, London, Scolar Press, 1972, pp. 19–42, esp. p. 36.

11. More to Conway, 31 March 1663 and Baxter to Glanvill, 18 November 1670, in Jackson I. Cope, *Joseph Glanvill: Anglican Apologist*, St Louis, Washington University Press, 1956, pp. 15, 102 n.36; Lamont, *Baxter and the Millenium*, p. 45; Glanvill, *Scepsis Scientifica*, London, 1665, sig. c^r. Compare T.H. Jobe, 'The Devil in Restoration Science', *Isis*, 72 (1981), 343–56, esp. pp. 345–6; Charles Webster, *From Paracelsus to Newton*, Cambridge, Cambridge University Press, 1982, p. 93.

12. Charles Webster, *The Great Instauration*, London, Duckworth, 1975, p. 255; Andrew Wear, 'Puritan Perceptions of Illness in Seventeenth Century England', in Roy Porter (ed.), *Patients and Practitioners*, Cambridge, Cambridge University Press, 1985, pp. 55–99, esp. pp. 60–7 on the continuing medical role of the reformed priesthood; Peter Elmer, 'Medicine, Religion and the Puritan Revolution', in Roger French and Andrew Wear (eds), *The Medical Revolution of the Seventeenth Century*, Cambridge, Cambridge University Press, 1989, pp. 10–45, esp. pp. 14–16, on the attack by physicians on priestly therapy.

13. Macdonald, *Mystical Bedlam*, p. 207; More to Hartlib, 30 December 1649, in Alan Gabbey, 'Cudworth, More and the Mechanical Analogy', in Richard Kroll, R. Ashcraft and P. Zagorin (eds), *Philosophy, Science and Religion in England 1640–1700*, Cambridge, Cambridge University Press, 1992, pp. 109–27, esp. p. 114; Glanvill, *Blow at Modern Sadducism*, p. 20. On earlier debates see Kocher, *Science and Religion*, pp. 127–45; on the Restoration body–spirit continuum see Simon Schaffer, 'Godly Men and Mechanical Philosophers', *Science in Context*, 1 (1987), 55–85; on Glanvill's fight with the physicians see Harold J. Cook, 'Henry Stubbe and the Virtuoso Physicians', in French and Wear (eds) *Medical Revolution*, pp. 246–71, esp. p. 252.

14. The episode is recalled in the county history of Daniel Lysons and Samuel Lysons, *Magna Britannia*, 6 vols, London, Cadell and Davies, 1817, vol. 5, pp. 27–8; documented by Joseph A. Silverman, 'Anorexia Nervosa in Seventeenth Century England as Viewed by Physician, Philosopher and

Pedagogue', *International Journal of Eating Disorders*, 5 (1986), 847–53 and Noel Malcolm (ed.), *The Correspondence of Thomas Hobbes*, Oxford, Oxford University Press, 1994, p. 703; and fully analysed in Janet Wadsworth, 'Martha Taylor – the Fasting Maid of Over Haddon', *Derbyshire Miscellany*, 8 (1978), pp. 77–87, whom I follow here.

15. For the contrast between Martha Taylor and her surroundings, see H.A., *Mirabile pecci*, London, T. Parkhurst, 1669, pp. 5–6, 23–4, 26. For the miners and tithes, see W. Page (ed.), *Victoria County History: Derbyshire*, London, Dawsons, 1970, vol. 2, pp. 332–3. Defoe's comments are in Pat Rogers (ed.), *A Tour Through the Whole Island of Great Britain*, Harmondsworth, Penguin, 1971, pp. 463–8.

16. *Mirabile pecci*, pp. 9–11; Nathaniel Johnston to Timothy Clarke, 29 June 1669, in Birch, *History of the Royal Society*, vol. 2, p. 389.

17. Details of the watch are in Thomas Robins, *Newes from Darbyshire or the Wonder of all Wonders*, London, Thomas Passinger, 1668, p. 3; T. Robins, *The Wonder of the World*, London, Thomas Passinger, 1669, p. 2; *Mirabile pecci*, p. 65. Devonshire's arrival at Over Haddon is described in Thomas Hobbes to John Brooke, 20 October 1668, in Malcolm, *Correspondence of Hobbes*, p. 701. For the watchers' names see Wadsworth, 'Martha Taylor', p. 80. For government report, see *Calendar of State Papers (Domestic) 1668–9*, London, HMSO, 1894, p. 145 (4 January 1669).

18. Defoe, *Tour*, p. 461.

19. John Reynolds, *A Discourse of Prodigious Abstinence*, London, R. White for Nevill Simmons and Dorman Newman, 1669, p. 34; *Mirabile pecci*, p. 65. For Wheatcroft, see Dorothy Riden (ed.), 'Autobiography of Leonard Wheatcroft', *Derbyshire Record Society*, 20 (1993), 71–117, esp. p. 85. For the use of Hobbes's *De mirabilibus pecci carmen* in this case see *Mirabile pecci*, sig. A3.

20. John Gratton, *Journal of the Life of that Ancient Servant of Christ ...* , London, J. Sowle, 1720, pp. 6, 20, 31–2. Gratton's remark that Taylor 'pretended to live without meat' does not necessarily imply he doubted her. In seventeenth-century usage the term could simply mean 'to claim'.

21. Adrian Wilson, 'Participant or Patient? Seventeenth-Century Childbirth From the Mother's Point of View', in Porter (ed.), *Patients and Practitioners*, pp. 129–44, esp. p. 135; Barbara Ritter Dailey, 'The Visitation of Sarah Wight', *Church History*, 55 (1986), 438–55, esp. pp. 448–9; Macdonald, *Mystical Bedlam*, p. 108. For Willughby's presence see Birch, *History of the Royal Society*, vol. 2, p. 391; for his kinsman see Wadsworth, 'Martha Taylor', p. 80. For the deathbed see Mary O'Connor, *The Art of Dying Well: The Development of the Ars Moriendi*, New York, AMS, 1966; Philip Aries, *The Hour of our Death*, New York, Knopf, 1981, pp. 18–19, 108–9; Dailey, 'Visitation of Sarah Wight', pp. 438–45; Beth Ann Bassein, *Women and Death*, Westport, Greenwood Press, 1984, pp. 35–9. For domesticity in female conversions, see Phyllis Mack, *Visionary Women: Ecstatic Prophecy in Seventeenth-Century England*, Berkeley, University of California Press, 1992, p. 225. For Taylor's appearance see Robins, *Newes from Darbyshire*, p. 4.

22. Mack, *Visionary Women*, p. 34.

23. For such pamphlets see Jerome Friedman, *Miracles and the Pulp Press During the English Revolution*, London, UCL Press, 1993, p. 14. The

citation is from Robins, *Newes from Darbyshire*, p. 4. Robins describes himself as 'B. of D.', which is interpreted as 'ballad-maker of Derby' in Reynolds, *Prodigious Abstinence*, p. 34 and elsewhere as 'bachelor of divinity'.

24. Robins, *Wonder of the World*, p. 8; Hobbes to Brooke, in Malcolm, *Correspondence of Hobbes*, p. 702; Reynolds, *Discourse*, p. 34. Compare Mack, *Visionary Women*, p. 106.

25. Robins, *Newes from Darbyshire*, p. 6; *Mirabile pecci*, pp. 51, 28–32, 25.

26. *Mirabile pecci*, pp. 2–3, 16–17.

27. Ibid., pp. 46–9, 57–8, 76.

28. Caroline Walker Bynum, 'The Female Body and Religious Practice in the Later Middle Ages', in Michel Feher (ed.), *Fragments for a History of the Human Body*, 3 vols. New York, Zone, 1989, vol. 1, pp. 160–219, esp. p. 162, and *Holy Feast and Holy Fast*, pp. 83–4, 211.

29. For Taylor's comment see *Mirabile pecci*, 28–32. For male propaganda see Rudolph M. Bell, *Holy Anorexia*, Chicago: Chicago University Press, 1985, p. 168; for the problems of female authorship see Elaine Hobby, *Virtue of Necessity: English Women's Writing 1649–1688*, London, Virago, 1988, p. 1–25.

30. For Riverain see Rudolph, 'Histoire mémorable', pp. 18–20. For saints and nutrition see Frank Bowman, 'Of Food and the Sacred', *L'Esprit Créateur*, 16 (1976), 111–33, esp. p. 119 and Brigitte Cazelles, *Le Corps de Sainteté*, Geneva, Droz, 1982, p. 83; for deliberate fasts, see Aviad Kleinberg, *Prophets in their Own Country*, Chicago, Chicago University Press, 1992, pp. 19–20; for Church regulation of canonization, see Kleinberg, *Prophets*, pp. 28–31; Benedicta Ward, *Miracles and the Medieval Mind*, Aldershot, Wildwood House, 1987, pp. 184–7; Bell, *Holy Anorexia*, pp. 158–9; Vandereycken and van Deth, *From Fasting Saints to Anorexic Girls*, pp. 50–51.

31. On translation see Kleinberg, *Prophets*, pp. 17–18; Jean-Pierre Albert, *Odeurs de sainteté*, Paris, Ecole des Hautes Etudes en Sciences Sociales, 1990, p. 242; on the sealing of all orifices see Bynum, *Holy Feast*, p. 211. For debates about the proper celebration of the Eucharist in the New World, where bread and wine were not available, see Janet Whatley, 'Food and the Limits of Civility', *Sixteenth Century Journal*, 15 (1984), 387–400, esp. p. 389.

32. Albert, *Odeurs de Sainteté*, pp. 79, 183, 242; Constance Classen, David Howes and Anthony Synnott, *Aroma: the Cultural History of Smell*, London, Routledge, 1994, pp. 52–4. For Herbert see 'The Odour', in F.E. Hutchinson (ed.), *Works of George Herbert*, Oxford, Clarendon, 1941, p. 174. For 'dead souls' see Nigel Smith, *Perfection Proclaimed: Language and Literature in English Radical Religion 1640–1660*, Oxford, Clarendon Press, 1989, p. 94.

33. For canonists' scepticism of saints' smell, see Kleinberg, *Prophets*, p. 35. For Browne's *Musaeum clausum* see Geoffrey Keynes (ed.), *Miscellaneous Writings*, London, Faber and Faber, 1931, p. 142 and for aerial food see *Pseudodoxia epidemica*, vol. 1. pp. 242–51.

34. Richard Baxter, *Autobiography*, J.M. Lloyd Thomas (ed.), London, Dent, 1925, pp. 202–3; Richard L. Greaves, *Enemies Under His Feet: Radicals and Nonconformists in Britain 1664–1677*, Stanford, Stanford Univesity Press, 1990, pp. 142–51, 180–1; Douglas R. Lacey, *Dissent and Parlia-*

mentary Politics in England 1661–1689, New Brunswick, Rutgers, 1969, pp. 56–61; William Lamont, *Richard Baxter and the Millenium*, London, Croom Helm, 1979, pp. 131–2, 220–6. For Parkhurst's arrest see *Calendar of State Papers (Domestic) 1668–9*, pp. 409, 411.

35. Geoffrey Nuttall, *The Holy Spirit in Puritan Faith and Experience*, Oxford, Blackwell, 1946, p. 57; Sprat, *History of the Royal Society*, p. 362. In general, see George Williamson, 'The Restoration Revolt Against Enthusiasm', *Studies in Philology*, 2 (1933), 571–603; T.G. Steffan, 'The Social Argument Against Enthusiasm 1650–1660', *Studies in English*, 21 (1941), 39–63; George Rosen, 'Enthusiasm: A Dark Lanthorn of the Spirit', *Bulletin of the History of Medicine*, 42 (1968), 393–421; Michael Heyd, 'The Reaction to Enthusiasm in the Seventeenth Century', *Journal of Modern History*, 53 (1981), 258–80. For Sprat's position see Paul Wood, 'Methodology and Apologetics: Sprat's *History of the Royal Society*', *British Journal of the History of Science*, 13 (1980), 1–26 esp. pp. 16–21 and Michael Heyd, 'The New Experimental Philosophy: A Manifestation of Enthusiasm or an Antidote to It?', *Minerva*, 25 (1987), 423–40, esp. pp. 434–5.

36. K.L. Carroll, 'Quaker Attitudes Towards Signs and Wonders', *Journal of the Friends' Historical Society*, 54 (1977), 70–84, 71–6; B. Reay, 'Quakerism and Society', in J.F. Macgregor and B. Reay (eds), *Radical Religion in the English Revolution*, Oxford, Oxford University Press, 1984), pp. 141–64, esp. pp. 148–9; for Restoration mitigation of miracles, see Christopher Hill, *The World Turned Upside Down*, New York, Viking, 1972, pp. 202–3.

37. Peter Elmer, 'Medicine, Science and the Quakers', *Journal of the Friends' Historical Society*, 54 (1981), 265–86, esp. pp. 272–4; Thomas, *Religion and the Decline of Magic*, pp. 148–9.

38. For Puritan fast days see Thomas, *Religion and the Decline of Magic*, p. 135 and for black fasts ibid., p. 612. For fast sermons and Cudworth see Gabbey, 'Cudworth, More and the Mechanical Analogy', pp. 115, 125 n.32.

39. *Mirabile pecci*, p. 36. For Wight see Geoffrey Nuttall, *James Nayler: A Fresh Approach*, London, Friends' Historical Society', 1954, pp. 9–10, 14; Alfred Cohen, 'Prophecy and Madness: Women Visionaries During the Puritan Revolution', *Journal of Psychohistory*, 11 (1984), 411–30, 420–2; Barbara Ritter Dailey, 'Visitation of Sarah Wight', *Church History*, 55 (1986), 438–55. For Worsley and Boate see Webster, *Great Instauration*, p. 64. For an Oxford resurrection in 1650, in which William Petty and Thomas Willis were involved, described as a *Wonder of Wonders*, see Friedman, *Miracles and the Pulp Press*, pp. 26–9 and Robert Frank, *Harvey and the Oxford Physiologists*, Berkeley, University of California Press, 1980, p. 50.

40. For Hatfield see Nuttall, *Nayler*, pp. 13–14; Cohen, 'Prophecy and Madness', pp. 419–20. For Farnsworth in East Anglia see T. Llewellyn-Edwards, 'Richard Farnworth [sic] of Tickhill', *Journal of Friends' Historical Society*, 56 (1992), 201–9, esp. p. 205. For the resurrection episode at Worcester in 1655–7, see C.D. Gilbert, 'Some Incidents in Early Worcester Quakerism', ibid., 57 (1994), pp. 5–12. Farnsworth's attack on Robins is *England's Warning Piece Gone Forth*, London, 1653.

41. B.R. White, 'Henry Jessey: A Pastor in Politics', *Baptist Quarterly*, 25

(1973), pp. 103–5; Lamont, *Baxter and the Millenium*, pp. 30–31; Friedman, *Miracles and the Pulp Press*, pp. 245–52; Thomas, *Religion and the Decline of Magic*, pp. 110–12; Richard L. Greaves, *Deliver us from Evil: The Radical Underground in Britain, 1660–1663*, Oxford, Oxford University Press, 1986, pp. 211–16; Michael McKeon, *Politics and Poetry in Restoration England*, Cambridge, MA, Harvard University Press, 1975, pp. 194–6.

42. For Reynolds on miracles see *Discourse*, sig. A2ᵛ; for his career see A.G. Matthews (ed.), *Calamy Revised*, Oxford, Clarendon Press, 1934, new edn 1988, p. 409 and Baxter, *Autobiography*, p. 206.

43. For Reynold's medical chemistry see *Discourse*, pp. 16–17, 27–8; for priest and physician see Geoffrey Nuttall, 'A Transcript of Richard Baxter's Library Catalogue', *Journal of Ecclesiastical History*, 3 (1952), 74–100, esp. pp. 94–5; Baxter, *Autobiography*, p. 15; Lamont, *Baxter and the Millenium*, p. 36; Reynolds to Baxter, 23 July 1670, in N.H. Keeble and G.F. Nuttall (eds), *Calendar of the Correspondence of Richard Baxter*, 2 vols, Oxford, Clarendon Press, 1991, vol. 2, p. 95. For Willis's work of the early 1650s, see Frank, *Harvey and the Oxford Physiologists*, pp. 165–9. For Puritan critiques of priests who practised medicine, see Elmer, 'Medicine, Religion and the Puritan Revolution', 14–15. Thanks to David Harley for advice on this problem.

44. Thomas Hall, *Histriomastix*, London, 1654, p. 203: for Hall see Elmer, 'Medicine, Religion and the Puritan Revolution', pp. 30–2. Reynolds's arguments against the Quakers are in Thomas Taylor, *Ignorance and Error Reproved, Being an Answer to Some Queries that One John Reynolds Wrote to Two of the People Called Quakers*, 1662; London, T. Sowle, 1697, pp. 10–37 (citations from pp. 13, 37, 8). For Baxter on scripture and inspiration against the Quakers, see Nuttall, *Holy Spirit*, pp. 26–33 (citation from p. 32).

45. Reynolds, *Discourse*, p. 4–5. For 'prodigious abstinence' see Vandereycken and van Deth, *From Fasting Saints to Anorexic Girls*, pp. 98–103.

46. Ibid., pp. 5, 36. For Baxter on miracles in the 1650s, see Gilbert, 'Incidents in Early Worcester Quakerism', pp. 7–8.

47. Reynolds, *Discourse*, pp. 4, 36.

48. Ibid., pp. 30, 8, 21, 35. See Everett Mendelsohn, *Heat and Life*, Cambridge, MA, Harvard University Press, 1964, pp. 49–66; Audrey B. Davis, *Circulation Physiology and Medical Chemistry in England 1650–1680*, Lawrence, Coronado Press, 1973, pp. 81–90; Frank, *Harvey and the Oxford Physiologists*, pp. 110–11, 166–9, 198–200.

49. Reynolds, *Discourse*, pp. 25–7, 7–8, 29.

50. Ibid., p. 7; Richard Baxter, *Of the Immortality of Mans Soul*, London, 1682, p. 71, cited in John Henry, 'Medicine and Pneumatology: Henry More, Richard Baxter and Francis Glisson's *Treatise on the Energetic Nature of Substance*', *Medical History*, 31 (1987), 15–40, esp. p. 35. Henry notes the similarity between the views of Willis, Lower and Baxter on fire in the blood. For another version of the relation between 'the Spirit of God' and 'the life and radicall heat of spirits', see Browne, *Religio Medici*, p. 100.

51. Harold J. Cook, *The Decline of the Old Medical Regime in Stuart London*, Ithaca, Cornell University Press, 1986, pp. 162–80; Michael Hunter, *Science and Society in Restoration England*, Cambridge, Cambridge Uni-

versity Press, 1981, pp. 41–2, 49–50; Roy Porter, 'The early Royal Society and the Spread of Medical Knowledge', in French and Wear (eds), *Medical Revolution*, pp. 272–93.

52. Hobbes to Brooke, in Malcolm, *Correspondence of Hobbes*, pp. 701–3; *Calendar of State Papers (Domestic) 1668–9*, p. 145.

53. Fairfax to Oldenburg, 28 June 1669, in A.R. Hall and M.B. Hall (eds), *Correspondence of Henry Oldenburg*, 14 vols, Madison and London, University of Wisconsin Press and Mansell, 1965–86), vol. 6, pp. 67–71 and Birch, *History of the Royal Society*, vol. 2, pp. 386–7. See Nathaniel Fairfax, 'Anatomical Observations on a Humane Body, Dead of Odd Diseases', *Philosophical Transactions*, 2 (1667), 546–51; William Durston, 'An Extract of a Letter ... Concerning a Very Sudden and Excessive Swelling of a Womans Breasts', *Philosophical Transactions*, 4 (1669) 1047–9; Porter, 'The Early Royal Society', pp. 277, 286. For Fairfax on spirits see his *Treatise of the Bulk and Selvedge of the World*, London, Robert Boulter, 1674, p. 141.

54. Johnston to Clarke, in Birch, *History of the Royal Society*, vol. 2, p. 390 (my translation). For Clarke see Frank, *Harvey and the Oxford Physiologists*, pp. 172–3; Porter, 'The Early Royal Society', p. 275; Cook, *Decline of the Old Medical Regime*, p. 143. For precedents for such an interrogation, see Vandereycken and van Deth, *From Fasting Saints to Anorexic Girls*, p. 52.

55. Johnston to Clarke, in Birch, *History of the Royal Society*, vol. 2, pp. 390–1. For Taylor's mother see *Mirabile pecci*, p. 5.

56. Hobbes to Brooke, in Malcolm, *Correspondence of Hobbes*, p. 702. For Brooke's interests see ibid. pp. 798–9. For Johnston on *Leviathan*, see his *The Excellency of Monarchical Government especially of the English Monarchy*, London, T.B. for Robert Clavel, 1686, pp. 4–5, 27 and for the attack on portents see ibid., p. 428.

57. Johnston to Clarke, in Birch, *History of the Royal Society*, vol. 2, pp. 391–2. For the 1669 charter see Michael Hunter, *Establishing the New Science*, Woodbridge, Boydell and Brewer, 1989, pp. 21, 175.

58. Hobbes, 'An Historical Narration Concerning Heresy', in William Molesworth (ed.), *English Works of Thomas Hobbes*, 11 vols, London, John Bohn, 1839–45, vol. 4, pp. 385–408, esp. p. 407; Hobbes to Brooke, in Malcolm, *Correspondence of Hobbes*, p. 702. For Hobbes's earlier illness see Hobbes to Sorbière, 17 November 1647, ibid., p. 164; for his predicament in 1668 see Robert Willman, 'Hobbes on the Law of Heresy', *Journal of the History of Ideas*, 31 (1970), 607–13.

59. Browne, *Religio Medici*, p. 107. For Taylor's death see Wadsworth, 'Martha Taylor', p. 83.

CHAPTER EIGHT

Plague, Prayer and Physic: Helmontian Medicine in Restoration England

Ole Peter Grell

In 1665, when London experienced what turned out to be the last outbreak of plague, Helmontian physicians and practitioners used the occasion to promote aggressively their particular type of medicine. They considered the epidemic to be a golden opportunity for the trial they had cherished for years, between their remedies and those of their Galenic collegues within the College of Physicians. The trial, however, turned out to be more than a test of two competing natural philosophies and types of medicine, it became as much a test of two faiths. As such it was a confrontation between on the one hand those who considered themselves to be truly Christian practitioners, who through divine inspiration and experiments sought to retrieve the remedies and cures God had made available to Man in Nature, and on the other 'ungodly' Galenic physicians, who were not only considered medically redundant, but also seen to be irreligious by their Helmontian rivals. For the Helmontians the epidemic in 1665 provided the ideal occasion for such a trial to be conducted in public and adjudged by God, the only and ultimate judge of all things.

Before turning to this event it is worth emphasizing that plague undoubtedly was the most terrifying disease which affected England in the seventeenth century. Major epidemics devastated urban communities at irregular intervals from 1603 until 1665. Such outbreaks often killed between 10 and 12 per cent of the urban population in less than six months. Thus more than 80,000 died in the metropolis in 1665 – almost 20 per cent of the city's population. Even if health regulations and their enforcement could demonstrate some limited success over time, plague continued to be perceived as near impossible to cure. Undoubtedly the lack of understanding of the disease, what caused it and how it was transmitted, added to the dread and the feeling of impotence it generated. Consequently, a religious rationale and approach to the outbreaks continued to play a prominent part in the response it generated.

Little, however, had changed in the perception of plague in post-Reformation England. It continued to be seen as a primarily supernatural disease, sent by God to punish man for his sins and contemporary terminology continued to equate sin with disease. In an age where most religious and social responses were based on readings of the Bible, which had become widely available in the vernacular as a consequence of the Reformation, plenty of evidence for such views could be found in the Scriptures, especially the Old Testament where it constitutes the typical punishment portrayed as one of the three arrows of war, famine and pestilence released by God to punish his people.[1] As such it proved particularly popular among English Puritans or Calvinists who considered themselves to be God's chosen people, the new Covenanters, as can be seen from the influential tract published by the Puritan minister, William Gouge, entitled, *Gods Three Arrows. A Plaister for the Plague*.[2]

By the start of the seventeenth century, God had gradually come to be perceived as working mainly through secondary causes, according to the Law of Nature, and natural explanations of epidemic disease, with their Galenic emphasis on contagion and miasma, had come to form part of a useful circular explanation. Thus, as Paul Slack emphasizes in his magisterial study, *The Impact of Plague in Tudor and Stuart England*, supernatural and natural explanations came to form 'two interlocking parts of a single interpretative chain' which provided a rationale for plague.[3] Consequently, religious remedies such as prayer and repentance continued to come first. This undoubtedly found its most visual and prominent expression in the weekly, public fasts which were instituted in connection with major epidemics in the sixteenth and seventeenth centuries, consisting of a day of abstinence, supplemented with a lavish offering of sermons and prayers in the local parish churches. Only when added to such godly remedies could medicine be properly used and have any hope of success. Medicine was considered part of God's Creation and accordingly could only work through the grace of God.

By 1665, this picture was beginning to change. The dominant religious or supernatural element in the explanations of, and approach to, plague appears to have been on the wane. By then weekly fasts had been replaced with monthly ones. If the frequency of such public religious expressions is anything to go by then the significance of religion in connection with plague was certainly on the decline. Furthermore, while during the plague epidemics of 1625 and 1636 more than half of all the works published on this subject had been of a purely religious and devotional nature offering spiritual consolation, by 1665 the religious element of the published plague-literature had dwindled to around a third of the total output.[4]

The fact that plague demonstrated a much clearer social bias in the seventeenth century as compared with the previous century may also have served to dilute the religious emphasis in connection with epidemics. It is noteworthy that by 1665 the mortality rates in the poorer parishes and suburbs to the south and north-east of London were double those in the centre.[5] Furthermore the sheer cost of professional medical advice, would have guaranteed that the patients of most physicians were recruited predominantly from the upper echelons of society, residing in the centre. Consequently, English physicians of the seventeenth century would have had considerably less direct experience of plague than their predecessors of the sixteenth century, because far fewer of their patients caught or died of the disease. Obviously, the hand of God had to play a less prominent role in the plague-tracts written by physicians towards the middle of the seventeenth century.

In this connection it should also be borne in mind that whereas the earlier literature had been divided over the role of the supernatural, religious causes of plague as opposed to the role of natural causes, the controversy in 1665–66 was mainly about the efficacy of traditional Galenic remedies as opposed to the new alchemical ones recommended by an influential group of Paracelsian/Helmontian physicians. This controversy was accompanied by another conflict or rather campaign against the English practice of strict household isolation. Here, however, antagonists such as the Helmontian physician George Thomson and the Galenist, Fellow of the College of Physicians, Nathaniel Hodges could find some common ground. Still their arguments against isolation differed substantially in origin. Thomson based his objections to the strict enforcement of long-term household isolation on his Hermetic, neo-Platonic natural philosophy which considered itself rooted in God's original revelations to Adam. Thus, Paracelsian/Helmontian physicians claimed to be the only true, Christian practitioners as opposed to the heathen and corrupt Galenists they sought to replace. Consequently, the need to show Christian charity to one's suffering neighbours by providing them with medicine and nursing had to take precedence over the wider social interest of the Commonwealth which might justify strict quarantine. Nathaniel Hodges's argument for a 'softer' approach to household isolation, on the other hand, was based solely on the common-sense assumption that the psychological effect of being locked up with plague-infected members of one's household might prove detrimental to one's general health and thus make people easier prey to plague. Thomson would have agreed with Hodges, even if his epistemology and practical arguments in favour of a milder regime differed substantially from those of his antagonist, such as his claim that isolation could destroy the Archeus which helped protect against infection. This, however, was not an agreement which could be extended to their overall natural philosophy. As opposed to Hodges and the overwhelming majority of the members of the College of Physicians, Thomson considered his Paracelsian/Helmontian medicine to be 'ordained in these last times by special providence of God, for the comfort and relief of distressed Man'.[6]

Paracelsianism even in its religiously modified and politically adjusted form, such as that expressed by the Dane, Peter Severinus, in his influential work *Idea Medicinæ* (1571) had only made a very limited impact in England before the outbreak of the Civil War.[7] Only during the late 1640s and 1650s did it begin to gain ground, thanks not least to the influence of the medical ideas of Jan Baptista van Helmont, whose collected works, *Ortus medicinae* were posthumously edited and published by his son, Franciscus Mercurius van Helmont, in 1648. The growing significance of Paracelsian/Helmontian medicine in England was clearly in evidence by the 1650s when this approach was vigorously promoted by the circle of scholars connected with Samuel Hartlib in particular. The popularity of Helmontian medicine with Puritan physicians of the Cromwellian period, many of whom, such as George Starkey, used it as a vehicle to attack the College of Physicians's monopoly on medicine, has been convincingly demonstrated by Charles Webster.[8] Webster, however, has been unable to provide a similarly convincing explanation for the attraction of Helmontian medicine for royalist, 'Anglican' physicians, such as George Thomson, who was to become a leading light in the society of chemical physicians which actively challenged the monopoly of the College of Physicians in the years immediately after the Restoration. Webster's claim that 'Anglican Hermeticists' concentrated 'on a less practical and more esoteric range of Hermetic writings', than did their Puritan colleagues, may have to be modified for this group, especially its leading exponent, George Thomson.[9]

In this chapter I attempt to provide an explanation for the religious rationale which encouraged Thomson's advocacy of a neo-Platonic/Helmontian natural philosophy. This, in turn, will also help explain Thomson's close collaboration with such ex-radical/Puritan figures as George Starkey and Marchamont Nedham. But more importantly I emphasize the continued significance of religion in connection with plague epidemics in Restoration England. I argue that in spite of the general trend towards a more factual and natural approach to plague during the epidemic of 1665 a religious interpretation and reaction to plague continued to characterize the approach of one particular and influential group of medical men, namely those Helmontian physicians, such as George Thomson, who constituted the driving force behind the society of chemical physicians.

George Thomson, born to prosperous parents in 1619, appears to have aimed at a medical career from his early years. However, the death of his father and the outbreak of the Civil War caused him to interrupt his medical studies in London. He left for France and may well have continued his studies there until he returned in 1644 intent on settling in Oxford. Instead Thomson joined the royalist army and took part in Prince Maurice's successful campaign in the west of England until he was captured at Newbury in October 1644.[10] Having been released from prison Thomson was examined by the censors of the College of Physicians in order to obtain a licentiate membership. However, he found the fees demanded by the College prohibitive. Thus his later antagonism to the College and its Galenic medicine might well have been fuelled by this personal experience. Instead Thomson gained professional recognition by obtaining an MA from the University of Edinburgh and an MD from the University of Leiden which he was awarded in 1648. It is more than likely that Thomson was introduced to the ideas of Van Helmont during his stay at Leiden.[11] Upon his return from the Netherlands he began to practise at Romford in Essex, outside the College's jurisdiction, and not until after his splenectomy experiment in 1656 does he appear to have settled in London where he remained until his death in 1677.[12]

In 1665 Thomson published his first attack, *Galeno-Pale*, on his Galenist adversaries within the College of Physicians. This pamphlet was written before plague had broken out in the city of London. In his general attack on the members of the College Thomson makes a statement which, with hindsight, was to have a somewhat prophetical character: 'What we pray should our City have done, if some Epidemical contagous Disease, as the Plague, had reigned amongst us sith they (*the Galenists*) (according to their Masters Dictates) would all have run out of it.'[13] William Johnson was less fortunate with his defence of the College of Physicians. In his tract he underlined that since 'our Galenists' have actively fought the disease during earlier epidemics it is unlikely that they 'should now run from their colours, if the like danger should happen'.[14] Johnson's high expectations of his colleagues were to be disappointed while Thomson's negative predictions were proved right by the reaction of most London physicians to the plague of 1665. They followed in the footsteps of most of their predecessors among the fellows and licentiates of the College and fled the city. A few, however, stayed behind and ministered to plague victims, among them William Johnson who fell victim to the disease and died proving that he, at least, had the necessary moral rectitude.[15] The question of flight and the obligation of physicians to stay and treat the plague-stricken became an important point constantly raised by Helmontian physicians such as

Thomson and Starkey in their subsequent attacks on their Galenist adversaries during 1665–66. Consequently members of the College of Physicians must have felt an urgent need to justify their reaction upon their return to London. Samuel Pepys, however, showed little if any sympathy for the excuses made by Dr Jonathan Goddard at the first meeting of the Royal Society after the epidemic. According to Pepys, Goddard did his utmost to convince them that since most of the important patients of the physicians had fled the city the physicians had been at liberty to follow them.[16] Even Nathaniel Hodges, who stayed in London and attended the sick, had to admit that most physicians had 'retired' from the city, but as he pointed out, they had done so 'not so much for their own Preservation, as the Service of those whom they attend'.[17]

George Thomson dedicated *Galeno-Pale* to the recently appointed Archbishop of Canterbury, Gilbert Sheldon. A most fortuitous choice bearing in mind that later events were to show Sheldon as a man who did not abandon his post or shy away from his responsibilities in times of crisis: Sheldon was among those leading government figures who stayed in London during the plague of 1665.[18] Thomson justified his choice by pointing out that Sheldon belonged to a group of 'Mæcenas of Hermetic Philosophy' and added:

> And all things duly pondered where can Chymical Physick better shelter itself against Maligners and Opposers of it, then under the wings of Divinity, on which it ought to attend as an Hand-maid? Yea, there should be a Synergie, and conspiration of all Arts and Sciences to advance Theology, which makes the better Part of us happy.[19]

Considering that Gilbert Sheldon had topped the list of religious and political dignitaries who supported the creation of a patented society of chemical physicians in the spring of 1665 the choice was hardly surprising.[20] But more importantly it served to draw attention to the fact that a Christian, Helmontian natural philosophy and medicine constituted an important supplement to theology and religion, and that true religion and medicine were mutually dependent. The godly, Helmontian physician had 'a Commission from the Angel Raphael' and was endowed with the gift of healing as opposed to others (i.e. Galenists).[21] By referring to Raphael which means 'God has healed' in Hebrew, Thomson evidently wanted to make an important point while showing off his Christian humanist credentials![22] For Thomson medicine depended as much on true godliness as the true church depended on a Christian, Helmontian medicine. Thus he posed the question: 'How can the Soul act aright when there is an Atonie, Ametrie and Dyscrasie in the Body?' In his answer Thomson implied that by curing the diseased body the

Helmontians could help the soul come to its senses. This could be achieved by searching for 'those great Arcanas in Nature, which the good Creator hath ordained for the preservation and reintegration' of body and soul.[23] This was in fact a theme Thomson returned to several times in his later writings.

In the main, however, *Galeno-Pale* was a comprehensive attack on the heathen, Galenic medicine promoted by the College of Physicians. Thomson portrayed the Galenic medicine it advocated as a scholastic self-indulgent and corrupt enterprise which only served to glorify individual members of an organization urgently in need of reform. In particular he scorned the Galenic corruption of anatomy:

> Our Antagonists raise no small dust, and make no little noise with their dissecton of Bodies, which were much to be commended, if they did not spend more time then needeth, rather for ostentation, and to get a fame abroad, than for any notable improvement in the Cure of poor miserable Man.[24]

Only when anatomy was intended as an aid to therapy, was it a truly 'Pyrotechnical Anatomy', and could be considered a worthwhile enterprise for the godly physician. Galenic anatomy which sought to establish the exact location of disease in the body was ridiculed by Thomson. Ironically he refers to an unusual dissection:

> which indeed was boldly attempted (though in vain) by an industrious Galenist of late years, who cut up a Pestilential Body, to find out in what part the Plague did principally reside, to the loss of his own life, perhaps for want of some Arcanum which an Helmontist could have given him. Anatomy we stand up for, as much as any, without which we are certain a Physician must necessarily be much defective in Physic.[25]

Considering that George Thomson was to perform the first documented dissection of a plague victim later that year this proved a particularly poignant example. Furthermore Thomson's outspoken criticism of contemporary anatomy did not preclude a realization that anatomical knowledge and experience was necessary for physicians. It was not anatomy as such he was opposed to, but only the form it had taken in the hands of 'discredited' Galenists trained in a scholastic tradition.

Other dangerous and corrupt Galenic practices such as phlebotomy ought not only to be changed, but should be abandoned, especially when treating plague victims, since it weakend the vital spirits. According to Thomson this central element in Galenic therapy was no less than 'Satan's device and plot to destroy mankind'.[26]

Here, however, the Helmontians could draw on the support of other less unorthodox physicians such as the Utrecht professor of medicine, Isbrand van Diemerbroek, whose *Tractatus de Peste*, first printed in

Arnhem in 1644, but reprinted in Amsterdam in 1665 in connection with the outbreak of plague there, became something of a standard authority in England after the plague had reached London.[27] Thus, Diemerbroek is the most quoted authority in the manuscript, entitled *Loimographia, or an Experimentall Relation of the Plague, of What Hath Happened Remarkable in the Last Plague in the City of London* (1666), written by the learned apothecary, William Boghurst.[28] Furthermore, part of the fourth book of Diemerbroek's work, which contains 120 case stories of plague, was translated into English in 1666. This English edition consisted of a selection of 27 of these case stories, 16 of which ended fatally, among them a surgeon who 'foolishly' interfered with Diemerbroek's treatment by bleeding himself.[29]

In order to prove the superiority of godly, Helmontian medicine over heathen Galenism, Thomson in all his writings emphasized the original demand of Van Helmont that the Galenists should consent to a trial of their remedies and those of the Helmontians in front of independent assessors.[30]

In his reply to William Johnson Thomson vigorously defended himself against the accusations of being a dangerous religious and political fanatic, claiming to have risked his life in the royalist cause during the Civil War and pointing out his 'Loyalty, fidelity to the crown of England, and a healthy desire to promote the Peace, unity, Order and Conformity of Church and State'.[31] He was, in other words, despite his Paracelsian/Helmontian natural philosophy a loyal subject of the Crown and an orthodox member of the Church of England. Printed with Thomson's reply to Johnson was a letter from his 'cordial friend and brother',[32] George Starkey, which made direct reference to the growing epidemic in London and the obligations of the godly physicians. Starkey wrote:

> But this I may, and shall not doubt to affirm, that this hand of God, in case it continue upon us, and increase among us will prove a signal note of distinction, between Physicians elected, and sent forth by God, and those mercenary Hirelings, who either run unsent, or were created by the Schools.[33]

Starkey had no doubt that the physicians who strove piously to serve God 'in doing their duty faithfully and effectually, and charitable serving their Neighbour to the comfort of the Patients, and credit of themselves, the merciful God will hear'.[34] This religious and professional duty of the physician to stay and care for the afflicted was a position with which Thomson and other supporters of the society of chemical physicians could fully associate. In his first work concerned with the plague, *Loimologia*, Thomson confirmed this view:

> For my part, although I could enjoy my ease, pleasure, and profit
> in the Country, as well perhaps as any Galenist; yet I would rather
> chuse to loose my life, then violate in this time of extream neces-
> sity, the band of Charity towards my neighbour, and dedecorate
> that illustrious profession I am called to, in hopes to save my self
> by a speedy discession, a remote procession, and a leisurely reces-
> sion, according to that infamous, and insidous advice which Galen
> hath given his Disciples.

Adding:

> To visit, relieve and exhilerate any one whom God hath wounded
> with this Pestilential Arrow, is the part of a truly religious Samari-
> tan; as to flie from him, or keep aloof, when he may preserve or do
> him good, is onely proper to some distrustful wicked Priests, Levites
> and Galenists.[35]

The metaphors used by Thomson are significant. While the Helmontian
physicians are shown as true and caring representatives of New Testament Christianity the Galenists are identified with the Jewish priesthood (Levites) who had sought to destroy Christianity and had been
instrumental in bringing about the crucifixion of Christ.

Thomson's choice of titles for this plage tract, *Loimologia*, and the
subsequent work, entitled *Loimotomia* published in 1666,[36] are also of
significance in this context. To my knowledge George Thomson is the
first English author to use the Greek word for plague, loimos, in a title.
By using it he clearly wanted to convey the message that the Helmontian
medicine he was promoting was part of the Christian humanist renaissance.

The recovery of Thucydides's history had been an important event in
Renaissance humanism. Thus in 1629 Thomas Hobbes appeared in
print for the first time with a translation of Thucydides's *Peloponnesian
War*, which proved popular and went through several editions in the
first half of the seventeenth century.[37] In this work Thucydides provides
a vivid description of the plague in ancient Athens, referring to a verse
predicting that 'a Dorique Warre shall fall, and a great plague withall'.
In order to make his translation of the subsequent passage comprehen-
sible to his English audience Hobbes had been obliged to include the
Greek word 'loimos'.

> Now were men at variance about the word, some saying that it was
> not loimos (i. the plague) that was by the Ancients, mentioned in
> that verse, but limos (i. famine). But vpon the present occasion the
> word loimos deseruedly obtained. For as men suffered, so they
> made the verse to say.[38]

Furthermore, loimos also carried strong Christian and apocalyptic con-
notations having been used by Luke to describe the pestilence God
would send in the last days in order to test the faith of the godly.[39]

In *Loimologia* Thomson took the opportunity to encourage the magistracy to take action against those physicians who had fled the city. Upon their return they should be compelled to visit the sick. Thomson added that he would be only too pleased to accompany them visiting some infected patients. Ironically Thomson suggested that they could then take the pulse of these patients, look at their tongues and 'peep into Urinals and Close-stools'. Such actions were, of course, part of traditional Galenist therapeutics which these physicians, according to Thomson, had always been keen on performing 'when there was least need of them'. He then returned with some relish to his earlier criticism of contemporary anatomy:

> Yea, and because they boast they are such excellent Anatomists, we will disect together a Pestilential body, that they may (if they can) inform me better where the subject of that disease is: and for Prevention and Caution, they shall take their Preservatives and sanatives, and I mine; and let the world judge whom God favours most, and who fares best.[40]

Thomson clearly intended to take full advantage of the situation which the outbreak of plague had provided. Now was the time to have the long awaited comparative trial of Helmontian and Galenic remedies. Faced with the plague independent assessors were no longer necessary. God would be the arbiter and the general public the jury. At this stage, however, Thomson was only advocating a dissection of a plague victim in order to have a reliable test of the efficacy of the respective medical remedies.

For Thomson and his colleagues within the society of chemical physicians the plague of 1665 proved a godsend in more than one sense. First, the hand of God provided them with an opportunity to promote their particular brand of natural philosophy and medicine. They were not slow in making use of this opportunity. In June 1665 they published a broadsheet or 'Advertisement' promoting their chemical remedies which they pointed out had not been copied out of old medical books, unlike the Galenic advice lately published by the College of Physicians. Instead their medicines had been developed specifically for the present plague, which differed from previous plagues in other countries. They also took the opportunity to remind the public of the Christian nature of their remedies:

> Which Medicines so prepared we here offer to our Countrymen, not doubting but that the great God, who hath given us a heart and light to search in to the mysteries of *Nature* and the *mysterious nature* of diseases will so second our endeavours by his special blessing, as to make us and our *Remedies* as his own hands, to secure the sound, and save the sick from this devouring Maladie.[41]

Second, having challenged his Galenist opponents to a test of remedies, exposed to the dangers of infection, while dissecting a plague victim, Thomson eventually performed a dissection of a 'pestilential body' on his own. This proved a unique event even if rumours seem to have persisted in London that some of Thomson's Helmontian colleagues, such as Thomas O'Dowd and George Starkey, who died while attending their patients during the plague, might have caught the disease while performing a dissection of a plague victim; similar rumours, however, also circulated about Galenist members of the College of Physicians, who died while attending their patients in the city. It is more than likely that such rumours had been fuelled by George Thomson's repeated references to this particular type of dissection, and they appear to have been no more than hearsay.[42]

But why did Thomson decide to perform this particular dissection which he had been so scathing about in his previous works? Was it simply in order to prove that Helmontian remedies were effective in treating or preventing plague? This can hardly have been the case, considering both the title and the frontispiece which George Thomson chose for his pamphlet. As if the title *Loimotomia: or the Pest Anatomized*, does not tell us enough, the frontispiece, which shows the dissection of the plague victim, leaves no room for doubt. Thomson wanted to demonstrate the learning and ability involved in the only proper form of anatomy: 'pyrotechnical anatomy' (Figure 8.1). In his preface to the reader he underlined his ambition to pursue the 'Therapeutical Truth', adding:

> that I was restless till I had the full view of the inward parts of the pestilential Body, whereby my Judgement was confirmed in some things, and my Intellectuals instructed in others. I have acted many years formerly, but especially now of late, when there was most need, the part of Physician, Chirurgion, and Apothecary, as becomes every honest able Man Lawfully called to this Noble Faculty.[43]

Apart from telling us that the dissection is the central element of this work, the frontispiece graphically demonstrates the continued significance and interdependence of religion and medicine for Helmontian medicine in post-Restoration England. In one picture we are shown the patient or victim of the epidemic, clearly recognizeable by the many black spots on his body, who is in the process of being dissected by George Thomson. Thomson is portrayed standing at the head of the body holding his surgical knife, while a similar figure is shown standing at the feet of the body, folding his hands in prayer while directing his gaze towards heaven. The plague-infected body lies in a coffin placed on a catafalque with a dish containing burning sulphur placed next to

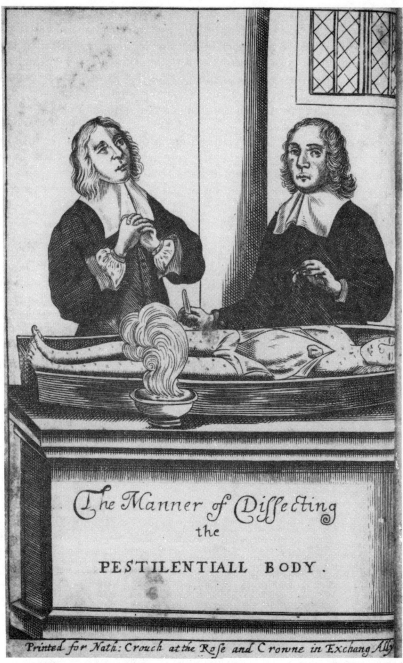

8.1 Title-page of George Thomson's, *Loimotomia: or the Pest Anatomized*, London, 1666.

it. This dish is in accordance with the Helmontian practice which recommended the use of sulphur to fumigate infected houses.[44]

The inscription on the catafalque: 'The Manner of Dissecting the Pestilentiall Body' together with the subtitle of the pamphlet: 'the Pest Anatomized', emphasizes the significance of this particular anatomical event: apart from advocating the proper Helmontian approach, this dissection constitutes the first documented dissection of a plague victim by any English physician.

George Thomson gives a detailed account of his dissection in chapter 5 of *Loimotomia*. The anatomized corpse belonged to a young man of around 15, a servant, whom Thomson seems to have been unable to help despite successfully curing his master, a certain 'lusty proper man by name Mr William Pick'. Having been instrumental in Mr Pick's recovery Thomson had requested permission to dissect the body of the deceased servant, as he explained for his own instruction 'and the satisfaction of all inquisitive Persons to which having given him some perswasive reasons to that purpose' Mr Pick quickly agreed.[45] From Thomson's description of the event we may assume that the figure who is seen praying in the frontispiece is supposed to be the servant whom Mr Pick ordered to assist him in the dissection. The way this figure is dressed, however, would indicate that this may not necessarily be the case. Considering that both figures are shown as wearing the same, scholarly clothes, and that they look like identical twins, an interpretation which sees the Helmontian physician, George Thomson as appearing twice in the same picture, seems far more likely.

First, Thomson is portrayed as praying to God for spiritual guidance and direction in his imminent and major undertaking. This was an essential act for a Helmontian physician such as George Thomson. Without spiritual insight and inspiration any hope of understanding and eventually finding a cure for this major scourge of contemporary society was doomed to fail.

Second, Thomson is depicted half-way through his dissection of the young servant, having his surgical knife in his right hand while holding in his left hand 'a white congealed matter' which he had extracted with his fingers from 'the right cavity of the heart' (the gap in the heart, created by Thomson's incision, is clearly visible on the frontispiece). Evidently, this was a particularly crucial moment of discovery in Thomson's dissection of this plague victim since it merited depiction. Furthermore Thomson offered a detailed explanation of this peculiarity built on Helmontian principles which saw the key to the disease as lying in the 'Archeus' or vital spirits of man and viewed the disease as spreading through a poisonous fermentation:

> To render a sound reason of this albified coagulation in this right Ventricle of the heart, may perhaps puzzle a good Physiologist. For in all those cadavers I ever saw dissected, this hollow receptacle did still contain a blackish blood condensed, arising from a stopping of the Circulation of it first in that place. Now the most probable cause (as I conceive, with submission) of this unwonted white substance, may come from a sumption of meer crude milk, which an indiscreet Nurse had given this youth not long before he died, part of which passing out of the stomach little altered, might be conveyed, upon a pinch and stress to preserve life, through the *Venæ lacteæ* in the Mesenterie, or some shorter passage, into the subclavian vessels, and there entring the right cavity of the Heart, be changed according to the capacity of the Matter by a virulent preternatural ferment into this seeming glandulous flesh.[46]

By performing this particular dissection Thomson had been able to demonstrate that plague did not reside in any particular part of the body. Instead he had been able to show that it was a kind of poison which infected the stomach and the spleen, causing these organs to ejaculate 'virulent black Effluviums' to the head and heart. Furthermore, Thomson, who had himself caught the plague while performing the dissection, was able to observe that this effluvium was 'causing a dizziness in the one, and a tedious oppression in the other'.[47] Having been unfortunate enough to catch the disease while 'dabbling incogitantly in the cadaverous gore' this misadventure provided Thomson with a golden opportunity to prove the efficacy of his Helmontian remedies. Thus he cured himself taking the best of his medicines in large quantities which, through his experiments, he had already assured himself were 'safe and effectual' before the disease made him delirious.[48]

Thomson concluded the description of his dissection with an attack on the Galenists and the College of Physicians for their lack of Christian compassion:

> These Pseudiatori are prone to corrupt the *Text*, and to deprave the genuine Sense of any Physical Experiment, which through fear, and want of appropriate Remedies, they dare not venture upon for the benefit of their distressed Countrey. For they enter in at the Back-door, and run away at the Fore-door, on whom the gift of Healing was never bestowed, because they never sought aright, for that reason they could never obtain such a favour from Heaven, to be protected by Divine Preservatives from the stinking noysom Breath of this mortiferous Basilisk: wherefore they maliciously backbite those that perform any thing above themselves, calling that a Pre-sumption, that tends to the preventing a Consumption and Devas-tation of a whole Nation.[49]

By taking on such a dangerous inquiry and, furthermore, by catching the disease Thomson had been able to show the providential nature of his Helmontian medicine. God had heard the godly physician's prayer and given him guidance in his study of the Book of Nature. This divine blessing of his undertaking had made it possible for Thomson to retrieve some of the remedies which God had originally made available to Man when he created the world, but which had been forgotten after the Fall. In accordance with the early Protestant reformers such as Martin Luther and John Hooper in England the Helmontian physicians of the Restoration period were strongly opposed to flight. It was the Christian obligation of the physician to love his neighbour and offer his services to those who had fallen victim to the plague. This meant that in the first instance the physician's duty lay with the sick individual as opposed to the healthy and the Commonwealth.[50]

Thomson and his Helmontian friends undoubtedly shared their Christian spirituality with many of the early reformers. Where the reformers considered themselves to have saved the Word of God – the Bible – from the scholastic corruption of Rome, the Helmontians saw themselves as doing the same for the Book of Nature. The complementary nature of their undertakings – one taking on the scholastic theology of Catholic Church, the other opposing the scholastic, Galenic medicine of the College of Physicians – is evident. The emphasis these Helmontian physicians placed on the obligation of doctors to remain and attend the plague-stricken was obviously a direct consequence of their religious and natural philosophical outlook. They may not have been alone among English physicians of the seventeenth century in having this view, but it is remarkable how few supporters can be found for it outside their ranks.

In 1665 both the apothecary, William Boghurst, and the astrologer, John Gadbury, were opposed to flight by medical men when faced with epidemics. Both, however, were familiar with and interested in Paracelsian/Helmontian medicine and may well have gained their inspiration from such sources.[51] Furthermore, it is significant that the emphasis of Thomson and Starkey on the physician's Christian obligation to stay is missing not only from Gadbury's and Boghurst's arguments against flight, but also from those of the physician Gideon Harvey, who only went as far as to say that 'physicians can never discharge their Duty with greater Applause than by contributing their aid to popular Diseases'.[52]

Similarly in connection with the epidemics of 1625 and 1636 two physicians, Francis Heering and Stephen Bradwell, both members of the College of Physicians, had argued against the use of flight. Heering would undoubtedly have agreed with Bradwell's statement: 'But I will not teach to flee; far too many with Dedalus put on wings in the last visitation, that with Icarus dropt down by the way.' People should stay but avoid social contact as much as possible: 'Stay then, you that are

Rich, to helpe the Poore, and you that haue skill in Physicke to helpe the sick.'[53]

It is noteworthy that both Heering and Bradwell were familiar with Paracelsian medicine and alchemical remedies and were guardedly advocating their use. Bradwell mentioned his grandfather, John Bannister, who had published a recipe book which included many Paracelsian remedies, and emphasized that with regard to the plague 'all these Symptomes must be looked to very diligently and skilfully. As for the Sores, there are many good and known medicines, and hands skilful enough in Chymigical ways'.[54]

Accordingly it seems reasonable to interpret this revival of the Christian obligation to attend the sick rather than give priority to the Commonwealth and the healthy, which had been strongly supported by the first generation of Protestant reformers, as being dependent on the interest in Paracelsian/Helmontian medicine and natural philosophy which increased dramatically by the late 1640s.

As Charles Webster has shown us this concern was closely associated with the Puritan, millenarian expectations of the period.[55] That explains the reactions of such unorthodox physicians as Marchamont Nedham and George Starkey, but does not assist us much in understanding the views of a royalist supporter of the Church of England such as George Thomson.

Thomson certainly shared the millenarianism of those of his ex-Puritan friends and colleagues who had been active during the Commonwealth, as appears from his above-mentioned statement in *Galeno-Pale*, that God had ordained Helmontian medicine 'in these last times'. He also shared their eirenicist ambition for a unification of all the good Protestant churches, in his case within a comprehensive Church of England, based on what can best be described as a minimalist, anti-dogmatic theology.[56] This was, of course, a scheme similar if not identical to that strongly supported by the Hartlib circle which had found a leading exponent in John Dury. In fact, such an eirenical unification of the Protestant churches had been considered a necessary precondition for bringing about the golden age which most of the reformers had been praying for. The religious heterodoxy and lack of significant medical reforms which characterized the Interregnum eventually served to disappoint most of those who had worked for 'the great instauration'. The frustrations of the 1640s and 1650s generated a sense of failure and disappointment which caused some of the leading Helmontians such as John Webster and Noah Biggs to withdraw from public life and pursue their experiments in private, while others such as George Starkey and Marchamont Nedham projected their hopes for a golden age and a Christian renewal in medicine on to the Restoration of the monarchy and the Church of England.[57] By the late 1650s these former radicals had come full circle and attached their Helmontian colours to a religious and political unification of the Commonwealth which could only be brought about by the Restoration of the monarchy and the Church of England. By transposing their hopes to the Restoration and working actively for its realization they were able to join hands with George Thomson.

Thomson gave the following expression to these aspirations:

> I should not question by means of wholsome Chymical Physick to make Men of more sound Religion. Atheism, Hypocrisie, Prophaness, Debauchery, might in some measure be lesened, quailed, and restrained, by power of a Mastering Discipline of the Intellectual Soul made more apt to understand the Truth of things, by means of the organs of the Body, Blood, and Spirits well clarified.
>
> By Virtue of our Hermetic Physick the Head, Heart and hands of Hierophants might be purified. Their Exemplary Dumb and deaf Preaching up of Vice throughout the World, be corrected. Circumstances and Punctilios in Religion lovingly, calmly proposed, debated, and Accepted. And those fierce eager Altercations about Adiophora laid aside.[58]

Through the application of such remedies Thomson hoped to bring the sects, such as Anabaptists, Quakers and Independents to realize their mistakes, and instead focus on the essentials of their Christian faith. This would help them to see the truth and cause them to reunite within the newly restored Church of England.

Bearing this in mind, George Thomson's decision to dedicate his first work to the Archbishop of Canterbury, Gilbert Sheldon, becomes triply important. First, by pointing to Gilbert Sheldon's interest in neo-Platonic natural philosophy and his attraction to Helmontian medicine which could serve as a 'hand-maid' for true godliness, Thomson had drawn attention to their shared objective in promoting a truly harmonious Christian community. That Thomson's claims about Sheldon's Hermetic interests had substance are confirmed by his antagonist, Nathaniel Hodges. Later in 1665 Hodges tried to counterbalance the effects of Thomson's dedication by dedicating his own vindication of the Galenist position to the Archbishop. Here he admitted that Gilbert Sheldon favoured alchemical medicine and Hermetic natural philosophy.[59] Indications of Sheldon's position can also be gleaned from the sermon he preached before Charles II in Whitehall on 28 June 1660. Here Sheldon pointed out:

> That *all Deliverance comes from (him from) the Lord* 'twere needless to multiply Proofs out of *Scriptures*, which are but the registers of his *Providence*, and you cannot look besides them there. And 'tis no less apparent unto *Reason*; for that (*with great clearness, and*

by degree of evidence even beyond knowledge, as those old Philosophers *Hermes* and *Iamblicus* express it) finds that *there is a
God*, and from thence (with as great evidence) demonstrates a
Providence. So that should I lead you out of the Church into the
Schools of Philosophers, Poets, Historians, Writers of all sorts
among the Heathens, you would find them by the very instinct and
impression of Nature, acknowledging the same truth ...

Unfortunately, according to Sheldon, there were many Englishmen who
were 'more heathenish than the Heathen, that will not allow God to
govern in his own House, that deny him any care of things below'.[60]
Not only does Sheldon specifically refer to Hermes and another less
well known neo-Platonic philosopher, Iamblicus, who had been particularly concerned with magic and theosophy, in this sermon, but his
attack on those 'atheists' who did not detect God's hand in nature could
only have encouraged the chemical physicians in their attack on the
heathen, Galenic medicine of the College of Physicians.

   Second, Sheldon also emphasized the Christian obligation to lead a
pious life and actively demonstrate love of one's neighbour. Faith and
gratitude to God was best shown though acts, helping the sick and the
poor. In Sheldon's words: 'We relieve him in the poor, visit him in the
sick, cloath him in the naked, redeem him in the prisoner: *For in that
we do it to these we do it to him (Matth. 25.45)*.'[61]

   Third, in Gilbert Sheldon Thomson would also have found a supporter who fully endorsed his eirenic, non-dogmatic Protestantism which
sought to unite the sects within the Church of England, espousing a
'liberal' Arminian theology. This, for instance, had been an important
point in Sheldon's sermon of June 1660 where he had urged religious
tolerance and understanding in the wake of the Restoration:

   And therefore I beseech you, take care that we strip our selves of
   all unruly passions, that we may have peace within, peace from
   turbulent revengeful affections: For unless we have this, what's
   outward peace worth? Certainly no more to thee then health in the
   City when the Plague is in the bosome.[62]

Sheldon, who had been a close friend of the Socinian/Arminian philosopher, William Chillingworth, and been a member of the Great Tew
Circle, was undoubtedly an Arminian in both theological and ecclesiastical terms. As such Sheldon had not supported the clericalism and
rigorous, so-called Arminian uniformity, introduced by Archbishop
William Laud in the 1630s. His own eirenicism and the 'liberal' Arminian
theology which characterized the gathering at Great Tew would have
served to antagonize him to the Laudian policy of 'thorough'. Not
surprisingly Sheldon appears to have been distrusted by the Laudian
party and received no preferment under them.[63]

Sheldon's attack on the irreligion of the age was echoed by Thomson. Referring to Sir Thomas Browne's work, *Religio Medici*, George Thomson offered the following observations:

> In my Minority I had been a little amazed to hear the Religion of Physicians indifferently, yea flightingly, Ironically spoken of. So that I have not without some indignation, Vindicated it: perswading my self, that there were many, who like Dr. Brown, were able to assert it practically. But coming to greater Maturity in the Observation of Things, I found, for the most part, that really True, which before I apprehended was precipitately spoken by the vulgar.

Pointing the finger firmly at the Galenists he added:

> Besides, how is it possible they should be aquainted in the least with a Deity, who are so grosly ignorant of the Aitiologie of things in Nature. Needs must they be stone Blind as to any right apprehension of an Omnipotent Creator, a Wise Supporter, Disposer, and Governor of all things.[64]

Thus only the godly physician, via his diligent study of the Book of Nature and assisted by divine revelation, could hope to find remedies which might cure not only the sick but also the body politic. Here it would appear that Thomson was prepared to consider his Helmontian medicine as more than just a 'hand-maid' in bringing about the longed for golden age which in turn depended on the formation of an eirenic and non-dogmatic, Arminian Church of England in a politically united kingdom.

> All things rightly weighed my Prospect plainly discovers the Nation wants good store of true Philosophical Physicians to purine the Blood, to invigorate the Archeus, to coroberate the Stomach: then the exorbitancie in Religion and evil Manners, which an Indirect Method of Curing has brought upon us, might sooner be rectified. For this Henry Stubbe is quite mistaken in his thoughts, that a Society of Experimentors should at all debauch the world, sith they can best detect the Fountain of those enormous evils which have been perpetrated in Church and State, through the misapprehension of crasie Brains, and dislocated fancies.[65]

Evidently, for Thomson Helmontian natural philosophy and medicine was not only able to cure the sick body of its afflictions, even when plague-stricken, but also the body politic of all its political and religious ills. As such, Hermetic natural philosophy and medicine had become more than just a helper in advancing true religion. For Thomson it had in fact, become the way to cure both body and soul of the individual, as well as of the nation as a whole. Helmontian medicine might, in other words, provide what theology had been unable to deliver: peaceful coexistence within the framework of an Arminian, eirenicist Church of

England in a stable monarchy. If the efficacy of medicine depended on divine inspiration and guidance of the physician, so in turn did a true Christian theology and the salvation of the nation depend on a Christian Hermetic natural philosophy and medicine.

Notes

1. See for example Exodus 5:3, Leviticus 26:25.
2. W. Gouge, *Gods Three Arrows. A Plaister for the Plague*, London, 1631.
3. P. Slack, *The Impact of Plague in Tudor and Stuart England*, London, 1985, p. 29.
4. Slack, *Impact of Plague*, pp. 240, 244.
5. See Slack, *Impact of Plague*, pp. 153, 166 for the changes in the pattern of plague.
6. G. Thomson, *Galeno-Pale: Or, a Chymical Trial of Galenists*, London, 1665, p. 4; quoted in C. Webster, 'The Helmontian George Thomson and William Harvey: The Revival and Application of Splenectomy to Physiological Research', *Medical History*, 15 (1971), 156.
7. For Paracelsianism in England in the late sixteenth and early seventeenth century, see A.G. Debus, *The English Paracelsians*, New York, 1965.
8. See C. Webster, *The Great Instauration. Science, Medicine and Reform 1626–1660*, London, 1975, esp. pp. 273–88. For a critique of the Webster thesis, see P. Elmer, 'Medicine, Religion and the Puritan Revolution', in R. French and A. Wear (eds), *The Medical Revolution in the Seventeenth Century*, Cambridge, 1989, pp. 10–45; see also C. Webster, 'Puritanism, Separatism and Science', in D.C. Lindberg and R.L. Numbers (eds), *God and Nature: Historical Essays on the Encounter Between Christianity and Science*, Berkeley, 1986, pp. 192–217; and O.P. Grell, 'Protestantism, Natural Philosophy, and the Scientific Revolution', in *Studies in History and Philosophy of Science*, 23 (1992), 519–27, esp. pp. 523–7.
9. Webster, *Instauration*, p. 282. The scholarly interest in Helmontian-Galenist controversy in Restoration England has been considerable, see H. Thomas, 'The Society of Chymical Physicians' in E.A. Underwood (ed.), *Science, Medicine and History*, 2 vols, Oxford, 1953, vol. 2, pp. 56–71; P.M. Rattansi, 'The Helmontian-Galenist Controversy in Restoration England', *Ambix*, 12 (1964), 1–23; C. Webster, 'English Medical Reformers of the Puritan Revolution: A Background to the "Society of Chymical Physitians"', *Ambix*, 14 (1967), 16–41; and most recently H.J. Cook, *The Decline of the Old Medical Regime in Stuart London*, London, 1986, pp. 145–80 and his 'The Society of Chemical Physicians. The New Philosophy and the Restoration Court', *Bulletin for the History of Medicine*, 61 (1987), 61–87.
10. For Thomson's career, see C. Webster, 'The Helmontian George Thomson and William Harvey', pp. 155–6. Thomson refers to his service under Prince Maurice in his dedication to his brother, Prince Rupert, of his pamphlet, *The Direct Method of Curing Chymically*, London, 1675; for Prince Maurice's campaign, see C.V. Wedgwood, *The King's War 1641–1647*, London, 1966.

11. See H. Beukers, 'Clinical Teaching in Leiden From Its Beginning Until the End of the Eighteenth Century' *Clio Medica*, **21** (1987–88), 139–52, and Webster, *Instauration*, p. 276.
12. Webster, 'George Thomson', pp. 155–6.
13. G. Thomson, *Galeno-Pale: Or, A Chymical Trial of the Galenists*, London, 1665, p. 11.
14. W. Johnson, *Some Brief Animadversions Upon Two Late Treatises*, London, 1665, p. 12; quoted in Rattansi, 'Helmontian-Galenist Controversy', p. 18.
15. See Rattansi, 'Helmontian-Galenist Controversy', p. 21.
16. Quoted in O.P. Grell, 'Conflicting Duties: Plague and the Obligations of Early Modern Physicians Towards Patients and Commonwealth in England and the Netherlands', in A. Wear, J. Geyer-Kordesch and R. French (eds), *Doctors and Ethics: The Earlier Historical Setting of Professional Ethics*, Amsterdam, 1993, pp. 131–52.
17. N. Hodges, *Loimologia or, an Historical Account of the Plague in London in 1665*, London, 1720, (published in Latin in 1671), p. 23.
18. V. Staley, *The Life and Times of Gilbert Sheldon*, London, 1913, pp. 157–9.
19. Thomson, *Galeno-Pale*, A2r–v.
20. Thomas, 'The Society of Chymical Physitians', pp. 62–3. Likewise, one of the pivotal figures behind the society of chemical physicians, Thomas O'Dowde, dedicated his first work published in 1664 to Gilbert Sheldon, see T. O'Dowde, *The Poor Man's Physician, Or the True Art of Medicine*, London, 1664; see also Cook, 'Society of Chemical Physicians', p. 70.
21. Thomson, *Galeno-Pale*, A2v.
22. According to the pseudepigraphical books ascribed to Enoch the Archangel Raphael is said to have healed the earth when it was defiled by the sins of the fallen angels, Enoch 10:7.
23. Thomson, *Galeno-Pale*, A2v.
24. Thomson, *Galeno-Pale*, p. 26.
25. Thomson, *Galeno-Pale*, p. 26.
26. Thomson, *Galeno-Pale*, pp. 93–4; quoted in Cook, *Old Medical Regime*, p. 150.
27. I. van Diemerbroek, *Tractatus de Peste, In Quator libros distinctus*, Amsterdam, 1665; see also W. Frijhoff, 'Gods gave afgewezen. Op zoek naar genezing van de pest: Nijmegen, 1635–36', in M. Gijswijt-Hofstra (ed.), *Geloven in genezen. Bijdragen tot de sociaal-culturele geschiedenis van de geneeskunde in Nederland*, *Volkskundig Bulletin*, **17** (1991), 143–70. Diemerbroek's advice against blood-letting was opposed by Thomas Sydenham, see Rattansi, 'Helmontian-Galenist Controversy', p. 20, n. 93.
28. W. Boghurst, *Loimographia. An Account of the Great Plague of London in the Year 1665*, J. F. Payne (ed.), London, 1894.
29. I. van Dimerbroek, *Several Choice Histories of the Medicines, Manner and Method Used in the Cure of the Plague*, London, 1666.
30. See for instance *Galeno-Pale*, p. 42.
31. G. Thomson, *A Gag for Johnson. That Published Animadversions Upon Galeno-Pale*, London, 1665, pp. 13, 17.
32. These words were used by Starkey in his preface (letter) to George Thomson's, *Loimologia. A Consolatory Advice, and Some brief Observations Concerning the Present Pest*, London, 1665. For Starkey, see W.R.

Newman, *Gehennical Fire: The Lives of George Starkey, an American Alchemist in the Scientific Revolution*, Cambridge, MA, 1994.

33. Thomson, *A Gag for Johnson*, p. 53 (G. Starkey, *An Epistolar Discourse to the Learned and Deserving Author of Galeno-Pale*, London, 1665).

34. Thomson, *A Gag for Johnson*, p. 59 (Starkey, *Discourse*).

35. Thomson, *Loimologia*, pp. 2, 9.

36. Thomson, *Loimotomia: Or the Pest Anatomized*, London, 1666.

37. For the recovery of Thucydides, see Q. Skinner, *The Foundations of Modern Political Thought*, 2 vols, Cambridge, 1978, vol. 1, p. 84. For Hobbes's translation, see R. Tuck, *Philosophy and Government 1572–1651*, Cambridge, 1993, p. 281.

38. T. Hobbes (trans.) *Thucydides, Peloponnesian Warre*, London, 1648, p. 110. As a measure of the influence of Hobbes's translation it is noteworthy that Clarendon read Thucydides in this translation, see H. Trevor-Roper, *Catholics, Anglicans and Puritans. Seventeenth Century Essays*, London, 1987, p. 184, note. I am grateful to Dr Simon Goldhill, King's College, Cambridge for drawing Hobbes's translation to my attention.

39. Luke 21:11. Thomson's use of loimos proved popular. His antagonist, the Galenist Nathaniel Hodges, later used the title *Loimologia* for his description of the plague published in 1671; while the apothecary, William Boghurst, used loimos in his manuscript description of the plague, entitled *Loimographia* which he finished in 1666. In this work Boghurst referred specifically to Thucydides and his description of the plague in Athens, see *Loimographia*, p. 8.

40. Thomson, *Loimologia*, p. 10.

41. Advertisement cited in Thomas, 'The Society of Chymical Physicians', p. 57.

42. For the unreliability of these contemporary rumours, see R.S. Wilkinson, 'George Starkey, Physician and Alchemist', *Ambix*, 11 (1963), 121–52, esp. pp. 144–9. Thomson refers to these rumours, emphasizing that he alone conducted the dissection of the plague victim, and that Starkey caught the disease from one of his patients, see Thomson, *Loimotomia*, pp. 103–4.

43. Thomson, *Loimotomia*, To the Reader.

44. See Slack, *Impact of Plague*, p. 249.

45. Thomson, *Loimotomia*, pp. 70–7. The account of the dissection is reprinted in W.G. Bell, *The Great Plague in London in 1665*, 2nd edn, London, 1951, Appendix II, pp. 335–8.

46. Bell, *Great Plague*, pp. 337–8.

47. See G. Thomson, *A Check Given to the Insolent Garrulity of Henry Stubbe*, London, 1671, p. 23. For the role and significance of the spleen in Helmontian medicine, see W. Pagel, 'The Smiling Spleen', in H. Lloyd-Jones, V. Pearl and B. Worden (eds), *History and Imagination. Essays in Honour of H. R. Trevor-Roper*, London, 1981, pp. 81–7, esp. pp. 84–6.

48. Thomson, *A Check to Henry Stubbe*, p. 23.

49. Thomson, *Loimotomia*, p. 105.

50. Grell, 'Conflicting Duties', pp. 131–52.

51. For Boghurst, see *Loimotomia*, p. 3 where he states that: 'Many able persons might have saved mee this labour, and have done it better, especially if they had not been timorous, and, like Foxes in a storme, run to

the next borough'; for Boghurst's references to Van Helmont, see pp. 8–9. After praising astrology Gadbury goes on to say: 'Howbeit, Physick is a Study I exceedingly love and honor, and its Learned and legal professors (whether Galenists or Chymists) I truely reverence'; see J. Gadbury, *Londons Deliverance Predicted*, London, 1665, A2v.

52. G. Harvey, *A Discourse of the Plague*, London, 1665, p. 1.

53. S. Bradwell, *Physick for the Sicknesse Commonly Called the Plague. With All the Particular Signes and Symptoms, Whereof the Most are too Ignorant*, London, 1636, C3v, A3r. See also F. Heering, *Certaine Rules, Directions, or Advertisments for this Time of Pestilentiall Contagion*, London, 1625, A3v.

54. For Heering and Bradwell's interest in Paracelsian medicine and alchemical remedies, see Debus, *English Paracelsians*, pp. 78–9, 145. See also Bradwell, *Physick for the Sicknesse*, G4r–v.

55. Webster, *Instauration*.

56. Peter Elmer has emphasized the significance of eirenicism for many of the medical reformers of this period, although Elmer seems reluctant to draw any precise religious and political conclusions from this observation, see Elmer, 'Medicine, Religion and the Puritan Revolution', pp. 34–45.

57. For Starkey's disappointment and active support of the Restoration, see Wilkinson, 'George Starkey', pp. 138–9; for Nedham, see Cook, *Old Medical Regime* pp. 145–7. For the 1640s and 1650s, see Webster, *Instauration*, pp. 273–323.

58. G. Thomson, *The Direct Method of Curing Chymically*, London, 1675, pp. 186–7.

59. N. Hodges, *Vindiciæ Medicinæ et Medicorum or an Apology for the Profession and Professors of Physick*, London, 1665, A4v. Hodges justified his dedication to Gilbert Sheldon by appealing to the shared 'professional' interests of the Church of England with the College of Physicians and their mutual difficulties and sufferings during the Interregnum, see A3v; see also Cook, *Old Medical Regime*, p. 159, and Cook, 'Society of Chemical Physicians', p. 70.

60. G. Sheldon, *David's Deliverance and Thanksgiving. A Sermon Preached Before the King at Whitehall Upon June 28, 1660, Being the Day of Solemn Thanksgiving for the Happy Return of His Majesty*, reprinted in Appendix IV in Staley, *Gilbert Sheldon*, pp. 217–64, for quotation, see p. 229. Apart from this sermon, the one printed out of only three preserved, very little is known of Sheldon's theology and natural philosophy. Ronald Hutton has recently summarized the prevalent view of him as 'devout as any and eloquent as most' but not 'a theologian nor a pastor but an organizer of men, a holy bureaucrat rather than a holy warrior', see R. Hutton, *The Restoration. A Political and Religious History of England and Wales 1658–1667*, Oxford, 1985, p. 145. The most recent biography of Sheldon appears to have misunderstood Sheldon's religious views totally, portraying him as 'a complete conservative in religious matters', see V.D. Such, *Gilbert Sheldon, Architect of Anglican Survival, 1640–1675*, The Hague, 1973, p. 9. As pointed out by Robert Beddard, such a description makes a mockery of Sheldon's theological liberalism with its appeal to prudence, as well as reason. Sheldon's theological liberalism and eirenicism is emphasized by the words he chose to use in his will, thanking God for calling him 'by his Gospel and grace to his knowledge

and obedience, abhorring all sects, sidings and tyranny in religion, holding fast and true orthodox profession of the Catholique faith of Christ', quoted in R.A. Beddard, 'Sheldon and Anglican Recovery', *The Historical Journal*, **19** (1976), 1016; see also p. 1007. Furthermore, it is noteworthy that Sheldon took a considerable interest in one of the prominent figures in the circle of educational reformers which had gathered around Hartlib in the 1650s, the mathematician John Pell, securing a parsonage for him in Essex in 1661, and later, after having become archbishop, making him one of his two Cambridge chaplains, see *Aubrey's 'Brief Lives'*, A. Clark (ed.), 2 vols, Oxford, 1898, vol. 2, pp. 123–4, 127.

61. Sheldon, *David's Deliverance*, p. 260.
62. Sheldon, *David's Deliverance*, p. 262.
63. For Gilbert Sheldon and The Great Tew Circle, see the excellent chapter by H. Trevor-Roper, 'The Great Tew Circle', in his *Catholics, Anglicans and Puritans*, pp. 166–230.
64. Thomson, *The Direct Method*, pp. 187–8.
65. George Thomson, *A Check to Henry Stubbe*, p. 44.

CHAPTER NINE

Of Physic and Philosophy: Anne Conway, F.M. van Helmont and Seventeenth-Century Medicine

Sarah Hutton

> I could not read your letter to Bennett, wth out being sensibly
> affected wth your kinde expressions and something astonished, y^t
> notwithstanding my ten yeares exclusion from ye world, you should
> still retaine ye memory of me, and a feeling concern for my sufferings,
> it commonly hapning y^t ye greatest afflictions by long continuance
> grows unregarded, and expectation of a change beeing long frus-
> trated, the patience is tired and then pitty ceases in persons uncon-
> cerned, thogh to those under ye pressure of great sufferings the
> weight is much augmented by continuance as our strength to beare
> does daily decrease.[1]

So wrote Lady Anne Conway to her brother-in-law, Sir George Rawdon,
in 1674. This letter is a rare instance of Anne Conway giving expression
to her feelings about the long and unrelieved pain which had afflicted
her since her teens. At the time of writing, five years before she died, the
increasing intensity of her incurable illness had meant that she was
more or less housebound at her husband's country estate, Ragley Hall,
in Warwickshire. Her husband, Edward, third Viscount Conway and
Killultagh, was a busy man of affairs who spent much time away from
home attending to his estates in northern Ireland and political affairs in
London. Lady Conway's isolation at Ragley is attested in this letter, her
family having become so accustomed to her being an invalid that they
had almost forgotten her. The letter does however mention the very few
loyal friends who stood by her to the end: her former tutor and friend,
the Cambridge Platonist, Henry More, who maintained a lifelong correspondence with her, and the physician of her last years, Francis Mercurius
van Helmont.[2] Of the latter her letter continues:

> To your kinde enquiry after what ease I find from Monsieur van
> Hellmont, I must give this account, my paines and weakness does
> certainly increase daily, but yett I doubt not, but I have had some
> releef (God bee thanked) from his medicines, I am sure more then I
> ever had from ye endeavours of any person whatsoever else, but
> yett I have had much more satisfaction in his company, he yas yett

ye patience to continue wth mee in my solitude, wch makes it ye
easier to mee, none of my own relations having ye leasure to afford
mee y^t comfort, and indeed I think very few friends could have
patience to doe it in ye circumstances that I am in, wch makes my
obligations to him so much ye greater.

It seems clear from this that Van Helmont had more to offer his patient
than mere medicines. Indeed, by this time, the great hopes she had had
of his finding a cure for her affliction had already been dashed. But it is
evident his care, concern and companionship were extremely important
to her, not to say efficacious in themselves. What is not so apparent
from this letter is that the impact of Van Helmont on Anne Conway's
life went far beyond the medical. For when he arrived at Ragley Hall in
1670, he came as the purveyor of more than medical learning. And he
encountered a patient who had more inside her cranium than a headache. Anne Conway was one of the most highly educated women in
Britain at this time, and an independent thinker in her own right. Van
Helmont's learned baggage included not just his own pharmacopœia of
cures, but religious and philosophical views which excited the interest
of his patient, and helped bring about profound changes in her religious
and philosophical outlook.

Historians of medicine are not, perhaps, accustomed to examining
the role of doctors as the transmitters of non-medical ideas, or to
exploring the impact of doctors on the non-clinical lives of their patients. Nor is it standard to consider the impact of the clinical circumstances of a patient on his or her outlook. In this chapter I explore the
interaction of medicine and the intellectual life of the seventeenth-
century by examining the case of Anne Conway, and in particular her
relations with the younger Van Helmont.[3] In so doing, I must acknowledge that the doctor–patient relationship of Anne Conway and Van
Helmont was not typical of its period, for, as a female practioner of
philosophy, she was a most unusual woman for her time. Van Helmont
too was an independent in point of medical theory and practice, educated outside the universities and largely by his father, Jan Baptista van
Helmont. At the same time, it has to be acknowledged that, in the
seventeenth century, apparently non-medical thinking cannot be divorced from what is to us obviously medical: Van Helmont's medical
concerns, his theory and practice as a physician, were deeply interconnected with aspects of his thinking which would not nowadays be
recognized as medical: his cabbalism, millenarianism, his linguistic theories and his religious views. Likewise, it can be argued that Lady Conway's
experience of pain was a significant determinant in the development of
her mature philosophy.

The Conway Letters and seventeenth-century medicine

In the annals of medical history, Lady Conway figures as a famous patient. We are fortunate in possessing two important contemporary documents of her illness: the account by Thomas Willis in his *De anima Brutorum* (*Two Discourses Concerning the Soul of Brutes*)[5] and the letters which she exchanged with Henry More throughout her adult life (now published as *The Conway Letters*).[6] The potential of this correspondence as a source in the history of medicine, has been under-exploited. As one might expect any collection of intimate letters, especially one covering such a long period (in this case about 30 years), will mention health, either in passing or as a topic of discussion. And indeed, at this day-to-day level, *The Conway Letters* does not disappoint. Among other things, the letters give vivid insight into the everyday experience of patients: the search for medical help, the 'cures', explanations of success or failures of treatment, comments on practitioners and so on. We hear of jaundice afflicting Lord Conway's mother (p. 142), and of a dropsical malady affecting Lady Conway's sister (p. 443) and of 'the plague' (p. 272). There are reports on the breast cancer from which Henry More's niece died (pp. 398ff) and a detailed description of the 'Squinancy' or 'quinsy' which nearly killed John Finch, as well as of the treatment which saved him (pp. 89–90). Henry More reports outbreaks of smallpox (pp. 195–7), of 'chills and feaver' (p. 195), of quartan fever (p. 230). He mentions ailments afflicting him (e.g. an infected foot, 'obstructedness of my arm', pp. 205, 208, 398). Occasionally he describes symptoms both his own and those of others, ranging from a touch of fever which he suffered (p. 194) to a detailed account of the urine of 'my Cousin Hall' (pp. 387–8).

More himself endeavoured to treat himself, avoiding doctors wherever possible: 'they can do nothing in any disease where nature would not repair itself with the help of due diet and exercise' he observes (p. 92), preferring to preserve his health through a combination of careful diet and fresh air. 'Ease of mind, fresh aire and diet, may leasurely do that, which Physick could not effect so suddenly' (p. 80). The exception is 'acute diseases wherein letting of blood or some such like safer Remedy is seasonable' (p. 92). He does, however, acknowledge that he did submit to treatment as a kind of insurance policy in extreme circumstances: 'I am resolvd to take Physick when emergencyes require, that I may fall with credit' (ibid.). In one case he attributes his succesful recovery of health in part to a medicine, but largely to 'the moistness of this Spring'.[7] More also believed that 'the heating my spiritts with study' preserved him from a fever that afflicted other fellows of Christ's College, Cambridge.[8]

Anne Conway, being a high-class patient, was treated by the top doctors of her age. But her elevated social status did not prevent her from consulting healers of various kinds. Apart from the younger Van Helmont, she was, at different times, the patient of Theodore de Mayerne, William Harvey, Thomas Willis, Sir Francis Prujean, Thomas and Luke Ridsley, Frederick Clodius, and the Warwickshire physician, John Ward.[9] In addition to these worthy professionals, she consulted healers: two are mentioned – Matthew Coker and Valentine Greatrakes, known as the 'great Irish stroker'.[10] She was also the recipient of plenty of free advice from her brother, John Finch, who, after graduating from Cambridge, went to study medicine in Padua. From Willis's account, we learn that she submitted to all manner of treatments, some of them pretty drastic: 'she tryed the Baths, and Spaw-waters almost every kind and nature; she admitted of frequent Blood-letting, and also once the opining of an Artery; she had also made about her several issues, sometimes in the hinder part of her Head, and sometimes in the forepart, and in other parts' and on one occasion, she 'endured from an oyntment of Quicksilver, a long and troublesome Salivation, so that she ran the hazard of her life'.[11] Willis gives us no more detail besides naming the types of treatment Lady Conway received at the hands of the medical profession, and The Conway Letters do not, unfortunately, give us any details, beyond the fact that we are frequently informed that Lady Conway is 'in physick'. They also confirm that she seems to have nearly died of mercury poisoning at the hands of Hartlib's son-in-law, Frederick Clodius.[12]

The letters do give some information about some of the other 'cures' she was recommended to try, including tobacco and coffee amongst modern novelties, as well as a mysterious 'red powder' from Wales, a 'blew powder' prescribed for 'the headache' by one Dr Johnson, and salt of vipers (p. 89). In 1664, she asked her husband to obtain a medicine from Robert Boyle: she asks him 'to take his directions if you can procure his medison, for the taking of it, both for the time he would have it to be continued, and the quantity, as also what vehicle he thinks most proper to give it in' (p. 230), but we are not told what the medicine was. When she was pregnant in 1658, her husband went to great lengths to obtain an 'eagle stone' which was said to have helped Lady Chichester when she was in labour. Some detail emerges about this amulet: it was white, 'about the bigness of an egg' with 'little black streaks in it'; it is described as 'a German stone, such as are commonly sold in London for 5 shillings apiece', and Lady Conway's view was that the bigger the more effective. She wore it on her arm like an amulet (p. 154). In her search for a cure, Anne Conway visited Bath to take the waters, but without effect. And in her desperation she journeyed to Paris with a view to undergoing trepanning. Henry More accompanied her to Paris and, according to More's biographer, Richard Ward, it was he who dissuaded her from going through with this desperate remedy.[13] On her way through Rouen she called on a Dr Bochart but he was not in town when she was there.[14]

From *The Conway Letters* we can glean a certain amount about how people in the seventeenth century tried to get medical advice. The Conways may have been somewhat exceptional in so far as they had close contacts in the medical world, not just as patients, but because of their interests: Anne Conway's father-in-law dabbled in alchemy and collected books. He was a friend of Sir Kenelm Digby and well acquainted with Sir Theodore de Mayerne who helped him in his book-collecting activities. Lord Conway senior also knew William Harvey, which probably explains how his daughter-in-law came to be Harvey's patient.[15] Her brother, John Finch, who studied medicine at Padua and was for a time professor of anatomy at Pisa, was a source of expert medical advice from within her family.

As far as learned medicine is concerned, it is not perhaps surprising that people turned to learned men for advice on obtaining medical help. But it is, perhaps, notable that they did not necessarily consult members of the medical profession, but rather any trusted learned figure of their acquaintance. Thus it is that the Conways sought advice from Henry More, doctor of divinity, about possible doctors of medicine, in exactly the same way that they consulted him about suitable clergymen to fill the livings of which they were patrons. Nor was it just the practice of well-connected aristocrats to consult masters of metaphysics on the matter of experts in physic. When More's niece, Mrs Ladde, became ill with cancer, it was to uncle Henry, the Cambridge don, that the family turned for advice. He wrote to Van Helmont on her behalf, with the result that within a year of the original appeal, she was furnished with Van Helmont's most efficacious medicines. What these were, we are not told, but they did have some effect – so much so that Mrs Ladde refused to take them, and died, as she would probably have done anyway, a year later.[16]

To consult a doctor of souls on choosing a suitable doctor of medicine makes sense, when one considers that the connections between metaphysics and medicine were not then as remote as they might seem today, at least not to the metaphysician. This is particularly true in the case of Henry More, notwithstanding his own policy of avoiding doctors. More's eclectic neo-Platonic philosophy enabled him to provide a coherent explanation of the efficacy of non-medical healing. For More metaphysics and natural philosophy were closely intertwined. He was an eager follower of the latest developments in natural philosophy in the seventeenth century. Furthermore, he insisted that many of the explanatory weaknesses of the Cartesian mechanical philosophy (e.g. how motion is passed from one body to another; sympathetic vibration of strings, tidal phenomena)[17] could only be accounted for by the action of spirit, in particular what he called the *Principium Hylarchicum*, or Spirit of Nature.[18] Thus it is that he can provide a 'spiritual' explanation in the case of the healing powers of Matthew Coker, one of the healers who figures in the Conway story. In 1654 More defended Coker against the charge that he works 'by the power of the Devill'. At the same time he denies that Coker can perform miracles. Coker's power of healing is, he says, 'partly naturall and partly devotionall'. Coker's 'long temperance and devotion' have meant that 'the blood and spirits of this party is become sanative and healing ... a true elixir'. Coker works his cures by a sort of transfusion of spirit:

> therefore he laying his hands upon diseased persons, his spiritts run out of his own body into the party diseased, and actuate and purify the blood and spiritts of the diseased party, which I conceive they do with more efficacy, if he add devotion to his laying on of his hands, for that setts his spiritts afloat the more copiously and animates them the more strongly, and they being no spiritts of a melancholy man but thus refin'd sublimated, they are the more feirce and strong in their motions, and more effectuall for the kindling of life and spritt in such dead and diseased limbs as he is said to have healed.[19]

A similar explanation might have been given to explain the success of the healer, Valentine Greatrakes, although there is no letter on the subject by More.

Lady Conway's incurable illness brought her and her contemporaries forcefully up against the limitations of contemporary medical knowledge. In view of the fruitlessness of the attempts to find a cure it is perhaps surprising that the More/Conway correspondence only rarely contains expressions of overt distrust of the medical profession. The exception is Frederick Clodius who was recommended to Lady Conway by More but, it seems, was almost responsible for poisoning her with mercury.[20] More commonly one reads the occasional expression of self-distrust on the part of friends and counsellors. Henry More comments almost despairingly, 'this malady has non-pluss'd so many Physicians and medicines, that it makes a man have a little heart to propose anything'.[21] In these hopeless circumstances, prayer and faith in God seems to be all there is to offer. And that is what More does in abundance:

> The best advice I can give you is that which I endeavour after myself as much as I can, that your phansy add nothing to the torture of your sense, and to resigne yourself wholly to the will of

God, useing the best meanes you can for the removall of your present affliction.[22]

Anne Conway apparently accepted this advice. In the letter from which I quoted at the beginning, she writes with unbearable resignation: 'God Almighty, who disposes all things for ye best, can and I hope will afford y^t support, y^t hee sees needful for ye sustaining of y^t affliction wch hee has allotted for mee, I desire to bee humbled under His righteous hand wholly resigned to His good pleasure.'[23] In view of the chronic pain which she suffered for most of her life, her own letters are extraordinarily reticent about her condition.[24] When she does mention her affliction, her tone is almost apologetic, as when she wrote to More from Ireland in 1664:

> I still endure those violent paines (which I alwayes thought would be accounted intollerable by a stronger body then ever I had) and that more frequently then ever. I cannot dissemble so much as not to professe myself to be weary of this condition ... I am troubled my complaints should fill so great a part of my letter ... I could not forbear the giving you this account of my present condition, which otherwise I should have omitted, being hugely apprehensive of giving any occasion of trouble to you ... [25]

Francis Mercury van Helmont

The last physician to treat Anne Conway was the aforementioned Francis Mercury van Helmont. Son of the famous physician, Jan Baptista van Helmont, Francis Mercury represents no academic medical tradition, but rather the version of Paracelsian medicine practised by his father. He was not given an academic education but was instructed by his father who, being no Galenist, distrusted university medicine. Francis Mercury made his name in the medical world by editing the collected writings of his father, which appeared as *Ortus medicinae* in 1648.[26] His own success as a physician was confirmed when he was rewarded for his services with the title of baron by a grateful Elector of Mainz. Assessing Van Helmont on the basis of his writings is difficult because he published his thoughts piecemeal and usually with the aid of admirers and followers who recorded his discussions and published them with his permission. As a result his writings are sometimes attributed to others who were in effect no more than amanuenses.[27] His *Observationes circa hominem eiusque morbos* (Amsterdam, 1692) is described as 'per Paulum Buchium Med. Doct.'[28] and was translated into Latin by another medical aquaintance, Johannes Conrad Amman, author of two books on teaching the deaf to speak.[29] The problem of authorship surrounding

Van Helmont's works is further complicated by the fact that some of his own writings have been taken to be by Jan Baptista. This appears to be the case with his *One Hundred and Fifty Three Chymical Aphorisms* (1688, translation, 1690). This confusion may have arisen because he edited his father's writings. The most comprehensive account of his thought, 'Some Observations of Francis Mer: van Helmont', covers alchemical, religious, metaphysical and autobiographical topics and was dictated to Dr Daniel Foote in 1682, but was never published.[30] As these examples show, Van Helmont depended largely on his medical acquaintances for publishing and translating his writings. This is true even of some of his more metaphysical and unorthodox religious writings. For example, *Seder Olam*, a work which deals with the transmigration of souls, was translated into English by Dr John Clarke.[31]

Apart from the manuscript 'Some Observations', no single work by Van Helmont contains the full range of his thinking but his writings overlap and may be combined to construct a consistent natural philosophy with important metaphysical and religious implications.[32] He rejects the concept of body of 'our Moderne Philosophers' proposing a monistic vitalism in place of dualistic mechanism: a resounding theme of his writings is that 'whatever is, is a Spirit'.[33] With support from appropriate biblical texts he argues that there are two principles in nature, fire and water, the former warm and vivifying, the latter cool and rest-procuring. All things contain within them a male principle and a female one: fire being male and water female. There are three types of fire: natural, solar and artificial. The 'watery essence' is a manifestation of soul. All created things are in a state of continuous change, a 'Never-ceasing Revolution' as beings ascend and descend the ontological scale and 'work out themselves to their true perfection'. This constant state of transformation is possible because body and spirit, of which all things are constituted, are in fact one and the same substance:

> spirit & matter differ only gradually, & by consequence are mutually convertible into one another ... and so from Spirits condensed, ariseth light, and from light condensed ariseth Water, & from Water condensed ariseth other corporeall and sensible beings. By this ascent, y^t wh^{ch} is more immediate ariseth out of water is a certain stony concretion, wch vulgarly is termed ye quicksand etc.[34]

The overall pattern of this 'revolution' or conversion is meliorative both in terms of the purification of substance and the regeneration of souls.[35] Van Helmont explains pain suffered in life as part of the process of regeneration necessary for salvation. The religious conclusions which he derives from these doctrines are decidedly heterodox: he denies both *creatio ex nihilo* and the eternity of hell – advocating instead universal salvation achieved through a series of reincarnations.[36]

Underlying Van Helmont's philosophy of spirit is the alchemical doctrine of transmutation which he develops into general principle of natural metamorphosis. Another source for his views is kabbalism which lent support for his theory of substance as spirit and purification through suffering as well as for his concept of God, his account of creation and his tenaciously held belief in the transmigration of souls. A third important source for Van Helmont was undoubtedly his father's natural philosophy: although the younger Van Helmont does not employ the conceptual vocabulary of his father (terms like 'gas', 'blas' and the 'archeus'), in both general terms and specific details he adopts or reworks elements of the natural philosophy of his father, who also propounded a version of monistic vitalism as well as the theory that water is a primary substance, one of the *elementa primagenia*. And in the last quotation, Van Helmont refers to his father's concept of *quellem*, or quicksand, as the primary solid, discussion of which is more elaborate in his *Paradoxical Discourses* and *The Divine Being and its Attributes*.[37]

No doubt F.M. van Helmont developed his vitalistic monism in relation to his own experience as physician. In so far as the hypothesis in effect attributes to matter the properties of spirit, it can be set in relation to the work of other physicians of his time who considered the possibility that in living creatures, corporeal substance might be endowed with the power of perception or thought: Francis Glisson and John Locke are the most famous examples.[38] As far as Van Helmont's clinical management is concerned, there is one feature of his practice as a physician which appears to be peculiar to him and is connected with his monistic natural philosophy: in *The Spirit of Diseases*, he argues that diseases are psychosomatic in nature, 'that the Mind influenceth the Body in causing and curing of Diseases'. This, again, is a view which finds its origin in his father's account of disease. But with the younger Van Helmont it becomes the basis of treatment of illness through the alteration of the attitudes and feelings of the patient. Since diseases are the result of disordered passions (literally *dis*-tempers), they must be treated by bearing pain patiently and learning to love the disorder.[39] This was one feature of his clinical method which, according to him, did not meet with the approval of most doctors of his time.[40]

Much of Van Helmont's life was spent moving in German court circles, giving counsel both practical and medical in the courts of Heidelberg, Sulzbach and Hanover. This high-level existence was not without its dangers, however: in 1661 Philip Wilhelm Duke of Neuberg had him imprisoned by the Inquisition for, *inter alia*, disparaging Roman Catholicism, and attempting to set up a Hebrew school in Sulzbach. Van Helmont was fortunate in being released two years later without charge. But the incident is a pointer to the development of his personal spirituality away from the Catholicism of his birth towards Protestantism and philosemitism. Van Helmont's quest for religious eirenicism brought him into contact with a range of religious groups and stimulated his interest in the arcana of the Jewish kabbalah as a key to converting the Jews. His personal spiritual pilgrimage resulted in his conversion to Quakerism.[41]

Van Helmont and the Conways

Although Van Helmont did not enter Lady Conway's life until 1670, his fame had gone before him – nearly 20 years before in fact. In 1653, Lord Conway had written to John Finch in Italy to ask him to make enquiries about Van Helmont who was reputed to have the secrets of a universal panacea which Conway hoped might cure his wife.[42] John Finch expressed grave doubts about the possible efficacy of any universal elixir but suggested that the cure in question was that described by J.B. van Helmont in his treatise, 'Butler', which was the story of how an Irishman of that name cured a woman of a headache which had afflicted her for 16 years.[43] Finch made enquiries on behalf of his brother-in-law. Among others, he consulted the Venetian professor of anatomy, Molinetti, and the mathematician, Otto Tackenius. The reports seemed to confirm Finch's suspicions that the younger Van Helmont's greatness as a doctor resided in his reputation rather than his practice. Whether this conclusion reflects a predisposition to mistrust Van Helmont on Finch's part, or the professional jealousy of the Italians amongst whom Van Helmont had worked is not clear from his letter to Edward Conway. But he was prepared to make a five-day journey to Sarisburgh from Padua having heard that Van Helmont was in attendance upon the Elector of Luneburgh there. Finch apparently never managed to track Van Helmont down. He cannot have succeeded in discouraging his sister and brother-in-law from consulting Van Helmont (if, of course, that had been his intention), for they had not forgotten him when he arrived in England 17 years later and they lost no time in persuading him to pay a visit to Ragley Hall.

Van Helmont came to England in 1670 not as a doctor but as a diplomat – on a mission for Princess Elizabeth of the Palatinate, daughter of Charles I's sister, the 'winter queen', and correspondent of Descartes's. While in England, Van Helmont paid a visit to Henry More on behalf of the kabbalist scholar, Christian Knorr von Rosenroth. Van Helmont made a deep impression on More, who persuaded him to visit Lady Conway to offer her his medical advice. Thereafter Van Helmont stayed on as a permanent member of her household until her death in 1679.

As in the case of the other physicians whom Lady Conway consulted, we have no record of the treatment she received under Van Helmont's direction. Like all the medical men whose patient she had been, he did not succeed in curing her. His treatment seems to have given grounds for hope that he might, in its early stages. Four years later, in the letter from which I quoted at the beginning of this chapter, she acknowledged that she had 'some releef ... from his medicines, I am sure more then I ever had from ye endeavours of any person whatsoever else'.[44] In view of what we do know about Van Helmont's psychosomatic treatment of pain, it is possible the 'releef' he brought Lady Conway, in spite of being unsuccessful in his attempts to cure her, was perhaps psychological.

Whatever the clinical outcome of Van Helmont's treating Lady Conway, the extent of his impact on her is attested by her husband. In a letter to his brother-in-law, Sir George Rawdon, in 1676, he notes 'Van Helmont hath wrought himself extremely into my wife's good opinion, so as to think him the necessariest person in the world about her'. Furthermore, as this letter testifies, Van Helmont's influence extended well beyond the medical. To Lord Conway's embarassment and irritation, Van Helmont brought Lady Conway into contact with the then reviled and persecuted sect, the Quakers: 'To injure Monsr. van Helmont,' he writes 'is to injure my wife in sensibilest part, but it is from him that all the reproach of her being a Quaker and a thousand other stories proceeds, and she is content to bear it'.[45] In spite of assurances from Henry More 'that my wife is no Quaker', Anne Conway's introduction to the Quakers resulted in her conversion in the last year of her life, an extraordinary decision for a woman of her social class at that time.

Quakerism was not the only matter about which Van Helmont aroused Anne Conway's curiosity. He had not actually declared himself a member of the Society of Friends when he first met her, but at that time he came on the scene as iatro-chemist and Christian cabbalist with a profound interest in millenarianism. The letters which Henry More wrote to Anne Conway after he first met Van Helmont show that the first topic of mutual interest was the interpretation of the Apocalypse.[46] Van Helmont also introduced More to the actual Jewish Kabbalah (as opposed to the imaginary one he had confected in the 1650s)[47] thereby generating great excitement in both Henry More and Anne Conway. He put them both in contact with his friend the Christian cabbalist Christian Knorr von Rosenroth. More's resulting exchange with Knorr led to his contributing to the critical apparatus of the *Kabbala denudata* and to his having to revise his own assessment of kabbalah.[48] In discussions with More and Anne Conway, Van Helmont advanced his theory of the transmigration of souls. (These discussions are recorded in his *Two*

Hundred Queries ... Concerning ... the Revolution of Human Souls and *Cabbalistical Dialogue*).[49] But the area of Van Helmont's impact with which I am most concerned here is on Anne Conway's philosophy, an area where his influence was decisive. It is already well established that Anne Conway's philosophy owes much to the kabbalistic thought with which Van Helmont brought her into contact.[50] What I argue is that Anne Conway is also indebted to Van Helmont's medical and alchemical wisdom. These strands of Helmontian natural philosophy and cabbalism in Anne Conway's thought are intimately interconnected, since cabbalist wisdom appeared to contain, and therefore confirm, fundamental elements of Helmontian natural philosophy. Furthermore, these aspects of her thought are also connected with the radical religious choice of her last years, her sympathy with and ultimate adoption of Quakerism.

Anne Conway's *Principia philosophiae*

When Anne Conway studied philosophy with Henry More she had been schooled in Cartesianism. But in her one work of philosophy, *Principia philosophiae antiquissimae et recentissimae*, published by Van Helmont after her death, she rejects not just the materialists Hobbes and Spinoza, but the dualists, Descartes and More. In place of dualism she propounds a monistic ontology in which all things are composed of a single substance.[51] Body and spirit represent the extremes of a continuum of substance, the former being more condensed, the latter more refined. This substance is constituted of an infinite number of particles each of which is a living principle, endowed with perception and the capacity for self-motion. Anne Conway formulates this concept of substance in opposition to that of the new mechanical philosophy, which, to use her words, reduces corporeal substance to 'dull and stupid matter'. In her view, the mechanical account of bodies was insufficient to explain life and action. And a key characteristic of her conception of created beings is their capacity for change according to which created things may move up or down the ontological scale, becoming more spirit-like or more corporeal, depending on the direction in which they change. In this scheme, ascent entails not just physical refinement of substance, but movement towards the good. The process by which substance becomes more corporeal is a falling away from perfection in the direction of sin. Anne Conway's system is thus both an ontology and a soteriology. All creatures are free to choose their spiritual destiny. But, since God is good and just, absolute perdition is by definition impossible. The process of becoming more corporeal entails suffering, but it is redemptive and purgative suffering which helps regenerate fallen creatures. Accordingly, Conway denies the eternity of hell, proposing instead the Origenist doctrine of universal salvation.

The spiritualized universe conceived by Anne Conway bears striking similarities to Van Helmont's. Not only do they both propound similar theories of monistic vitalism, but they both propound meliorative accounts of change. Among other things, they share similar views of suffering as purgative and salvific. Both were critical of the new mechanical philosophy and they had a common interest in the Jewish kabbalah. But it is not just in general outline that Anne Conway's system of philosophy has parallels with Van Helmont. The detail of her account of natural bodies and the operations of nature have a decidedly Helmontian ring. This comes out particularly in the course of her arguments in chapters 6, 7 and 8 and prove that body and soul are one and the same substance. Here some of the examples she uses can only have come from Van Helmont. For instance, when arguing that natural things transform into one another, she not only appeals to the alchemical model of the transmutation of metals and the theories of the genesis of creatures out of the earth, but she appeals to the evidence of the production of stones from water. Here she cites the specific example of two types of river on a 'Mountain in Helvetia', one of which 'breeds the Stone, and the other is a proper remedy against it; so that one Water is changed into a Stone, and the other Water proceeds from that Stone'.[52] The doctrine that water is a primary substance whence other bodies evolve is a central Helmontian teaching. And Van Helmont also uses the specific example of the Swiss mountain in his *Divine Being and its Attributes*.[53] Another instance of Lady Conway using a Helmontian argument 'how a gross Body may be changed into a Spirit', is her use of the example of digestion: 'For all Motion wears and divides, and so renders a Thing subtile and Spiritual. Even thus in Man's Body, the Meat and Drink is first changed into Chyle, thein into Blood, afterwards into Spirits, which are nothing else but Blood brought to perfection ... .'[54]

In *The Spirit of Diseases* and the Daniel Foote manuscript, Van Helmont describes the same process of the production of spiritual essence by the digestion of food. Other such instances of Anne Conway using Helmontian examples can be found in her *Principles*. An instance of Anne Conway's extended use of Helmontian doctrines is her account of the composition of living bodies, which, according to her, are constituted of an active and a passive principle corresponding to spirit and body (that is congealed spiritual substance). The conjunction of these principles is compared to the conjugal union of husband and wife. Each principle is dependent on the other in some way, the body being the material vehicle or form of the spirit. The image of the spirit is the seed retained by the female and the nature of the living being that is formed in this way depends on which spirit is dominant:

> And therefore whatsoever Spirit is then strongest and hath the strongest Image or *Idea* in the Seed, whether it be the Masculine or the Feminine, or any other Spirit from either of these received from without, that Spirit is predominant in the seed, and forms the Body, as near as may be after its own Image, and so every Creature receives his External form.[55]

A similar account of spiritual conception or 'mutually received Images of Man and Wife' occurs in Van Helmont's *Paradoxical Discourses*.[56] The common source for many of these examples is the older Van Helmont – in particular, the theory that water is a primary element that can transform into other elements. And the last example is indebted to Jan Baptista's doctrine of the archeus, even though neither his son nor Lady Conway use that term.

It would be misleading to present Anne Conway's philosophy simply as Helmontianism in more systematic dress: my dwelling on the similarities between the two inevitably distorts the picture. But, certainly as far as the chapters on created substance are concerned, there are many parallels with Van Helmont. Arguably, Anne Conway's philosophy already had monistic tendencies before she encountered Van Helmont.[57] There is also a sense in which her individual circumstances may have helped to mould her philosophical understanding of the world. After all, her personal experience of unrelievable pain was such as to make it hard to deny that interaction of mind and body was too close to be explicable in dualistic terms – this is in fact a question which she poses in her treatise when challenging dualist separation of body and soul:

> Why is the Spirit or Soul so passible in corporal Pains? for if when it is united with Body, it hath nothing of corporeity, or a bodily Nature, Why is it grieved or wounded when the Body is wounded, which is of quite a different Nature? ... But if it be granted that the Soul is of one Nature and Substance with the Body, although it is many degrees more excellent in regard of Life and Spirituality ... then all the aforesaid difficulties will Vanish, and it will be easily conceived, how the Body and Soul are united together, and how the Soul moves the Body, and suffers by it or with it.[58]

Furthermore, her personal experience of suffering at the hands of a supposedly good God required more by way of explanation than Henry More's balm of patient trust in the strange workings of divine providence. Lurianic cabbalism offered a way of accommodating the suffering of the godly with the goodness and justice of God.

In Anne Conway's *Principles* the demonstration that spirit and body are one substance is expressed in terms which are echoed in the writings of Van Helmont. The question remains open as to whether it was the influence of Van Helmont which led Anne Conway to abandon the Cartesianism of her philosophical education, or whether Anne Conway influenced Van Helmont's philosophy of spirit. All the relevant writings of Van Helmont post-date Anne Conway's death but, on the evidence of her correspondence with More, she was not acquainted with the genuine Jewish kabbalah before she met Van Helmont. Furthermore, the roots of Francis Mercury van Helmont's vitalistic monism lie with the medical thought of his father – as I have already observed, many of the parallels between Conway and the younger Van Helmont have analogues in the writings of Van Helmont senior. This fact would suggest that many elements of Van Helmont's thought that are to be encountered in his later writings were already in place before he met Lady Conway. In this respect, the medical philosophy of Van Helmont *père et fils* provides the corroboration of her metaphysical arguments: Helmontianism provides the natural philosophy underpinning of her system. This being so, Francis Mercury van Helmont was at least the catalyst of change in directing Anne Conway away from the neo-Cartesianism of her teacher Henry More. But this does not rule out the possibility that the influence also went the other way.

As a metaphysical system, Anne Conway's philosophy represents a departure from the prevailing philosophy of her day, including the Cambridge Platonism of her teacher, Henry More. In its religious implications, although eirenicist, it is most unorthodox. In her personal religion, too, Anne Conway took a spiritual path that was out of the ordinary when she became a Quaker. Behind these three interconnected aspects of her intellectual life is the multifaceted presence of her most extraordinary doctor, Francis Mercury van Helmont.

Notes

1. Lady Anne Conway to Sir George Rawdon, 25 September 1674, *The Conway Letters*, M.H. Nicolson (ed.) revised edn S. Hutton, Oxford, Clarendon Press, 1992, p. 534.
2. On Van Helmont see A. Coudert, *Leibniz and the Kabbalah*, Dordrecht, 1995; 'Henry More, the Kabbalah and the Quakers' in R. Kroll, R. Ashcraft and P. Zagorin (eds), *Philosophy, Science, and Religion in England, 1640–1700*, Cambridge, 1992, pp. 31–59; Stuart Brown, 'F.M. van Helmont: His Philosophical Connections and the Reception of his Later Cabbalistical Philosophy', in M.A. Stewart (ed.), *Oxford Studies in the History of Philosophy*, p. 2; Bernadino Orio de Miguel, 'Leibniz y la

Tradicion Teosofico-Kabbalistica: Francisco Mercurio van Helmont' Diss. Universidad Complutense de Madrid, 1992, published Madrid, 1993. Also Anne Becco, 'Leibniz et François Mercure van Helmont: Bagatelle pour des Monades', *Studia Leibnitiana, Sonderheft*, 7 (1978), 119–41, p. 125.

3. Please note, that unless there is specific indication to the contrary, the name 'Van Helmont' refers to the son, Francis Mercury, and not to his father, Jan Baptista.

4. Allison Coudert comments at the end of the introduction to the new English translation of Anne Conway's *Principles*, 'Her philosophy is also a compelling example of the way an individual's circumstances help to shape his or her philosophy'. Anne Conway, *The Principles of the Most Ancient and Modern Philosophy*, trans. A. Coudert and T. Corse, Cambridge, Cambridge University Press, 1996.

5. *De anima brutorum quae hominis vitalis ac sensitiva est exercitationes duae* (London, 1672), pp. 203ff, 207ff. English version *Two Discourses Concerning the Soul of Brutes, Which is That of the Vital and Sensitive of Man*, pt 2, ch. 1 'Of the Headache'; in *The Remaining Medical Works of that Famous and Renowned Physician Dr Thomas Willis* (London, 1683), pp. 122, 134. Anne Conway was Willis's patient in 1665: see *Conway Letters*, p. 240. See also G.R. Owen, 'The Famous Case of Lady Anne Conway', *Annals of Medical History*, 9 (1937), 567–71; M. Critchley, 'The Malady of Anne, Viscountess Conway', *King's College Hospital Gazette*, 16 (1937), 44. On Willis see Kenneth Dewhurst (ed.), *Willis's Oxford Lectures*, Oxford, 1980 and the introduction to Willis, *The Anatomy of the Brain and Nerves*, William Feindel (ed.), Montreal, 1965.

6. See note 1.

7. *Conway Letters*, p. 94. Cf. p. 96. Here he expresses doubts about purging in his own case.

8. Ibid., p. 95. More warns Lady Conway against too much study and 'thinking too intensely', lest doing so exacerbate her condition. None the less he was convinced that her illness was 'not contracted by meditation and over much study' (*Conway Letters*, p. 80).

9. Ibid., *passim*. Also, Robert G. Frank, 'The John Ward Diaries: Mirror of Seventeenth-Century Medicine', *Journal of the History of Medicine*, 29 (1974), 147–79, n. 10. On Greatrakes, see N. Steneck, 'Greatrakes the Stroker: The Interpretations of Historians', *Isis*, 73 (1982), 161–77 and B. Kaplan, 'Greatrakes the Stroker: The Interpretations of his Contemporaries', ibid., pp. 178–85.

11. Willis, *Medical Works*, p. 122.

12. *Conway Letters*, pp. 91, 94–7, 102, 104.

13. R. Ward, *The Life of the Learned and Pious Dr. Henry More*, London, 1710, p. 206; *Conway Letters*, pp. 106, 116.

14. A.R. Hall and M. Boas Hall (eds), *The Correspondence of Henry Oldenburg*, Madison and London, 1965–86, vol. I, 1641–62, p. 214.

15. Lord Conway's high opinion of Harvey implies acquaintance with his medical work: 'he hath deserved extreamely well of all learned men for what he hath found out, or offered the world to enquire farther into: he is a most exelent Anatomist, and I conceive that to be his Masterpeece, which knowledge is many times of very great use in consultations, but in the practicke of Physick I conceive him to be to mutch governed by his

Phantasy, the excellence and strength whereof did produce his two workes to the world'. While acknowledging Harvey's medical thought in this way, and although he states emphatically 'I doe greatly esteeme and value him', Lord Conway warns, 'to have a Physitian abound in phantasie is a very perilous thing, occations in diseases are very often suddaine, therefore one ought to have a Physitian that should be governed only by his judgement' (*Conway Letters*, p. 30).

16. Ibid., pp. 246–8, 254, 260.
17. See Alan Gabbey, 'Henry More and the Limits of Mechanism', in S. Hutton (ed.), *Henry More, 1614–1687, Tercentenary Studies*, Dordrecht, 1990, pp. 19–35.
18. And to this end he appropriated the experiments of Sir Robert Boyle as evidence for the workings of the spirit of nature. (In other words he substituted his own spiritual explanation for the phenomena described by Boyle in his experiments.) See A.R. Hall, *Henry More*, Oxford, 1990, pp. 181–95; John Henry, 'Henry More Versus Robert Boyle: The Spirit of Nature and the Nature of Providence', in S. Hutton (ed.), *Henry More*, pp. 55–76.
19. *Conway Letters*, p. 101.
20. Ibid., pp. 94–7, 102, 104.
21. Ibid., p. 231.
22. Ibid., p. 100.
23. Ibid., p. 534.
24. An exception is the letter she wrote to Henry More after the death of her only child, and the illness which ensued (ibid., p. 181).
25. Ibid., p. 224.
26. *Ortus medicinae, id est initia physicae inaudita, progressus medicinae novus in morborum ultionem ad vitam longam ... edente authoris filio Francisco Mercurio van Helmont, cum ejus praefatio ex Belgico translata* (Amsterdam, Elzevir, 1648). This was translated into German by F.M. van Helmont's friend, Knorr von Rosenroth (*Aufgang der Artzeny-Kunst*, Sulzbach, 1683), into English by John Chandler (*Oriatrike, or Physick Refined*, London, 1664), and into French by Jean Leconte (*Les Oeuvres de Jean Baptiste van Helmont*, Lyons, 1670). On J.B. van Helmont, see Walter Pagel, *J.B. van Helmont, Reformer in Science and Medicine*, Cambridge, 1982, and Guido Giglioni, 'La teoria dell'immaginazione nell "idealismo" biologico di Johannes Baptista van Helmont', *La Cultura*, 29 (1991), pp. 110–45.
27. The means whereby Van Helmont's ideas came to be published is described in the preface of his *Paradoxical Discourses* (London, 1685), which recounts how two admirers sought him out first in Amsterdam, then in London, and recorded their conversations with him when they found him.
28. Buchius is also credited with writing down Van Helmont's *Het Godlyk Weezen* (Amsterdam, 1694) written 'naar de Gronden van Franciscus Mercurius van Helmont. In't Nederduytsch geschreven door Paulus Buchius Med: Doctr.': or, as the English version, *The Divine Being and Its Attributes* (London, 1693) states on the title page, 'according to the Principles of M[onsieur] B[aron] of Helmont. Written in Low-Dutch by Paulus Buchius Dr of Physick'. Buchius also brought out another edition with the title, *De verduisterde waarheid aan het Ligt gebracht* (Amsterdam, 1695).

29. J.C. Amman, *Surdus loquens, seu methodus, qua qui surdus natus est loqui dicere possit* (Amsterdam, 1692) – English translation by D[aniel] F[oote], *The Talking Deaf Man: Or a Method Proposed, Whereby He Who is Born Deaf May Learn to Speak* (London, 1694) – and *Dissertatio de loquela* (Amsterdam, 1700).

30. British Library (hereafter BL) MS Sloane 530.

31. *Seder Olam: Or the Order of Ages, Wherein the Doctrine is Historically Handled, Translated Out of Latin by J. Clark, M.D. Upon the Leave and Recommendation of F.M. Baron of Helmont*, London, T. Hawkins, 1694.

32. In what follows, I draw on *Paradoxical Discourses, The Divine Being and Its Attributes, The Spirit of Diseases* (London, 1694), *A Cabbalistical Dialogue* (London, 1682) and *Seder Olam*.

33. *Cabbalistical Dialogue*, p. 13. Cf. ibid., p. 8: 'every Substance it self which appeareth under the form of *Matter* ... was sometimes past a spirit, and as yet is fundamentally and radically such, and will sometime hereafter be such again formally'; and *Seder Olam*, sects 32 and 33; 'Observations', MS Sloane 530, fols 62, 94.

34. BL MS Sloane 530, fol. 94v.

35. *Paradoxical Discourses*, pp. 16–18, Cf. *Seder Olam*.

36. See in particular, *A Cabbalistical Dialogue* and *Seder Olam*.

37. *Divine Being*, pp. 168ff.

38. Francis Glisson, *Tractatus de natura substantiae energetica* (London, 1672), J. Locke, *A Treatise Concerning Human Understanding*, IV.3.6. On Glisson, see John Henry, 'Medicine and Pneumatology: Henry More, Richard Baxter and Francis Glisson's *Treatise on the Energetic Naure of Substance*', *Medical History*, 31 (1987), 15–40, and Guido Giglioni, 'Il *Tractatus de natura substantiae energetica* di F. Glisson', *Annali della Facoltà di Lettere e Filosofia del Università di Macerata*, 24 (1991), 137–79.

39. In his 'Observations' in MS Sloane 530, Van Helmont recounts how he acquired this insight into the treatment of pain and disease by loving them. See also, G. Sherrer, 'Philalgia in Warwickshire: F.M. van Helmont's Anatomy of Pain Applied to Anne Conway', *Studies in the Renaissance*, 5 (1958), 196–206.

40. He says his method 'would oblige them to abandon their accustomed method, and to new-model the whole system of their practice', *The Spirit of Diseases*, sig. A4[5].

41. On Van Helmont's Quakerism see Allison P. Coudert, 'A Quaker-Kabbalist Controversy: George Fox's Reaction to Francis Mercury van Helmont, *Journal of the Warburg and Courtauld Institutes*, 39 (1976), 171–89; A. Coudert, 'Henry More, the Kabalah and the Quakers' in R. Kroll, R. Ashcraft and P. Zagorin (eds), *Philosophy, Science, and Religion in England, 1640–1700*; W.I. Hull, *Benjamin Furly and Quakerism in Rotterdam*, Swarthmore, PA, 1933, p. 112.

42. *Conway Letters*, pp. 494–7. Lord Conway may have been prompted to ask his brother-in-law to locate the younger Van Helmont by the appearance in England of a pamphlet entitled *A Treatise of the Great Antidote of Van Helmont* (London, 1665) which describes an elixir emanating from J.B. van Helmont which claimed to be capable of 'effectually taking away the Seeds of all Diseases'.

43. J.B. van Helmont, 'Butler' in *Ortus medicinae*.

44. *Conway Letters*, p. 534.
45. Ibid., p. 535.
46. On More and the apocalypse, see my articles, 'Henry More and the Book of Revelation', *Studies in Church History*, 10 (1994), and 'Henry More, Isaac Newton and the Language of Biblical Prophecy', in *The Books of Nature and Scripture*, J. Force and R.H. Popkin (eds), Dordrecht, 1994.
47. H. More, *Conjectura cabbalistica*, London, 1653.
48. On More and the Kabbalah, see A.P. Coudert, 'A Cambridge Platonist's Kabbalist Nightmare', *Journal of the History of Ideas*, 35 (1975), 633–52.
49. *Two Hundred Queries Moderately Propounded Concerning the Doctrine of the Revolution of Human Souls and its Conformity with the Truth of the Christian Religion*, London, 1685 – reprinted in German in 1686 and in Latin, in the collection entitled *Opuscula philosophica* in 1690. *A Cabbalistical Dialogue*, first printed in Latin in the second part of volume 1 of *Kabbala denudata* (Sulzbach, 1677).
50. See Coudert, art. cit. supra n. 2; D.P. Walker, *The Decline of Hell*, London, 1964, p. 141, and the Introduction to the new translation of *The Principles of the Most Ancient and Modern Philosophy* by Coudert and Corse (see note 4 above).
51. Anne Conway's *Principia philosophiae antiquissimae et recentissimae de Deo, Christo et Creatura id est de materia et spiritu in genere* was published anonymously in Latin translation in the collection entitled *Opuscula philosophica*, Amsterdam, 1690. English translation of this Latin version, *The Principles of the Most Ancient and Modern Philosophy*, London, 1692. On her philosophy see S. Hutton, Introduction to *The Conway Letters*; S. Hutton, 'Ancient Wisdom and Modern Philosophy: Anne Conway, F.M. van Helmont and the Seventeenth-Century Dutch Interchange of Ideas', *Quaestiones infinitae, Publications of the Department of Philosophy, Utrecht University*, no. 9; R.H. Popkin, 'The Spiritualistic Cosmologies of Henry More and Anne Conway', in S. Hutton (ed.), *Henry More 1614–1687: Tercentenary Studies*, Dordrecht, 1990, pp. 97–114; and Stuart Brown, 'Leibniz and More's Cabbalistic Circle', ibid., pp. 76–95. For a different assessment of Anne Conway's relationship to Leibniz, see Carolyn Merchant, 'The Vitalism of Anne Conway: its impact on Leibniz's Concept of the Monad', *Journal of the History of Philosophy*, 7 (1979), 255–69.
52. Conway, *Principles*, p. 195.
53. *Divine Being*, p. 170.
54. Conway, *Principles*, p. 218.
55. Ibid., p. 189.
56. *Paradoxical Discourses*, pp. 15ff.
57. See my article, 'Anne Conway, Critique de Henry More' in *Archives de Philosophie*, 58 (1995), pp. 371–84.
58. Conway, *Principles*, p. 214.

CHAPTER TEN

The Reluctant Philanthropist: Robert Boyle and the 'Communication of Secrets and Receits in Physick'

Michael Hunter

Since attention was drawn to it by Margaret Rowbottom in 1950, Robert Boyle's earliest published writing has been widely cited as an almost emblematic statement of the Baconian impulse to the free dissemination of knowledge in mid-seventeenth-century England.[1] On the title-page of the volume of *Chymical, Medicinal, and Chyrurgical Addresses* to Samuel Hartlib in which it appeared in 1655, it is described as 'An Invitation to a free and generous Communication of Secrets and Receits in Physick', and in this short essay Boyle made a powerful plea for the unrestricted circulation of information. What is especially important about it in the context of this volume is its overt stress on the religious imperative to such free communication. Though subsidiary considerations were invoked, the most significant impulse was a spiritual one. 'The more diffused, and the less selfish and mercinary our good actions are, the more we elevate our selves above our own, and the neerer we make our approximations to the perfections of the Divine nature', Boyle wrote. Moreover, the merits of such charity were especially urged in connection with medicine. Noting how Christ 'did far seldomer employ his omnipotence to feed the hungry, then he wrought miracles to heal the diseased', Boyle wrote: 'certainly the almes of curing is a piece of charity, much more extensive than that other of relieving'. In his tract, he attempted to answer a range of selfish and prudentialist reasons for withholding useful medical data, particularly the prestige attached to secrets and the extent to which knowledge made common was thereby devalued. Such considerations seemed to him insignificant compared with the overriding, Christlike obligation to put such information at the disposal of those who needed it.

The dissemination of useful medical recipes was thus presented as an act of charity, the special significance of which as a religious virtue was often stressed in the context of the increasing emphasis on practical morality which typified religious attitudes of the day, and which is often associated with the rise of Latitudinarianism.[2] Indeed, in the fullest extant account of the ethos of charitableness in late seventeenth-century England, R.B. Schlatter has pointed out how charity was seen at this time as more than a kindly gesture: rather, preachers insisted that it was something which Christians had a real obligation to provide.[3] Isaac Barrow, for instance, thought charity 'the main point of Religion', considering 'the liberal exercising of bounty and mercy, to be the necessary duty, the ordinary practise, and the proper character of the truly pious man'.[4] Moreover, charity was central to Boyle's religious persona throughout his life.[5] As Bishop Gilbert Burnet put it in the sermon that he preached at Boyle's funeral:

> His Charity to those that were in Want, and his Bounty to all Learned Men, that were put to wrastle with Difficulties, were so very extraordinary, and so many did partake of them, that I may spend little time on this Article. Great Summs went easily from him, without the Partialities of Sect, Country, or Relations; for he considered himself as part of the Humane Nature, and as a Debtor to the whole Race of Men.[6]

Both Burnet and other posthumous commentators on Boyle stressed how the dispensing of medication to his relations, tenants and friends was a key part of his charitable activity. Burnet explained of Boyle's chemical work, 'It was a Charity to others, as well as an Entertainment to himself, for the Produce of it was distributed by his Sister, and others, into whose hands he put it.' This was echoed by Thomas Dent, rector of Stalbridge, who emphasised how Boyle kept a laboratory 'not only for Experiments, but to prepare medecines for his friends, & the poor, of which he was most freely communicative; & used to attend the present, with money, if he heard any person was necessitous'.

It is interesting that – presumably unconsciously – Dent echoes the title of Boyle's 1655 essay, and the same is true of Boyle's friend, Sir Peter Pett, in *his* posthumous memoir of Boyle. Pett considered that Boyle had 'made the many moral vertues that were in him, the more conspicuous & useful to the World by his skill in physic, & in his free communication of his excellent & successful medicaments'. More striking still is the commentary on this that Pett gave, for, by way of parallel with Boyle, he felt it appropriate to cite the sentiments of the early seventeenth-century Italian cleric, Giovanni Ciampoli. Pett noted how Ciampoli had claimed of Christ that, in order to ensure that his apostles were obeyed, 'in effect he made them Doctors of physic', since 'No power is greater then that of Medicine, because no humane good is greater then health'.[7] Boyle himself echoed this Christlike analogy for the provision of health in the first section of the second part of his *The Usefulness of Natural Philosophy*, published in 1663:

> when I consider the character given of our great master and exemplar, in that scripture, which says, *That he went about doing good, and healing all manner of sickness, and all manner of diseases among the people*; I cannot but think such an imployment worthy of the very noblest of his disciples.[8]

As such texts testify, there is no doubt that Boyle was active in purveying medication to those who needed it. If his enthusiasm for collecting recipes may have owed something to the anxiety about his own health which he repeatedly voiced from the early 1650s onwards, he was happy to place this expertise at the disposal of others who needed it. Thus he speaks of medicines which he had administered, 'which God hath been so far pleased to bless on others, as to make them relieve several patients, and seem (at least) to have snatched some of them almost out of the jaws of death'.[9] Elsewhere, he specifically refers to 'the experience of my own prescriptions, which charity led me to provide for the indigent (particularly when I was living in the country among my tenants)', an evident reference to the 'Stalbridge' period of his life, prior to his move to Oxford in the 1650s and thence to London.[10] It is clear that, throughout his life, he exemplified in almost ideal form the role model of the philanthropic, paternalistic, lay purveyor of medicine.[11]

For Boyle, an experienced author who in the course of his life published a whole range of books on scientific and religious topics, a natural extension of this charitable activity might have seemed to be to publish a collection of recipes, thus using the printing press to further the aim of free communication that he had advocated in his 'Invitation'. In this, he would have been following the example of various medical writers during the interregnum and Restoration periods, when medical knowledge was more widely disseminated in printed, vernacular form than ever before.[12]

In fact, Boyle *did* bring out a work entitled *Medicinal Experiments*, a collection of 'choice and safe Remedies, for the most part simple, and easily prepared', which he considered worth printing for the use of the public. But, although Boyle worked on this in the last decade and a half of his life, perhaps the most significant thing about this work is that it was not until after his death that it was properly published, after a prehistory of private publication during his lifetime which is revealing in itself. Moreover, manuscript evidence reveals that this delay was due not least to considerable indecision on Boyle's part as to whether it was proper for him to publish a recipe collection of this kind at all – despite the strong charitable imperative to do so of which he was only too aware. It is on this dilemma and its implications that I dwell in this chapter.

By way of background, it is first necessary to go back to Boyle's major published work on medicine, the relevant section of his *The Usefulness of Natural Philosophy*, published in 1663. Ostensibly, the aim of this work was to illustrate the value to medicine of techniques and findings from natural philosophy, with instances ranging from the role of chemical analysis to the applicability of corpuscular explanations in a medical context. Boyle also took up a position in the virulent medical debates of the day, balancing his reservations about the therapy of Galenic physicians with a cautious attitude towards the practice of their empirical rivals. But, in the course of illustrating his views on these themes, Boyle provided a vast amount of data, including details of a number of recipies that he had come across and tried: this facet of the book burgeoned as Boyle wrote it, reaching a climax in a book-length appendix in which Boyle expounded at length the preparation and application of various novel and effective remedies.[13] It is clear that the book was popular with its audience – and unpopular with medical conservatives – at least partly because of the information of this kind that it contained. As Boyle later wrote of the medicines there divulged: 'they have been prosperous to many patients, and not altogether unuseful to some noted physicians; and have procured me from both more thanks, than I pretended to, besides inviting encouragement to further communications'.[14]

On the other hand, though Boyle was happy in retrospect to take credit for this aspect of the book's content, it had caused him some anxiety at the time. In part, this was because of a general problem about *Usefulness* of which Boyle was aware, namely the danger of the work's tenuous thematic thread being overwhelmed by a proliferation of data. In addition, specifically regarding medical recipes, Boyle stated: 'it may appear somewhat below me, in a book, whose title seems to promise you philosophical matters, to insert I know not how many receipts'. Yet in this case, he did not allow such objections to prevail, explaining how 'I thought, that Christianity and humanity itself obliged me not to conceal those things ... how despicable soever they may seem to a speculative philosopher'. He went on to note how, in recording such data, he had such eminent examples as Pliny, Bacon and Mersenne; in particular, he cited in justification of the fact that he had 'alledged the testimonies of others, and divers times set down processes or receipts, not of my own devising' the example of various physicians, and especially that of the French doctor, Lazare Rivière or Riverius, who 'hath not been ashamed to publish together a good number of receipts, given him by others, under the very title of *Observationes communicatae*'.[15]

Between the publication of *Usefulness* and the period from which *Medicinal Experiments* originated a further development had occurred which needs to be briefly sketched here. This is that Boyle planned a sequel to *Usefulness*, developing the passages in that work that were implicitly critical of the orthodox therapy of his day in a more overtly reformist direction; this treatise was to have been called 'Some Considerations & Doubts about the Vulgar Method or Practice of Physick'. Though only synopses and fragments of its text survive, enough is extant to give a sense of its content and approach, which was undoubtedly more aggressive than its predecessor, excoriating the shortcomings of Galenic medical practice and its intellectual rationale. In the end, however, Boyle suppressed it for various reasons; that to which he gave most prominence was the hostility of professional doctors, who 'were not well pleased, that a person not of their profession should offer to meddle with it, though with a design of advancing it'.[16]

Only in the 1680s did Boyle return to publishing on medical topics, and the works that he brought out at this time eschewed such confrontation, instead comprising uncontroversial material derived from the suppressed work, or ancillary studies focused on the medical implications of Boyle's 'general' scientific programme. Thus his *Memoirs for the Natural History of Human Blood* (London, 1684) drew on his work of the 1660s in exploring the 'natural history' of the blood; his *Of the Reconcileableness of Specifick Medicines to the Corpuscular Philosophy* (London, 1685) vindicated a corpuscularian explanation of how specifics achieved their effects; and his *Medicina Hydrostatica: or, Hydrostatics applied to the Materia Medica* (London, 1690) demonstrated the value of the calculation of specific gravity in detecting adulteration in drugs and the like.[17] Only one of the writings published at this point dealt with recipes, *The Advantages of the Use of Simple Medicines proposed by Way of Invitation to it* which was annexed to *Of the Reconcileableness* in 1685: this provided a battery of arguments in favour of simple, as against compound, medicines – that they were easier and cheaper to prepare, that it was easier to foresee their result, and that potential complications due to the interraction of ingredients could be avoided. On the other hand, only in passing did this book give details of the recipes whose use it advocated.[18]

Meanwhile, however, Boyle had clearly continued to collect recipes of the kind that he had divulged in *Usefulness*. Lists of his writings from the 1660s include 'Communicated Observations Physiologicall & Medicall', while others dating from the early 1680s have such items as 'A Short Collection of Parable Medicins', 'A Short Collection of Medicins for the Eyes' and 'Severall Receipts chiefly Chymicall'.[19] What is more, at some point in the early 1680s, Boyle wrote a lengthy 'Introductory

Preface' for a collection which he evidently intended to publish, entitled
'Receipts Chymical, and Medicinal communicated to the Author'. This
survives as a whole only in a Latin translation, though drafts for two
sections of the English text survive.[20] Boyle's solicitude for it is revealed
by the fact that it was the one work that he singled out for specific
reference in a undated memorandum which evidently lists matters that
needed to be dealt with prior to his death.[21] But he suppressed it,
probably not least because of the sharpness of his language in it, much
of it dealing with issues to do with medicine and its availability. It also
includes a few pieces of information not divulged elsewhere, for instance concerning Boyle's medical practice, or the fact that he was
unable to swallow pills (an argument for recording alternative medica-
tions to get around such individual idiosyncracies). Other points recur
in altered form in the preface to the second volume of Boyle's *Medicinal
Experiments*, published after his death, including an account of his own
ill-health. Presumably the recipes that it prefaced included those which
were to be published in the later collection. In addition, it is conceptu-
ally linked to *Simple Medicines*.

If the intended collection for which the preface was intended proved
abortive, however, Boyle did start to get his recipe collection into circulation during his lifetime, though this occurred in a rather circuitous
manner. It evidently began – perhaps in 1680 – with Boyle's dispatch of
a collection of 'five decades' of recipes (i.e. 50) to a correspondent in
New England, Dr William Avery, 'who earnestly desired of me some
receipts, that, being parable or cheap, might easily be made serviceable,
especially to the poor, in that country; where European books of physic
are too great rarities, and several remedies, here known, are not in
use'.[22]

Evidently the approach from Avery provided Boyle with the necessary
stimulus to make public a selection of the recipes that he had long
collected, and in 1688 he had an edition of the collection 'printed but
not publish'd' so that he could distribute it to selected contacts. He
makes it clear that he bought the whole impression himself, 'without
excepting those copies, that are wont to be claimd & taken by those
that had to do with the presse'.[23] This evidently explains the work's
extreme rarity. No copy at all was seen by J.F. Fulton during the many
years that he spent preparing his *Bibliography of Robert Boyle*; after
the appearance of that work, a single copy turned up in the British
Library, which was fortunately photographed for the University Micro-
films series, 'Early English Books 1641–1700', because that copy has
itself since disappeared again. The book was entitled *Some Receipts of
Medicines, For the Most Part Parable and Simple. Sent to a Friend in
America* (London, 1688) (Figure 10.1).[24] Boyle explains that he had it

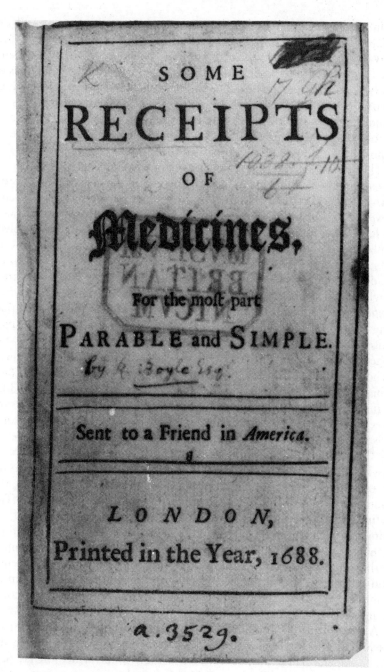

10.1   Title-page of Robert Boyle's *Some Receipts of Medicines, For the Most Part Parable and Simple*, London, 1688.

printed thus in order both to save transcribing multiple copies of the recipes and to assess 'whether 'twere adviseable to retaine them in their privacy, or to let them appear in publick'; the copies were then distributed 'gratis; not only to physitians, & surgeons, but cheifly to divines & Ladyes, & other persons residing in the countrey that were wont out of charity to give medicins to the poore'. They were vouchsafed copies on condition that they divulged only individual recipes, not the book as a whole (this was to prevent the text being pirated); and they were to report back to Boyle on the success of the recipes contained in it.[25]

The reports he received seem to have been enthusiastic: 'I was from divers hands made acquainted with the good & sometym's extraordinary effects that sometymes one, & sometymes another of the Medecins have produc'd both in England & out of it', and none of them was said to have done harm.[26] But though his informants 'addressed themselves with much importunity to the noble author, to suffer things, which were of such general benefit, and so easily to be procured by the poor, to be made more public', he continued to prevaricate.[27] Only in the year after Boyle's death in 1691 was a volume published with the title *Medicinal Experiments*, though the publisher's advertisement for this insisted that 'the major part' had been printed while he was still alive.[28] This comprised a reprint of the five 'decades' of recipes published in 1688, together with five decades more, all in a larger format than the original, 'whos unusuall smallnesse, made it not only lyable to be despys'd, but, which is worse made it easy to be lost'.[29] This was followed in 1693 by a further volume, brought out under the auspices of Boyle's literary executor, John Locke, which included a lengthy preface which comprises Boyle's fullest published statement of his rationale in such activity.[30] A third and final volume – probably supervised by another of Boyle's executors, Edmund Dickinson – materialized in 1694, and all three volumes went through several editions over the next 40 years, the fourth of which, of 1703, added a 'supplement' to volume 2.[31] The entire text comprises a series of recipes, each headed by a note of the ailment which it was intended to cure, and sometimes accompanied by a short commentary on its effectiveness. It was consciously kept simple, with a high proportion of the recipes deploying everyday ingredients, and with quantities being given in words rather than in the form of symbols.[32] Hence at last, and posthumously, Boyle's project had come to fruition.

A good deal of our knowledge of these developments derives from various drafts for Boyle's published preface which survive among the Boyle Papers. These also reveal considerable ambivalence on his part about publishing a collection of this kind, and it is to a reconstruction of what can be learnt from these texts about Boyle's mixed feelings on the subject that I devote the remainder of this chapter.[33] Perhaps not surprisingly, one theme that comes across strongly is Boyle's sense of the philanthropic imperative to an enterprise of this kind, repeatedly described as 'a great exercise of charity', 'a work, if not of (strict) duty, yet certainly of charity and humanity' or 'so charitable [a] designe'; it was to his philanthropic motives that he attributed his reluctance to see recipes lost.[34] Moreover, he felt that the provision of such compendia ought to be more of a priority for the medical profession than was currently the case, and he was critical of doctors for failing to supply them, particularly of the comprehensive kind to which he aspired; indeed, he argued that, even insofar as collections of remedies *did* exist, they were very imprecise as to what was good for what, and were lacking in alternatives in case the best ingredients were unavailable.[35]

One problem was the extent to which the polemics which dogged contemporary medicine meant that authors were prone to separate chemical and Galenic medicines, and to prescribe the use of one to the exclusion of the other. Though Boyle himself seems in at least some of his collections to have separated the two,[36] he disapproved of the exclusive use of recipes of either kind. 'I estimate their value not by the times they were 1st introduc'd or generally imploy'd but for their fitnes to performe the worke they were design'd for', he wrote, and he used a military metaphor to press home the need for the greatest variety of weapons in the fight against illness, seeing it as absurd to eschew 'Guns and Granados & Bombs' because of their modernity as to 'despise the use of swords & pikes because imploy'd by the Ancients'.[37] He was also critical of the half-hearted way in which doctors often applied remedies of the kind which he was advocating, even when they used them. Equally important was his hostility to existing practice, echoing his argument in *Simple Medicines* that prescriptions were often unnecessarily elaborate and hence expensive, thus denying those who needed medication access to it when simpler and cheaper materials might as easily have been used.

This formed part of a more general argument in the unpublished prefatory material that the practice of medicine was unduly exclusive, and that insufficient was done to make medication widely available to those who needed it. Indeed, although addressed to a doctor, the original, Latin preface includes a swingeing attack on the closed shop of contemporary medicine and the way in which vested interests upheld this, indicating how strongly Boyle felt about such matters. Here, we find a perhaps unexpectedly radical streak in Boyle, aligning him with the social reform movement of the interregum and placing him somewhat at odds with the priorities of the fashionable medical establishment of his day. Boyle's argument was 'that it seems excessively hard for anyone to be restricted to the services of men of a single profession, in order to obtain (if he can) a thing so necessary as health'.[38]

He justified this by analogy to other professions where such exclusivity was unheard of: 'no-one is denied the freedom to build his own house, despite the fact that there exist professional architects, who never claim that this is a fraudulent proceeding', while 'it is within parents' rights to educate their children in their own houses, either under or without a tutor, or in any way that they wish, so that they are not compelled to banish them to public schools or academies, although there exist public teachers and professors'. Indeed, he argued that

> if the objection which we are criticising were to hold good, then the cultivation of the human intellect would be brought to a halt (if not entirely overturned). Indeed you will find few new inventions which serve to improve the quality of people's lives, that can be introduced and widely received without harm being done to some ancient profession ... We would have lacked the benefit of printing, if the printing-shops had been destroyed for fear lest they should reduce the profit of so many notaries, who sought their livelihood from the transcription of books (and perhaps piled up considerable wealth for themselves in so doing). What would this be? It would seem to smack of nothing less than barbarism in Europe! For, in most of the territories of the Turks, and in most of the regions of the Orient, printing-shops are either eliminated, or never allowed to set themselves up, for the sake of the calligraphers. Similarly, the use of cannon would have to be abolished, in case it created a problem for the makers of arrows ... Thus it seems reasonable, for the purpose of preserving human health, to subordinate the profit of a few doctors to the universal benefit of the human race.

There is a sharpness here that is unparalleled in Boyle's published writings, and it reveals a rather unfamiliar Boyle, which has been obscured by recent interpretations of him which have laid undue emphasis on his establishmentarian credentials.[39] Indeed, implicit in his decision to publish a collection of recipes was a sense that medicine should be more accessible than was currently the case, and that the poor, in particular, would be the beneficiaries of this. As he explained most fully in one of his drafts:

> Sickness that is a thing very uneasy even to the Rich is oftentimes not only Afflictive, but Ruinous to the Poor. For it too frequently happens that such Distempers as do not endanger their Lives, do yet deprive them of their Livelihood. And if a Day labourer or som other poor man, that must get his own living and perhaps his Familys too, by imploying his Limbs in his Manual Trade or his body in some other calling, be confin'd to his Bed, or kept from working, or hinder'd from following his calling; he must quickly be undone, by the very want of his usual & necessary Income. And He is ordinarily so little able to bear the charge of Physick, which he

will far more certainly find expensive than successful, and which
even when it dos at length prevail, dos not seldom make him
before he ceases to be a Patient begin to be a Begger.[40]

Elsewhere, he refers again and again to his motive as 'charity to the
poor & sick', 'for whose sake principally twas that I made my collection'.[41] Moreover, it is revealing that one draft of his preface was to
have begun: 'Tis hop'd this smal Collection wil not be censur'd as very
prejudicial to the profession of Physick for the Rich'.[42]

Here Boyle echoes the language of the medical reformers of the
interregnum, as seen in Nicholas Culpeper's attack on the learned mo-
nopoly of his day, or in the Durham county medical plan of 1655 which
David Harley has recently published.[43] Indeed, this was the context of
Boyle's own activities in the 1650s. Hartlib, for instance, saw the *Ens
Veneris* recipe which Boyle was to divulge in *The Usefulness of Natural
Philosophy* as 'Medicina Pauperum because for 5 shillings so much may
be prepared with it as may serve 100 poore people', and in *Usefulness*
Boyle had been especially keen on remedies which could be seen as '*a
medicine for the poor*'.[44] During the Restoration period, however, there
had been a trend away from such an ethos, towards a more socially
exclusive view of medical practice: this was due not least to the prolonged dispute between doctors and apothecaries, which led to a hard-
ening of positions and a greater stress by physicians on their status.[45] It
was evidently not least because he was conscious of being out of step
with such trends that Boyle was so forceful in his arguments about the
desirability of providing medication for the poor.[46]

In Boyle's attitude, there is an interesting parallel with the 'last treatise' of his friend, the Presbyterian divine, Richard Baxter: this was a
searing indictment of the poverty that resulted from rack-renting, which
its twentieth-century editor suggested remained unpublished in Baxter's
own time because his literary executors considered it too radical. Certainly, the repeated protests of this powerful work that it was not
advocating 'levelling' are indicative of the extent to which Baxter's
Gospel-based prescriptions were uncomfortable for the well-to-do.
Moreover amongst those whom Baxter criticized were doctors, along
with lawyers and others. 'Little do the rich and Lawyers and Physicians
thinke how precious a shilling is with the poore', he wrote, and the
provision of healthcare for the poor specifically exercised him: 'had not
approaching death and modesty forbidden me, I had (though no physician) published a Directory for every ingenious Minister to become the
parish physician for the poore'.[47]

Baxter's tract has been described as 'one of the few important works
of social criticism written by a divine of the period',[48] and Boyle's views
on medical provision may be seen in a similar light. Indeed, this was not

the only facet of the ethos of Restoration England with which Boyle was uncomfortable. His hostility to the way in which medicinal improvement was impeded by a closed shop was echoed by Sir Peter Pett's anecdote of how Boyle 'tooke notice to me how every great New Invention, necessarily crossing the private Interest of many particular persons, was thereby hindred in its birth and growth, by such interested persons'. Gilbert Burnet similarly recalled how Boyle withdrew from the Council for Foreign Plantations after his initial participation in its work, 'some upon private reasons or humours obstructing it'.[49] There is a tension here in Boyle's relations with the wider world which is elided by interpretations such as that of J.R. Jacob, in which Boyle is seen as a grand strategist, committed to forging an alliance of science, trade and empire which would 'harness private interests to the public good'. In fact, Boyle was only too aware of the potential tension between individual interests and what he perceived as the greater good of society, though he made his views more explicit in private documents than in anything he published.[50]

This is particularly clear in connection with medicine. If Boyle believed that a truly Christian attitude would lead to medical priorities that were exemplified by the publication of recipes, and which were at odds with the prevailing values of the medical establishment, only with great difficulty could he bring himself to say so publicly. None of the drafts so far quoted saw the light of day, and those that did were much more apologetic, as were many of the drafts that preceded them. Boyle was in no doubt that the impulse of charity ought to be sufficient justification for divulging the collection he had made. He returns again and again to this, yet each time it is in answer to counter-arguments which, in practice, inhibited him from doing so.

Indeed, for all the fighting language displayed in his suppressed preface, Boyle was in fact rather ambivalent towards the medical profession. The question of whether, despite his lack of medical qualifications, he should be writing on medicine at all had much concerned him earlier in his career: as we have seen, this formed the principal stated reason for his suppression of his critique of orthodox medical practice, and similar considerations are echoed here. Indeed, the published version of the preface actually begins with the words, 'Though physic be not my profession, yet I hope this small collection of receipts will not incur the censure of equitable and charitable persons, though divers of them are professed physicians'.[51]

In part, this was due to a genuine respect for medicine as an art, and its practitioners as skilled artists. Boyle was thus anxious to stress of his recipes – as he had earlier in *The Usefulness of Natural Philosophy* – that 'I do not pretend, that these should play the part both of medicines and physicians too'.[52] In addition, Boyle's drafts reveal that he was heavily dependent on doctors both for supplying him with recipes and for testing them for him, which made it harder publicly to criticize their profession than he perhaps initially anticipated. The juxtaposition of such considerations with the iconoclastic remarks already quoted bears witness to an unresolved tension in Boyle's attitudes, which needs to be taken into account in judging the validity of recent assessments of Boyle's relations with professional groups like doctors which have stressed the advantages to be derived from his status as an outsider.[53]

The role which Boyle *did* espouse was that of natural philosopher, but this, too, presented problems as far as the publication of recipes was concerned, in that such a collection was at odds with Boyle's conception of what natural philosophy should properly comprise. Contrary to recent claims that Boyle's primary stress was on 'matters of fact',[54] in fact his view was that natural philosophy should be characterized by the interpretative use to which empirical findings were put. It is this that explains why in *The Usefulness of Natural Philosophy* he apologized that it might 'appear somewhat below me' to insert 'I know not how many receipts' in a book ostensibly about 'philosophical matters'.[55] As Antonio Clericuzio has pointed out, Boyle distinguished himself from vulgar 'chymists' by the philosophical status that he claimed for his studies in this area.[56] It was thus that he differentiated natural philosophy from 'our vulgar chymistry' in *Usefulness*, criticizing the latter as being:

> as yet very incomplete, affording us rather a collection of loose and scattered (and many of them but casual) experiments, than an art duly superstructed upon principles and notions, emergent from severe and competent inductions, as we have elsewhere endeavoured more particularly to manifest.[57]

It is similarly interesting that in a reply to a 'Mr H.' which will be considered shortly, in which he justified himself against accusations of plagiarism, he did so partly on the grounds that 'the great use I make of Chymical as well as other Experiments is to prove or to illustrate some truth or notion in Philosophy'.[58] In publishing something as mundane as a collection of recipes, Boyle landed himself with a problem, since he could be accused of taking a rather retrograde step.

Linked to this was Boyle's conception of his own status, since, whatever the charitable impulse to publishing a collection of recipes may have been, he seems to have been concerned as to whether it was beneath his dignity to divulge such trivia. The published version of his preface explained – echoing his earlier comments in *Usefulness* – how 'as I was induced to what I had done by the dictates of Philanthropy and Christianity, so I was warranted by great examples, both in antient times and in ours', citing classical and more modern instances of eminent people who published collections of recipes, ranging from Democritus and Pythagoras to Louis XIV.[59] The reason for Boyle's anxiety on this score is made clear by various of his drafts. 'I thought it allowable for me, in gratifying my Philanthropy, to expose my self, as little as I well could, to the censure of indiscretion', he wrote. By way of defence of printing such material, he replied how the combination of 'the solicitations of severall well natur'd persons' and 'the impulses of Charity' 'prevayld over the Reluctancy which a natural tendernes for reputation had given me to suffer things that many will looke upon as tryfles to appear publickly in a criticall age'. Elsewhere he reiterated this, concluding that 'the designe of a work of Charity such as this is ought not to be to gain applause, but to do good'.[60]

Related to this was the issue of the reliability of the data that he was purveying, and here complexities appear in Boyle's views on trust and credibility in the purveying of information which are elided in the recent account by Steven Shapin.[61] For the whole point about the content of his collection was that it comprised 'Communicated Receits': in Boyle's own words, 'the greater mass of the following collection consists of prescriptions that have been communicated to me by others'.[62] Elsewhere he elaborated on this, echoing his comments in *The Usefulness of Natural Philosophy* about the precedent for such practices provided by the section devoted to 'communicated' material in Riverius' *Observationes Medicae* (1646), and explaining how 'most of them thô not all (som being of my own devising) came to my hands by way of discourse or of Barter or by som other way of Comunication ... & that not always very easily'.[63] This presented the problem of whether he should only publish those of which he was most confident, or indeed whether he should only make public those which he had tested himself. Clearly it was not very philanthropic to disseminate bad recipes; in addition, it might be all the more damaging to his reputation. As he put it:

> I hope the Reader wilbe too equitable to expect I should be responsible for every [one] of the Remedys that helps to make up the following Collection, for the very Title Prefixt to it of Communicated Observations intimates that I take (most, for I say not all of) them upon the credit of others. And therefore thô I have been careful to refuse room in this collection to severall highly commended Receipts because I distrusted the veracity of judgment of the Extollers yet I would not pawn my own credit for the goodness of particular medicines upon the truth of the characters [I received of others] & hop[e] I shall be judg'd to have perform'd my part on this occasion by haveing been wary in admitting these Receipts & faithful in delivering them.[64]

But the matter continued to worry him, perhaps because of the extent to which he knew that he was criticized at the time for too readily accepting the reports of others. Commenting on Boyle in connection with Burnet's intended life of him in 1692, the diarist, Abraham de la Pryme, wrote: 'Some condemns him for being too credulous and giving too much heed to the relations of his informers in philos[ophical] matters', though in his view 'this springs from nothing but ignorance and envy'.[65] The same concern was echoed in the context of chemical medicine by Hermann Boerhaave, who wrote of Boyle – referring to nostrums promoted in *Usefulness* –

> that taking the virtues of his preparations on the report of other people, he commends some of them too much, and attributes virtues to them which experience does not avow. For, as he did not practise physic himself, his way was, upon making any new preparation, to give it some physicians to make trial thereof; and they, it seems, out of complaisance, would speak more largely of it than it deserved. Hence, those profuse commendations he bestows upon the spirit of human blood and hart's-horn in phthisical, and on the *Ens Veneris* in rachitical cases.[66]

In an attempt to illustrate that he did not intend 'to impart an absolute Equality between them all',[67] therefore, Boyle devised an elaborate system of coding recipes as to both their excellence, and the number of times they had been tried; this was divulged in varius drafts and appeared in published form in the preface to the 1688 recension of his collection. Recipes were marked either 'A' which 'signifies, that the remedy it belongs to hath been, either by the affirmation of the physician, or other credible persons, that imparted it to me, or by trials, that I caused to be made of it, recommended as very considerable and efficacious in its kind', or 'B' for 'a second or inferior sort, but yet considerable for its good operations', or 'C' for 'those remedies that are of the lowest order, though good enough not to be despised'. Then, 'because I presume it may be expected, that I should give you some short character, of those, whereof I have had some kind of experience', he added either the figure '1', which 'denotes, that I have known but a single trial of it', or a cross, which 'imports, that the trials have been made two, or some few more times', while 'an asterisk (consisting of several lines crossing each other in one point) (*) signifies, that the trials, wherein it hath been found useful, were many, if not very many'. On the other hand, the latter failed to appear in the published text, while any classification at all was abandoned after the first volume.[68]

The strength of his feeling on the matter, however, is clear from the fact that he referred in an apologetic way to this attempted demarcation in yet another of his unpublished drafts, writing how, 'If I would have consulted my own reputation rather than the good of others' he would have been more selective: 'it had been more for my credit & that of the Receits too, if I had cull'd out the choicest such as those that are markt with an Asterick, or at lest with 2 Cross-Lines, and made my Collection to consist only of Them'. Against this, on the other hand, was the consideration that, even if differentiated from the best, the inclusion of mediocre recipes might be justified on the grounds that the best might not always be available: hence 'it may be act of discretion but not of charity to suppress medicins that thô of an inferior order may be useful ones'.[69]

Since so many of the recipes had been imparted to him by others as against being tested by Boyle himself, it might have seemed appropriate to record the names of those who supplied them. Indeed, it is implicit in the views of Shapin that the assurance of persons of appropriate status ought to have been a sufficient guarantee of their efficacy.[70] As Boyle put it:

> I know that one might request that the authors' names should be prefixed to other people's prescriptions and processes. Nor do I disagree: I thought it gentlemanly (I might say, only fair) to add mention of the names of those whose distinguished materials of this sort I had followed.

In fact, however, in none of the published volumes are the names given of those who supplied Boyle with the recipes that were included.[71] This, too, was something for which he felt obliged to apologize, explaining how he had

> receiv'd many of them from learned or ingenious Travellers some of whose names I never knew & as to divers of the rest when I came to make up my scatter'd notes, I found that by length of time their names which are things wont to be easily forgot, were slipt out of my memory.

Even in the case of informants whose identity he *did* know, however, and particularly of those 'whom their residence & practise in this place, may make it more fit for me to take notice of', he did not feel it desirable to divulge their names.[72] The reason for this is explained in his Latin preface, where he pointed out that practitioners who profited from patients' faith in the cures that they purveyed did not want the exact recipe for their nostrum to be identified as theirs in print, even if it were printed, lest it detract from their practice by encouraging patients to prepare it for themselves.[73]

On the other hand, Boyle clearly felt that, even if prudence dictated that the names of their originators be suppressed when the recipes were disseminated, it was nevertheless proper that the ownership of recipes should be recorded. To this end he devised a complex scheme for false attributions to be attached to recipes, to which he prepared a key which he claims that he entrusted to 'a discreet friend'. This apparently juxtaposed a column of the 'Fictitious' names used in his 'Collection of Receipts Processes &c and the Lists belonging to it' and a column of true names: 'so that any of these fain'd Names being affixt to the Ordinal Number in the Collection (reaching from 501 to 4000) the Process it belongs to is to be understood as imparted or recommended to me, by the Person whose faign'd name is, at length, or by Contraction, expres't in the margine'.[74] The advantage of this (in Boyle's words) was that

> if any of these worthy persons shall think it his Interest to challeng either one or more of the Receipts ascrib'd to him, he may freely do it, & not be defrauded of his right, And thô none should think fit to make such claims there may be this advantage in this way of proceeding, that a Reader who has try'd one or a few of the Receipts ascrib'd to a Person of such a faign'd name may without knowing who the Person is, make probable Estimates how far he is to relye on, or to value the other medicin imparted to me by the same Author.[75]

Hence one of the reasons for such records was to give readers a kind of convoluted measure of reliability. It was perhaps also a way out of the double-bind in which Boyle found himself, in neither having tested the medicines himself, nor being able to divulge the names of his informants. But in addition, it seems likely that Boyle was concerned about the related issue of plagiarism: he did not wish to claim as his own information which in fact remained the right of other people. It was for similar reasons that he seems to have felt some embarrassment about duplicating what was already in print in his collection of recipes, something for which he offered various reasons, notably his lack of familiarity with the field and its literature that he would have acquired had he been a professional.[76] Moreover, this concern has a long background on Boyle's part which is worth sketching here, since, even when it has been noted, it has been misinterpreted by those anxious to elevate him to an ideal type of natural philosopher of the period.[77]

Thus it was in fact Boyle who had been most active in promoting initiatives to discourage plagiarism at the Royal Society in the 1660s. A series of references to such issues in the letters that Boyle exchanged with Henry Oldenburg in these years largely tally with references to steps taken by the Society that are recorded in its minutes. In November 1664, Oldenburg commented on Boyle's recommendation 'concerning the registring of the time, when any Observation or Experiment is first mentioned', which he claimed that the Society had declared 'should be punctually observed', though no related reference appears in the minutes. In March 1665, it seems likely that it was Boyle who was behind the motion made by Oldenburg 'in the name of some member of the society' that a Fellow with 'a philosophical notion or invention, not yet made out' should have it sealed in a box 'till it could be perfected, and so brought to light, this might be allowed for the better securing inventions to their authors'; this was agreed subject to those who availed themselves of such protection reporting back to the Society after about a year.[78] Then, in 1667, a similar order was made, 'that a security might be provided for such inventions or notions, as ingenious persons might have, and desired to secure from usurpation, or from being excluded from having a share in them, if they should be lighted on by others', again following a discussion in letters between Boyle and Oldenburg, in which Boyle specifically requested that the matter should be raised without naming him. Moreover, the following February, Boyle is the only known person to have availed himself of this facility, with Oldenburg recording his receipt of data from Boyle to 'the same minute, it came to my hands' before passing it to the Society's President, Lord Brouncker.[79]

If Boyle was already in the vanguard in safeguarding the rights of authors in the 1660s, his solicitude about such matters intensified thereafter, particularly in the late 1670s: this followed various instances of what he saw as the improper use or presentation of his work by authors at home and abroad, as a result of which 'I may be suspected to have taken divers things from others, which indeed borrowed of me'.[80] Boyle retained this concern for the rest of his life: in his later years he availed himself of the Royal Society's facilities to deposit sealed packages, a number of which were opened after his death, while the Council Minutes of the Society record that on 21 January 1691

> Sir John Hoskins proposed from Mr Boyle that a proper person might be found out to discover Plagiarys and to assist Inventions to their proper Authors, Whereupon it was put to the Question by Balot whether the Council were of Opinion that it would be a useful Work if such a person could be found and it was carried in the Affirmative.[81]

Boyle's motives are revealed by a paper on this subject dating from the latter part of his life, in which he made clear that he deprecated plagiarism because he believed that it damaged

> the commonwealth of learning, especially by discouraging the industry of those many that do not undervalue fame, and by encouraging laziness in those numerous pretenders to the new philosophy, who will never take much pains to promote experimental knowledge, whilst they find it far easier to usurp experiments than to

make them, and think they may securely, by turning plagiaries, pass for philosophers.[82]

Recipes may seem different, but what is especially interesting is that Boyle seems himself to have been accused of plagiarism in the sense of 'being a Purchaser of the Experiments I have publish'd', and that this accusation focused on the very collection of *Communicated Observations*, Medicall and Chymicall that we have been concerned with here.[83] The charge was apparently made by one 'Mr H.' – possibly Oliver Hill, a maverick figure who had in fact been elected to the Royal Society on Boyle's recommendation in 1677, though he had not proved very popular there[84] – who accused Boyle of intending to publish as his own recipes that he had obtained from a Huguenot chemist, Monsieur L.S., and 'another Person or two'.[85] Boyle was detailed and slightly ambivalent in his response. To the accusation that he had bought recipes, he replied

> I should not think it mony mispent but employed to promote a publick good, if upon reasonable terms I should redeem any valuable Receits or Processes, that being imparted to others, may releive the sick; and yet unles so rescu'd, would probably be suffer'd to dye with their Possessors, or at lest remain in hands wherein they would be useles.[86]

On the other hand, in this case the implication was that he was abusing the charity which he had shown to Monsieur L.S. as to other Huguenot refugees – part of that general charitable activity on Boyle's part on which Burnet had laid such stress[87] – by publishing as his own data which really belonged to someone else. Clearly, this rankled with Boyle, even though he answered the accusation to his own satisfaction. It may well be that this episode, too, contributed to his reluctance to put into general circulation a collection which – even more than most of his works – depended on data which was specifically advertised as 'communicated'.

Hence there is much to be learnt from this episode. We are presented with a rather pusillanimous face of Boyle, which is elided by recent characterizations of him like those of J.R. Jacob and Steven Shapin. We see a man with stronger private views than he felt able to express publicly, more ambivalent about the state of affairs in Restoration England than their interpretations imply. We also see a man riven with anxiety about the advisability of making available material which he was convinced it was both his Christian duty, and in the public interest, to disseminate; a man uncomfortably aware of the extent to which his impulse to carry out charitable acts might be damaging to his 'reputation'. Such evidence reinforces the view of Boyle that I have presented elsewhere – of a man who can only be fully understood if we do justice to the convoluted, conscience-ridden side to his personality, and who is misrepresented by readings of him which present him too simplistically as a decisive intellectual strategist.[88] Equally significant, this study illustrates the extent to which the 'free communication' of recipes turned out in practice to be more problematic than Boyle had believed when he wrote his 'Invitation' to Hartlib in 1649 – due to issues of plagiarism, and to the high standards to which he aspired for the validation of empirical data. For as scrupulous a man as Boyle, it was harder than he initially expected to be Christlike in the context of Restoration England.

Notes

1. M.E. Rowbottom, 'The Earliest Published Writing of Robert Boyle', *Annals of Science*, 6 (1950), 376–89 (pp. 377, 380–81). On the link of the work to various documents dating from 1649, see R.E.W. Maddison, 'The Earliest Published Writing of Robert Boyle', *Annals of Science*, 17 (1961), 165–73.
2. Cf. C.F. Allison, *The Rise of Moralism*, London, 1966, John Spurr, *The Restoration Church of England 1646–89*, New Haven and London, 1991, esp. ch. 6; Isabel Rivers, *Reason, Grace and Sentiment*, vol. 1, Cambridge, 1991, esp. ch. 2.
3. R.B. Schlatter, *The Social Ideas of Religious Leaders, 1660–88* London, 1940; reprinted New York, 1971, pp. 124–45.
4. I. Barrow, *The Duty and Reward of Bounty to the Poor*, London, 1671, pp. 22, 46.
5. It is, however, curiously neglected in the recent analysis of Boyle's religiosity in Steven Shapin, *A Social History of Truth: Civility and Science in Seventeenth-Century England*, Chicago, 1994, p. 156ff, despite its close linkage with the genteel practices on which such stress is there laid.
6. As cited in Michael Hunter, *Robert Boyle by Himself and His Friends*, London, 1994, p. 52.
7. Ibid., pp. 55, 105, 82–3.
8. R. Boyle, *Works*, Thomas Birch (ed.), 2nd edn, 6 vols, London, 1772, vol. ii, p. 201.
9. Loc. cit.
10. 'Medica Praescripta' (see below, note 20).
11. See Dorothy Porter and Roy Porter, *Patient's Progress*, London, 1989, esp. pp. 41–2; Paul Slack, 'Mirrors of Health and Treasures of Poor Men: the Uses of the Vernacular Medical Literature of Tudor England', in Charles Webster (ed.), *Health Medicine and Mortality in the Sixteenth Century*, Cambridge, 1979, pp. 237–73, esp. pp. 258, 261. See also Lucinda Beier, *Sufferers and Healers*, London, 1987, esp. pp. 215, 223, and, on role models, David Harley, 'The Good Physician and the Godly Doctor: the Exemplary Life of John Tylston of Chester (1663–99)', *Seventeenth-Century England*, 9 (1994), 93–117.
12. See Charles Webster, *The Great Instauration: Science, Medicine and Reform 1626–60*, London, 1975, p. 264f. On earlier publications, see Slack, 'Mirrors of Health', pp. 246, 250–51.

13. *Works*, vol. ii, pp. 135ff, 215ff, and *passim*.
14. *Works*, vol. v, p. 116.
15. Ibid., vol. ii, pp. 199–200. See further below.
16. *Works*, vol. v, p. 583. For a study of this abortive work, including a transcript of the extant passages from it, see Michael Hunter, 'Boyle Versus the Galenists: A Suppressed Critique of Seventeenth-Century Medical Practice and its Significance', forthcoming, *Medical History*, **41** (1997).
17. See Hunter, op. cit. See also B.B. Kaplan, '*Divulging of Useful Truths in Physick': the Medical Agenda of Robert Boyle*, Baltimore, 1993.
18. *Works*, vol. v, pp. 109–29.
19. Boyle Papers (hereafter BP) 36, fols 59–60, 119–20; BP 8, fol. 64v (and various recensions of this which will be discussed in the forthcoming 'Pickering Masters' edition of *The Works of Robert Boyle*).
20. The title is from the 1684 list of Boyle's unpublished writings in BP 36, fols 59–60. For the Latin text see BP 17, fols 1–36 (hereinafter 'Medica Praescripta'); for the English drafts, BP 38, fol. 23, Royal Society (hereafter RS) MS 199, fols 32–7. The entire text will be published in the 'Pickering Masters' *Works of Robert Boyle*.
21. BP 36, fol. 178 (third item), referring specifically to the 'Large Preface to the Communicated Receits' alongside a more general concern about the 'oversight' of Boyle's writings. See also Boyle's reference to the 'Preface' to his *Communicated Observations*, Medicall and Chymical in his reply to 'Mr H.' of *c*.1690 (ibid., fol. 7), which he states 'has been long in the hands of a Person you know'.
22. *Works*, vol. v, pp. 312, 314. Cf. R.E.W. Maddison, 'The first edition of Robert Boyle's *Medicinal Experiments', Annals of Science*, **18** (1962), 43–7, and a letter from Boyle to Avery of 13 March 1680, now in the Massachusetts Historical Library, in which Boyle writes: 'since in the latter part of your Letter you are pleasd to desire some Receipts for feavors & some few other Diseases frequent in your Countrey: that this Paper of mine may not be altogether insignificant I inclose you in it some easy & parable Receipts for some of the Distempers by you mentioned & for some others besides.'
23. RS MS 186, fol. 119v (*but* replaces *if* deleted).
24. See the microfilm series 'Early English Books 1641–1700', Ann Arbor, Michigan, no. 1479: 15. See also Maddison, 'First Edition', pp. 43–4. The photograph of the title-page reproduced here (which was not used in the 1962 article) is derived from a negative preserved amongst Dr Maddison's papers at the University of Kent at Canterbury by kind permission of the Librarian. See also J.F. Fulton, *A Bibliography of the Hon. Robert Boyle*, 2nd edn, Oxford, 1961, p. 118: he had been alerted to the existence of the 1688 recension by Birch, who had access to a copy, since the 'Introduction' and 'Advertisement' are printed in *Works*, vol. v, pp. 312–4, a point not noted by Maddison. Cf. *Works*, vol. i, p. cxxiv.
25. RS MS 186, fols 119v–20 (*adviseable* replaces *meet* [?] deleted; *or* replaces *then* deleted; *give* replaces *adven*, deleted). Cf. *Works*, vol. v, p. 314.
26. RS MS 186, fol. 120v.
27. *Works*, vol. v, p. 314.
28. Edward Arber (ed.), *The Term Catalogues 1668–1709*, 3 vols, London, 1905, vol. ii, p. 403.

29. RS MS 186, fol. 121 (*unusuall smallnesse* replaces *little* deleted; *not only* is inserted).

30. See M.A. Stewart, 'Locke's Professional Contacts with Robert Boyle', *The Locke Newsletter*, 12 (1981), 19–44, esp. 39–41. Stewart points out that Locke's hand is apparent in the fact that the recipes in vol. 2 appear alphabetically according to ailment, an arrangement that is not in evidence in vol. 1 (and is abandoned in vol. 3).

31. Fulton, *Bibliography*, pp. 118–25.

32. Vol. 3 reverts to the use of symbols, however, as had also been the case with the 1688 edition: cf. Maddison, 'First Edition', p. 44. For a manuscript version of certain of the recipes in the first part of the work, with their published numbers in pencil, but without titles specifying what diseases they were good for, see BP 19, fols 138–9: here, too, symbols are used for quantities.

33. The principal surviving drafts are as follows: RS MS 186, fols 91ff (this overlaps most closely with the published version, though one presumes that Locke found and printed a further version which no longer survives in MS) and 119vff; RS MS 187, fols 139v–40; and RS MS 189, fols 58–61. Ibid., fols 50–51, overlaps in sentiment but appears to have a slightly different rationale (it may relate to the essay on parable medicines referred to below); RS MS 198, fol. 12 is a fragment; BP 18, fol. 75 appears to be a preface to a further collection. In addition, Boyle seems to have planned a separate essay on parable medicines, which he specifically refers to in *Works*, vol. v, p. 114 (cf. the lists of his writings in BP 36, fols 72, 73 and 122, and RS MS 186, fols 33v–4); this would have been about the rationale of such medicines, as against comprising an actual collection of them. The following MSS evidently belong to it: BP 18, fols 67, 70–71, 73–4, 76, 125; RS MS 186, fols 14v–15, 138v–9, 142v; RS MS 187, fols 38, 113–15; RS MS 189, fols 20v–22. The following MSS are also related: BP 38, fol. 13; RS MS 187, fols 134–5; RS MS 199, fols 6–7.

34. 'Medica Praescripta'; RS MS 189, fol. 50v; RS MS 186, fol. 105v.

35. *Works*, vol. v, p. 316; 'Medica Praescripta'.

36. E.g. *Works*, vol. v, p. 586ff; BP 17, fols 43–5; BP 38, fol. 13; 'Medica Praescripta'.

37. RS MS 186, fols 103v–5 (*their* is altered from *the* and *the* from *their*; *or places the* is deleted after *times*; *or generally imploy'd* is inserted; after *to*, *some* is deleted).

38. *Works*, vol. v, p. 113, and pp. 109–29 and *passim*; 'Medica Praescripta'.

39. Steven Shapin, *Social History of Truth*, ch. 4. See also J.R. Jacob, *Robert Boyle and the English Revolution*, New York, 1977; Steven Shapin and Simon Schaffer, *Leviathan and the Air-Pump: Hobbes, Boyle and the Experimental Life*, Princeton, 1985.

40. RS MS 189, fols 50–51 (after *very*, *even is* deleted; after *Ruinous*, *also* deleted; *is* is deleted, but has been reinstated for the sense; *not only Afflictive but* is inserted, replacing *also*, with *un* deleted after *not only* within it; *For* replacing *And* deleted; *Day* inserted; *labourer* altered from *laboring man*; after *Trade*, *of* replaces *or* deleted; *kept* inserted, replacing *his hindred* deleted; *from* followed by *his usual* deleted; *And* replaces *&* deleted; *bear the charge of Physick* replaces *feed Doctors*, *& pay Surgeons and Apoth* deleted; after *Physick*, *whos* deleted; *certainly*

replaces *assuredly* deleted; *than* replaces & deleted; *seldom* followed by *before* deleted; *be* altered from *become*).

41. RS MS 186, fols 119–20 (*twas* deleted after *sake*). Cf., e.g., BP 17, fols 43–5, where he urged those who profited from recipes 'to remember that the Poor has (in some measure) a share with them'.

42. RS MS 186, fol. 99v: *for the Rich* was subsequently deleted.

43. Webster, *Great Instauration*, pp. 267–72; Cf. ibid., pp. 256–64, 288–300. David Harley, 'Pious Physic for the Poor: the lost Durham County Medical Scheme of 1655', *Medical History*, 37 (1993), 148–66.

44. *Ephemerides*, s.v. 1653; *Works*, vol. ii, pp. 136, 201. Cf. ibid., pp. 123–4, 202, 225, 240.

45. See, e.g., Jonathan Goddard, *A Discourse, Setting Forth the unhappy Condition of the Practice of Physick in London*, London, 1670, reprinted in Thomas Park (ed.), *The Harleian Miscellany*, 10 vols, 1808–13, vol. viii, pp. 462–76; J.L. Axtell, 'Education and Status in Stuart England: the London Physician', *History of Education Quarterly*, 10 (1970), 141–59.

46. For parallel arguments in favour of establishing a dispensary for the sick-poor, with which the College of Physicians was to comply largely for strategic reasons in its struggle with the apothecaries, see Albert Rosenberg, 'The London Dispenary for the Sick-Poor', *Journal of the History of Medicine*, 14 (1959), 41–56; F.H. Ellis, 'The Background of the London Dispensary', ibid., 20 (1965), 197–212; and H.J. Cook, *The Decline of the Old Medical Regime in Stuart London*, Ithaca, 1986, p. 233f.

47. F.J. Powicke (ed.), *The Revd. Richard Baxter's Last Treatise*, Manchester, 1926, pp. 14, 29, 43 and *passim*. For an interesting reading of the context of this tract, see W.M. Lamont, *Richrd Baxter and the Millenium*, London, 1979, p. 306ff.

48. Schlatter, *Social Ideas of Religious Leaders*, p. 74.

49. Hunter, *Boyle by Himself and His Friends*, pp. 33, 58.

50. *Boyle and the English Revolution*, p. 147, and see the critique of this view in Hunter, *Boyle by Himself and His Friends*, pp. lxix and xcvii, n. 322.

51. *Works*, vol. v, p. 314.

52. *Works*, vol. v, p. 313, Cf. ibid., vol. ii, p. 242; vol. v, p. 129.

53. See Shapin, *Social History of Truth*, esp. pp. 180–82; Kaplan '*Divulging Useful Truths*', esp. p. 144; John Harwood, 'Science Writing and Writing Science: Boyle and Rhetorical Theory', in Michael Hunter (ed.), *Robert Boyle Reconsidered*, Cambridge, 1994, pp. 37–56, on p. 42.

54. Shapin and Schaffer, *Leviathan and the Air-Pump*, esp. ch. 2; Jan V. Golinski, 'Robert Boyle: Scepticism and Authority in Seventeenth-Century Chemical Discourse', in A.E. Benjamin, G.N. Cantor, and J.R.R. Christie (eds), *The Figural and the Literal*, Manchester, 1987, pp. 58–82, esp. 68ff.

55. *Works*, vol. ii, p. 199.

56. Clericuzio, 'Carneades and the Chemists', in M. Hunter, *Robert Boyle Reconsidered*, pp. 79–90, esp. pp. 81–2.

57. *Works*, vol. ii, p. 145.

58. BP 36, fol. 8.

59. *Works*, vol. v, pp. 314–15. For an overlapping version of this, see 'Medica Praescripta'.

60. RS MS 186, fols 97v–8, 119v–20 (*in gratifying* is altered from *to gratify*;

self replaces *discretion* deleted; before *appear*, *be* is deleted; before *a work*, *such* is deleted; *as* replaces *is* deleted; *to gain* replaces *an* deleted). For a parallel concern about how his natural philosophical concerns might not be conducive to his credit, see, e.g., *Works*, vol. i, p. 459; vol. ii, pp. 479–80; vol. iii, p. 6; vol. iv, p. 79; vol. v, pp. 598, 612.

61. Shapin, *Social History of Truth*, chs 5–6.

62. 'Medica Praescripta'. For Boyle's comparable concern about the use of 'communicated' data in his *Experimenta et Observationes Physicae*, see *Works*, vol. v, pp. 568–9.

63. RS MS 189, fols 59–61 (*way of* is followed by *Barter* deleted; *of* before *Barter or* and *by* after it are inserted, as is the bracketed phrase earlier in the sentence). Cf. Riverius, *Observationes Medicae*, London, 1646, pp. 321–451. In this connection, it is worth noting Boyle's apology for retaining the uncorrected style in which recipes had been given to him, most fully expounded in the 1688 preface: *Works*, vol. v, pp. 313–14.

64. RS MS 186, fol. 106. *Most, for I say not all* is inserted; *I received of others* is deleted but has been reinstated to make sense of the passage, while *one* has been inserted and *hope* has been altered from *hoping* to complete the sense. After *credit of others* the following has been deleted: *thô of the goodnes of some I am otherwise satisfy'd*. The remainder of the passage is such a patchwork of insertions and deletions that it has not been feasible to record them here. Cf. RS MS 187, fol. 140.

65. A. de la Pryme, *The Diary of Abraham de la Pryme*, Durham, Surtees Society, 1870, vol. 54, p. 24. On Burnet's intended life see Hunter, *Boyle by Himself and His Friends*, pp. xxxi–xxxii.

66. Hermann Boerhaave, *A New Method of Chemistry*, trans. Peter Shaw and Ephraim Chambers, London, 1727, p. 47.

67. RS MS 186, fol. 93v (*between* is followed by *all the particular* deleted).

68. *Works*, vol. v, p. 313; Maddison, 'First Edition', p. 44. Cf. RS MS 186, fol. 93v, where he explains that those marked 'A' are better than those marked 'B', 'as far as I can judg by the Characters given them by the Imparters', and RS MS 187, fols 139v–40, which also has '1', '2' and '3' as well as 'A', 'B' and 'C': but the draft ends before the significance of the numerals has been explained. For references to Boyle's own trials of recipes in his published *Medicinal Experiments*, see *Works*, vol. v, pp. 321, 357.

69. RS MS 186, fol. 97v–8 (*made* replaces *make* deleted; *may* is reinstated, after having been replaced by *would*; after *discretion*, *more* is inserted but deleted again).

70. See Shapin, *Social History of Truth*, esp. ch. 6.

71. 'Medical Praescripta'. The nearest that Boyle comes to divulging his sources are occasional references to the source of a medicine such as 'a charitable lady, of whose ingenious chaplain I procured this'; rarer still are formulae like 'The Lady *Fitz-Harding's* Eye-water': *Works*, vol. v, pp. 345, 380.

72. RS MS 189, fol. 60 (*or* replaces *&* deleted; *divers of the rest* is inserted, replacing *when long after*[?] deleted; after *time, that made me forget that [del.] their names* deleted; *by things* and *whom* are inserted). Boyle here states that he had 'elsewhere declar'd' (replacing *given* deleted) his reason for omitting the names of his informants, presumably referring to the relevant passage in the Latin preface cited in the next note. See also BP

17, fol. 45, in which his lack of time is blamed, and *Works*, vol. v, p. 610, where the lack of names is blamed on the negligence of his transcribers.

73. 'Medica Praescripta'. Cf. *The Usefulness of Natural Philosophy*, *Works*, vol. ii, p. 204. It is interesting to compare Boyle's concern in *Usefulness* about queering the pitch of tradesmen by divulging their secrets: *Works*, vol. iii, pp. 397–9.

74. RS MS 189, fols 59v–60; BP 36, fol. 16 (*Names* is followed by *of* deleted; *the Process it belongs to* is inserted). The latter may in fact relate to the communicated data that Boyle intended to publish in *Experimenta et Observationes Physicae* (see above, n. 62; at one point he thought of including recipes from his medical collection in this work; see RS MS 186, fol. 105v): I hope to elucidate this matter in a future publication.

75. RS MS 189, fol. 59v (*ascrib'd* replaces *refer'd* deleted; *not be* replaces *injoy the* and *have* deleted; *thô none should think fit to make such claims* *there may* is inserted, replacing *there would* (replaced by *will*) deleted; before *advantage, further* deleted; *who has* replaces *was* deleted; after *Receipts, belonging* and *ref* deleted; *probable* replaces *an* deleted).

76. *Works*, vol. v, p. 316; 'Medica Praescripta'; RS MS 189, fols 58v–9.

77. See Rob Iliffe, '"In the Warehouse": Privacy, Property and Priority in the Early Royal Society', *History of Science*, 30 (1992), 29–68, esp. pp. 34–5, who refers to the material deployed in the next paragraph but fails to bring out Boyle's initiatory role in such matters. Cf. Shapin, *Social History of Truth*, p. 183, who says that Boyle 'took his full part' in them, and Adrian Johns, 'Wisdom in the Concourse: Natural Philosophy and the History of the Book in Early Modern England', Cambridge PhD thesis, 1992, pp. 159–60 and ch. 4 and *passim*.

78. A.R. and M.B. Hall (eds), *The Correspondence of Henry Oldenburg*, 13 vols, Madison, Milwaukee and London, 1965–86, vol. ii, p. 319; Thomas Birch, *The History of the Royal Society of London*, 4 vols, London, 1756–7, vol. ii, pp. 24–5: there is a gap in the correspondence between Boyle and Oldenburg at this point. Note how concern on such matters recurs when the correspondence recommences in the summer: *Oldenburg*, vol. ii, pp. 484, 486.

79. *Oldenburg*, vol. iii, pp. 533, 540; vol. iv, pp. 94, 185, 193; Birch, *History*, vol. ii, pp. 212, 247. It is conceivable that the item in question was the document that is now BP 19, fol. 184, and the papers it accompanied: however, this is dated just a few days later, 24 February 1668.

80. *Oldenburg*, vol. iv, p. 94. See also Michael Hunter and Edward B. Davis, 'The Making of Robert Boyle's *Free Inquiry into the Vulgarly Receiv'd Notion of Nature*', *Early Science and Medicine*, 1 (1996), 204–71, on pp. 217–18.

81. Royal Society Copy Council Minutes, vol. ii, p. 108. See also ibid., p. 113; R.E.W. Maddison, *The Life of the Hon. Robert Boyle*, London, 1969, p. 202. For a contemporary reference to Boyle's practice in depositing papers, see Southwell to Cole, 9 November 1699, BL Add. MS 18599, fol. 90. See also, in a medical context, RS MS 186, fol. 103.

82. *Works*, vol. i, p. cxxvii. The original MS of this, now BP 10, fol. 98, is in the hand of Robert Bacon, who began working for Boyle in the 1670s.

83. Boyle's reply survives as BP 36, fols 7–8, but not the attack to which he was responding. The reference in the opening line to 'what you tell me Mr H objected' suggests that he may only have heard about it.

84. Birch, *History*, vol. iii, pp. 351, 363, 366–7, 371; see also M. Hunter, *Boyle by Himself and His Friends*, pp. lxxi–ii. The clue suggesting that 'Mr H.' may have been Hill is to be found in John Aubrey's life of Boyle in his *Brief Lives*, Andrew Clark (ed.), 2 vols, Oxford, 1898, vol. i, p. 120, where he writes: 'vide Oliver Hill's ... where he is accused of grosse plagiarisme'.
85. BP 36, fols 7–8. The doctor was conceivably James Feuillel la Saufray: see H.J. Cook, *Trials of an Ordinary Doctor: Johannes Groenevelt in Seventeenth-Century London*, Baltimore, 1994, p. 5.
86. BP 36, fol. 7.
87. See M. Hunter, *Boyle by Himself and His Friends*, p. 52.
88. Ibid., esp. pp. lxiii–lxxix; id., 'The Conscience of Robert Boyle', in F.A.J.L. James and Judith Field (eds), *Renaissance and Revolution*, Cambridge, 1993, pp. 147–59.

CHAPTER ELEVEN

The Theology of Affliction and the Experience of Sickness in the Godly Family, 1650–1714: The Henrys and the Newcomes

David Harley

The central role of providential theology in shaping the attitudes of devout Protestants in early modern England is well known to historians.[1] The desire to read the will of God prompted the writing of diaries and autobiographies which have proved excellent sources for the study of family life.[2] There have also been attempts to analyse the attitudes of the godly towards sickness and medicine, although the subject has yet to receive definitive treatment.[3]

Each distinct religious position throws up its own worldview, formed by the interaction of theology, social status and organization, and this normally leads to a distinctive attitude towards disease and healing, even if there is little explicit discussion of the subject.[4] Religious beliefs shape the interpretation of sickness and death, the choice of therapeutic systems and medical attendants, and sickroom behaviour, creating medical subcultures.[5] A history of medicine based on the economic rationality of the 'medical market-place' cannot readily accommodate this ethnographic dimension.

There is a need for a clearer understanding of the relationship between belief systems and the practices associated with the maintenance of health and the treatment of disease.[6] A greater degree of theological specification will be required, especially for the study of periods of rapid change such as early modern England. Previously neglected groups, such as Catholics, Baptists, and the High Church faction, need to be examined and compared with lukewarm Christians and the godly. The attitudes of Calvinists are more familiar but they are still in need of close case studies integrating the reception of religious ideologies and the mediated experiences of personal life. There is no reason to suppose that religious groups were perfectly homogeneous since many factors other than theology also shaped both attitudes and patterns of consumption.[7]

The subjects of this chapter belonged to two clerical families on the moderate Calvinist borderline between dissent and conformity, the Presbyterian Henry family and the Newcomes, part Presbyterian and part Low Church conformist.[8] The two families were closely linked during the late seventeenth century, but drifted apart after the death of several family members in the 1690s. The son of a minor courtier, Philip Henry took his MA at Oxford in 1652. He became a minister on the Welsh border until his ejection in 1661, and married a local gentlewoman. His son Matthew studied under Thomas Doolittle in Islington and at Gray's Inn, then became the leading Presbyterian minister in Chester until he moved to Hackney, shortly before his death in 1714. Philip Henry's four daughters married locally, and regularly visited and corresponded with their parents and brother.[9]

Henry Newcome the elder was the son of a clergyman and took his MA at Cambridge in 1651. He married into a Cheshire gentry family and served as a minister in the county until appointed preacher at the Collegiate Church in Manchester. After his ejection, he was one of Lancashire's leading Presbyterian ministers, while remaining friendly with many conformists. His sons Henry and Peter went to university, conformed, and became Low Church clergymen. Henry Newcome the younger returned from Oxford to the area, serving as parish priest first at the little parish of Tattenhall near Chester and then at Middleton near Manchester until his death in 1713. Although he was bitterly opposed to the schism, he remained on good terms with several nonconformists. Peter Newcome had some difficulties at Cambridge but obtained an Oxford degree through the help of his uncle, Elias Ashmole. He subsequently served as a parish priest, first at Aldenham and then in Hackney, where he was friendly with Matthew Henry.[10]

Calvinist families, such as the Henrys and the Newcomes, had a high regard for health, a great gift of providence to the godly: 'Health is one of those mercyes that come alike to all but w[he]n wee have it in a way of Obedience & close walking with God, 'tis quite another th[ing] to us then tis to them that have it in wayes of sin & disobedience.'[11] Thanks to God should be offered for this gift which fitted Christians to enjoy other blessings and to serve God more fully.[12] In order to preserve their bodily health, the godly attempted to follow the best available advice. The Henry family looked to Hippocrates and his modern followers, such as Lessius, for aphoristic guidance on the rules of health.[13] Henry Newcome the younger read a broad range of medical authors, such as Schröder, Sydenham and Willis, and met fortnightly with a neighbouring clergyman to discuss medicine. In a favourite funeral sermon, preached on six occasions, he employed his knowledge of anatomy and disease to remind his hearers of the frailty of their bodies. In his essay on maternal breast-feeding, he cited modern authors as well as Galen and Avicenna.[14]

Morality and the preservation of health went hand in hand. It was the duty of Christians not to sin against their bodies, refraining from all uncleanness: 'so like wise is gluttony, Drunkness, & all manner of excesses of those Kinds, also sixth-commandm[en]t sins, whereinsoever wee doe that which præjudices the health or takes away the life of the Body, directly or indirectly'.[15] Sobriety and temperance were conducive to longevity, not drunkenness and excess. 'Its a com[m]on saying, that <u>there are more old drunkards than old Physicians</u>, yet none will pretend that drunkeness contributes more to a long life than physick.'[16] The practice of religion required 'the moderation of our passions, temperance in diet & chearfulness in conversation'.[17]

Accordingly, the godly attended to their health as part of their duty of self-preservation. Philip Henry wrote from prison that he was taking care of his diet and avoiding strong drink, for fear of 'Feavorish distempers, wanting exercise'.[18] His son said of him that his 'constitution was but tender, and yet, by the blessing of God upon his great temperance, and care of his diet, and moderate exercise by walking in the air, he did for many years enjoy a good measure of health'.[19] Food, exercise, and merriment were to be taken only for health's sake: 'If mirth be a medicine (understand it of diversion and recreation) it must be used sparingly, only when there is occasion, not turned into food, and it must be used medicinally, *sub regimine*, and by rule.'[20]

Awareness of the effects of the non-naturals had religious as well as medical implications. Preaching before the Lord Mayor of London, Peter Newcome noted, 'The Natural Constitution and particular Complexion of Bodies, will be apt to incline Men to particular and suitable Sins'.[21] Since one's normal temperament was a source of temptation, it was necessary to ensure that the humours did not become peccant. Philip Henry took a close interest in his son's use of the rules of health, especially while he was studying in London.[22] Advising his father to come to Chester to take physic, Matthew Henry wrote, 'While the Lord is for the body sure wee must bee for it, especially while God is pleased so much to use it. pray think of it, better lay by a few weeks than bee laid by a great deal longer'.[23]

The godly were also attentive to the medical effects of their environment. A Sussex vicar, formerly Philip Henry's pupil, lamented his insalubrious situation: 'sweating & warmth & a good diet ... are the best preventing physic, next to the Divine p[ro]tection, ag[ain]st it'.[24] Philip Henry wrote to his son in London, 'wishing you some of our sweet aire, which is now more then at other times of the year perfum'd, instead of your offensive town-smels, against which you have need to arm your self, especially at first til you are us'd to them'.[25] The Henrys avoided contact with epidemics and exchanged news on current diseases.[26]

The incidence of epidemics was of especial interest as an indication of national judgements.[27] Philip Henry analysed the London mortality figures for plague years from 1592 to 1665 and the family common-place book contained notes on the plagues of Athens, Alexandria and Italy.[28] The godly considered both the divine and natural causes of epidemics but they deplored those who considered only the second causes. Henry Newcome the elder noted during a Manchester epidemic:

> They talk, *they have catcht this new disease,* and this is from the unwholesome weather, or an effect of the late Comet, and the extream frost, and the unwonted drought that followed it. Or I have catcht it of such a one, or I catcht cold, and so have brought it upon me; all this may be true; yet this is pitiful common talk.[29]

The natural causes of disease and health might be complex but the moral causes were easy to discern and needed urgent consideration.

Although righteousness was the moral cause of health and prosperity, there was no automatic efficacy. 'It would not consist with man's de-pendent state, not to allow room for God's providence to make what exceptions he pleaseth from the ordinary course of things.'[30] Christians should be content with the portion of sickness or health allotted to them. It is hard to accept sickness because it comes closer to the self than other afflictions and tends to disturb the mind, hindering the practice of religion. Nevertheless, sick bodies often house healthy souls, and God's promises are most comfortable to the sick.[31] When healthy, the godly knew that 'the highest degree of health is the next step to sickness ... tis good therefore to rejoyce with trembling & to bee making ready for changes'.[32]

Following Calvin, Philip Henry differentiated between three kinds of providence, 'universal, to all, special, to his church, p[ar]ticular, to ours[elves]'.[33] God's particular providences included callings, mercies and afflictions. God had 'many arrows in his quiver', punishing na-tions by war, plague, famine or decay of trade.[34] Personal afflictions could include sickness and death in the family, persecution and bank-ruptcy, even falling off a horse. For God, there were no accidents.[35] Philip Henry stressed that the greatest affliction, 'sufferd with the people of God in the cause of God,' was preferable to the most trivial sin.[36] The images used by the Henrys to express the soul's need for affliction were the need of the body for physic, of gold for refining in the furnace, of trees for pruning, of the child for discipline, of corn for threshing.[37] God could also warn his children. When Mary Hoghton, a baronet's sister, died in his house in 1710, Matthew Henry com-mented, 'This is a very awakening Providence. Death is come into my house where it has not been of neare 12 y[ears] and usually it strikes double'.[38]

All afflictions, whether of mind, body or estate, were sent by God as a correction for sin, for the good of the sinner. Those under affliction should be humbled and reformed by it, neither disregarding it nor despising it. The affliction would only be lifted when it had done its work of reformation, so the need was to 'get every affliction Sanctifyed, make it y[ou]r Business to get good by it'.[39] No one was entitled to complain that afflictions were excessive. When Matthew Henry's wife was ill after a miscarriage and his children had the smallpox, he commented, 'Stil my God is stil contending with me, & he doth me no wrong'. In any case, God sent afflictions not only to punish corrupt and sinful desires but also to manifest moderate and gracious ones. The godly should neither try to excuse themselves nor judge others in affliction.[40] Henry Newcome the younger stressed this in a funeral sermon for a man 'who in an Aneurisma lived long in great pain' and in a sermon he preached for men who died in accidents, suggesting five reasons for God to send great sufferings other than the punishment of great sinners.[41] Even after describing a monstrous birth, Philip Henry commented, 'I neither adde nor alter any th[ing] you have it as twas related to mee, nor doe I make any inference from it'.[42] Affliction was to be distinguished from the remarkable providences with which God punished notorious sinners, such as ungodly magistrates and persecuting clerics, sabbath-breakers and drunkards.[43]

God's medicinal afflictions were inevitably bitter to the taste, like purges made from ingredients such as aloes, 'troublesom to the tast but operative in the stomack'. They would be especially bitter to anyone who had 'no Tast of the grace & sweetness of Christ in an Affliction'. Nevertheless, God's medicines were prescribed to his children in due time, in the same way that 'Physicians observe the proper time for administering Physique, purging, Blood-letting, at spring or fal, new or ful moon,' and they were given in careful measure, 'as if send to Apothecary for Potion for a sick child, how exact in everyth[ing] to a grain, a dram, a scruple'.[44]

Although affliction was sent to the godly to do them good, they were not obliged to welcome it: 'Submit to an affliction we may without loving & being fond of it.' They were not expected to display stoical indifference: 'The countenances of good men that have peace & Joy within are made sad by sickness. there's no disputing ag[ains]t sense.' Those who despised an affliction were guilty of failing to consider its purpose and therefore despised its divine author.[45] Equally, godly patients should not grieve inordinately or 'murmure under sickness,' since God only sent it to wean them from the world and encourage them to seek forgiveness. Complaining would only make matters worse and provoke further affliction.[46] The ideal conduct was a middle way between these two extremes, acknowledging God's hand in every affliction, accepting it as just punishment, seeking out the particular sin that brought it, bearing it patiently, endeavouring to have it sanctified and then removed by the use of means, believing in the love of God and the goodness of the eventual issue: 'Take away the cause, and the effect will cease. When the patient becomes a penitent, see what a blessed change follows.'[47] Godly families prayed daily that their afflictions might be sanctified and the afflicted might be comforted.[48]

Illness was therefore 'a special time to see sin'. Henry Newcome the elder, preaching at Gorton chapel when the curate had recovered from sickness, remarked that 'a good man in sickness, is convinced of his neglect in going to the house of God, when he was in health and had opportunity, and longs to be restored that he may go and obtain something for after-time'. He suggested that, in sending sickness, 'God perhaps aims at that coldness in his ordinances'.[49] When there was illness in Matthew Henry's family, he searched for God's purpose: 'O that it may be good for my Family that my Family is afflicted! Moderate Counsels are hearken'd to, praised be God.' On recovery, he gathered friends 'to be witnesses of our thanksgiving to God for the return of Health to our family'.[50] When his sister-in-law died shortly after his mother, Henry commented, 'A surprizing Providence, what shal we say to it! Still Death strikes double. God speaks once yea twice. Wherefore hast thou set me up for a mark?'[51]

Since God had sent the affliction, all healing was in his hands: 'In the common instances of recovery from sickness, God, in his providence, doth but speak it, and it is done.'[52] In May 1693, Matthew Henry wrote to his father that his wife and his brother-in-law, Dr John Tylston, were recuperating, 'but both weak, and have the remains of their distemper, w[hi]ch I trust wil by degrees wear off, when, and as the Lord pleaseth'.[53] On recovering from sickness, it was essential to give thanks to God for one's cure. Philip Henry emphasized this after his own recovery: 'what I shal say to you, I have been endeavoring to preach first to my own heart, that first feeling what I speak, I may then the better speak w[ha]t I feel'. He stressed the need to confess the sins committed during sickness, such as impatience, and to keep all the promises made to God.[54] Shortly before his death, Philip Henry wrote to one of his children, recently recovered from sickness, 'We rejoice in God's goodness to you, that your distemper hath been a rod shaken only, and not laid on'.[55]

It may seem that the godly were unusually interested in the details of illness, something that was noted at the time by a Lancashire Anglican who mocked Richard Baxter for recording 'the most trifling and dirty parts of his Actions, even how well his Physick wrought'.[56] This impression derives from the intensity of their self-examination. Generally, they avoided detailed discussion of medicine, preferring to consider the meaning of affliction, in contrast to the worldly invalids described by Henry Newcome the elder:

> Their whole discourse is, *how they are held and handled*, where their pain is, and how it works them. And a story they can make of all passages, as if nothing else was minded by them. And they spend their time in groaning and complaining, and in using means to get up again.[57]

Physic and physicians were noted only as God's instruments. When Henry Newcome the younger fell ill, 'thro Gods blessing & Dr Bannes directions (who came at my desire to visit me) the feavour remitted'.[58]

The doctrine of means encouraged Calvinists to spare no effort in seeking a cure by the legitimate methods supplied by general providence: 'It is our duty when we are sick, to make use of such means as are proper to help nature, else we do not trust God but tempt him.'[59] Patients were expected to be patient, accepting the advice of their physicians. As Peter Newcome remarked, 'it is no Excuse for a sick Man to vindicate the irregularity of his Appetite by, to say, *It is his Inclination*; since it is wholly owing to the Depravity of his Inclination, which aggravates his Crime, in that he neglects such Medicines as might correct it'.[60] The godly were critical of the conduct of friends and relatives who failed to summon help until it was too late to help.[61] When Matthew Henry's cousin suddenly collapsed, every effort was made to revive her: 'We got Physicians and Surgeons to her, rubd her with spirits, us'd all the meanes we could be advis'd to, open'd two veines, But never discern'd any life.'[62]

The physicians consulted by the godly, although not always medical graduates, were usually pious practitioners of learned physic. Indeed, Samuel Benyon, who succeeded Philip Henry at Broad Oak, took an MD at Glasgow and cared for the medical needs of the Henry family, on a daily basis when necessary, even after he had moved to Shrewsbury.[63] Henry Newcome the elder mainly relied on Nathaniel Banne, an ex-clergyman who had obtained a Cambridge medical licence in 1666 and was awarded an MD by royal mandate in 1690, and John Cart, an ejected clergyman's son who had received a licence from the College of Physicians after leaving Cambridge without a degree. Henry Newcome the younger consulted Banne and John Tylston while he was in Cheshire. When he had moved to Middleton, he usually consulted William Holbrooke MB, a conforming member of a family of nonconformist clergymen and apothecaries. The presence amongst the Henrys and the

Newcomes of Dr Tylston, the favourite pupil of Thomas Sydenham, led to some rather modern therapy. When Henry Newcome the younger had a fit of ague in 1691, Tylston promptly cured him with cinchona, corrected with laudanum: 'it proved effectual thro: God's blessing to cure me and put me in a better state of health than I had been for many years before'. The use of cinchona and laudanum became routine amongst Newcome's family and pupils.[64]

Calvinist ministers had formerly condemned self-medication as verging on the suicidal.[65] This prohibition had relaxed by the late seventeenth century but Henry Newcome the younger, who conformed to the Church of England, was far more ready to indulge in domestic medicine than were his nonconformist relations and acquaintances. When he was taken with pain in the bowels and vomiting in 1683, he managed to relieve the symptoms with tobacco glisters before his physicians arrived: 'The more signally did I apprehend the mercy of God, who in so great danger relieved me, wth such unlikly means as I my self cou'd prescribe.'[66] His willingness to prescribe for his own ailments led him into danger on occasion, as when he was seriously weakened by cinchona and laudanum until saved by a chance visit from a physician who advised him 'to use only Kitchin Physick'.[67]

The godly preferred learned medicine, both because they were expected to employ the best available means and because of the analogy with learned preachers. However, despite the contempt of Anglicans and Presbyterians for the mechanic preachers of sects such as the Baptists and the Quakers, the godly did not altogether despise women practitioners and other empirics as long as they were honest.[68] They did avoid magical medicine, however: 'If wee are cast into a Prison of Affliction and break out by unlawful meanes, wee are in danger of being caught again & twill bee the worse.'[69] The sorcery of cunning folk was to be avoided, as were the charms associated with Platonism, popular religion and Roman Catholicism. Henry Newcome the younger and his father's nonconformist physician, John Cart of Manchester, took great pleasure in dissecting a religious amulet 'took from the Neck of a sick patient, given by a popish priest as an effectual cure for all diseases'. The patient threatened to sue them for destroying it. A similar conflict over a charm was reported to Matthew Henry by his friend, the Chester apothecary Ralph Sudlow.[70]

The godly were in favour of medicine, as means provided by God, but too many people were prone to 'the sin of Asa', trusting the means rather than God: 'if any th[ing] ayles the Body, if that bee sick, if that bee sore, send hither, send thither, far and near for help. What & no concernedness for the poor soul?' Christ was the only physician for sicknesses of the soul and needed always to be sought to for healing, so it was appropriate in any illness to send first for the minister rather than for the physician. However, resignation to death should not preclude the taking of medicine: 'The event of sickness manifests what Gods will is & till that be known our duty is to use means for a recovery, relying on God for his blessing & resolving to acquiesce in his determination.'[71] Only when death seemed inevitable did the godly refuse medication. Matthew Henry wrote an account of an elderly Nantwich farmer who had been preparing for death for over a decade. Feeling at last the approach of death, 'he would by no means have any Physician sent for, but said, it was Time for him to leave the World, and it did not become him at that Age to use a Physician'.[72]

A decade of preparation may seem morbid to modern tastes, as it did to many contemporaries. In his very first funeral sermon, preached in 1675, Henry Newcome the younger noted that 'however usefull the thoughts of death are, it is a melancholy subject & men like it not: but put it off as much as they can'.[73] For the godly, all of life was a preparation for death: 'he that repents every day, for the sins of every day, when he comes to die, will have the sins but of one day to repent of'. Henry Newcome the younger advised Christians to contemplate death daily: 'In thy serious thoughts set thyself every day within the prospect of thy winding sheet, lay thyself in thy Coffin, & walk into the Charnel house, till the sight of a skeleton bacome familiar & the King of terrors be disarmed.' Since 'dying work is hard work', no one should delay repentance until disabled by the approach of death. Only fools 'defer their repentance to a death-bed' and their sincerity might be doubted'.[74] The object of contemplating death was always to ready one's soul for the life to come. Matthew Henry summarized this attitude: 'We should be more thoughtful what will become of us after death, than how, or when, or where we shall die; and more desirous to be told how we may carry our selves well in our sickness, and get good to our souls by it, than whether we shall recover from it.'[75]

Although the art of dying was studied throughout Christendom, it was a particular interest of the godly in England.[76] The focus of this discourse was death and judgement but its purpose was the amendment of life. 'It is not the manner of dying but of living that distinguishes the death of the righteous from other men.'[77] Reminding congregations of the need for a timely preparation for death was thus an integral part of the reformation of life, so readily cut short by accidents and apoplexies. 'He that in confidence of an healthfull constitution or the old age of his ancestors promises himself many years to come, doth not so properly consider his latter end, as put it out of his thoughts.' Even when warned of the approach of death, all too many men 'will hope their physician mistaken & all the Prognosticks of an approaching dissolution fallible, rather then not promise themselves a recovery'.[78] Anyone who had received the 'comprehensive mercy' of a ripe old age possessed 'more space to work out his own salvation' and should seek out unrepented sins. 'W[he]n wee ly under any affl[iction] in old age wee must examin whether some sin did not provoke God – some miscarriage in yonger dayes – some youthfull prank.'[79]

The godly made an especial point of praying with their sick friends and relations. In 1709, Matthew Henry visited his friend, the licensed physician John Bruen, daily during a serious illness. When Henry was afflicted with urinary gravel, he thanked God for the solicitude of his friends. 'Visiting the sick ... is our duty. The sick bed is a proper place both for giving comfort and counsel to others, and receiving instruction ourselves.'[80] The diaries of the godly record the salutory lessons they had learned. In March 1707/8, Matthew Henry 'went to Saughton to vis. Jos. Smith, who is ill in one room, his wife in another, his maid dead, buried yester[day] one d[augh]t[e]r ill, a d[augh]t[e]r in law in childbed – many are the afflic[tions] of the righteous'. Such diligence could lead to conflict with the parochial clergy. Matthew Henry noted of an elderly nonconformist that he was 'a useful man, visiting the sick, the vicar formerly check'd him for it, but at his funeral prais'd him for it'.[81]

The godly did not simply exhort others to die well; they endeavoured to set a good example. They visited the deathbeds 'of good ministers and other good men', since nothing in their life became them like the leaving of it.[82] In December 1687, Philip Henry wrote at length to Henry Ashurst on the subject of dying well. The aim was to die safely with one's sins forgiven, comfortably with the promises of God in mind, and profitably by setting a good example: 'Thus I have written to you, Sir, a Funeral-letter, God knowes, perhaps my own. Tis certainly good to bee alwayes ready, seeing wee know neither Day nor hour.' In his next letter, he reported that he had been seriously ill: 'How quickly were the good lessons in my last of Dying by Faith made seasonable unto my self!'[83]

In his final illness, Philip Henry was stricken with severe pain in his back, breast and bowels:

> The means that had been used to give him relief in his illness were altogether ineffectual ... When the exquisiteness of his pain forced groans and complaints from him, he would presently correct himself with a patient and quiet submission to the hand of his heavenly Father, and a cheerful acquiescence in his heavenly will.[84]

In 1713, Matthew Henry suffered from diabetes, kidney disease and the stone yet when he drew up his spiritual account on New Year's Day he thanked God for 'the many mercies of the year past, a good measure of health'. As for the year to come, 'if it be my dying year, *welcome the holy will of God*'.[85] His death in June was blessed with an unexpected mercy: 'Whereas he expected to be Ground to the Dust by the *Stone*, or dissolved by the *Diabetes*', he simply slipped painlessly into sleep and death.[86]

Death was familiar throughout early modern society, so the godly were perforce acquainted with grief. At the end of 1702, Matthew Henry noted that it was three years since any of his close relations had died: 'Since I set out in the world, I never was so long without the death of children, or others near and dear to me.'[87] Those who did not feel bereavement deeply were 'justly stigmatized as without natural affection' and as exhibiting contempt for God's providence and the memory of the deceased.[88] The consolations offered might sometimes seem rather cold comfort. Henry Newcome the younger repeatedly told the families of young girls who had died of smallpox that 'it will never be very well with us, till we are delivered from the burden of the flesh'. His father told the bereaved, 'let us travel on and make haste after them to that rest into which they have entered, and which remains for all the people of God'.[89]

In the midst of joy, the godly expected grief. In 1689, the last of Philip Henry's daughters was married. He commented, 'Now we have a full lease, God only knows which life will drop first'. It was to be Matthew Henry's first wife, who contracted smallpox while in childbed. Philip Henry was concerned for all his children, none of whom had been through the disease, and publicly resigned them all to God, 'for good I am sure we have received, and shall we not receive evil also?'[90] The dying woman's response was, 'Well, when I come to heaven, I shall see that I could not have been without this affliction'. After her death, Matthew Henry was deeply distressed, despite the survival of his son. He tearfully told William Tong, 'I know nothing could support me under such a Loss as this, but the good Hope I have that she is gone to Heaven, and that in a little Time I shall follow her thither'.[91]

The response of the godly to sickness in the family was resignation to God's will, repentance and prayer. Early in August 1697, Ann Hulton was nursing both her mother, who had 'fits of vapors', and her sister Eleanor Radford, weak after childbirth. She wrote to her eldest sister, 'Bro. [Matthew] Henrys Letter will acquaint you how God hath dealt with us in these his ways of affliction & Correction ... this is the likeliest way to try us whether we can trust God or no, by ups, & downs'. Three of the four sisters fell gravely ill. Matthew Henry found it 'hard to submit'. When two died, he struggled to find 'a matter for praise and thanksgiving, even in this sad providence'.[92]

Providential doctrine supplied meaning for every misfortune, even if that meaning was sometimes hard to bear. Although sickness required an individual interpretation, bereavement affected the whole family. Having lost two brothers-in-law during 1699, Matthew Henry wrote to his mother on a cousin's death, 'We are still in the Furnace, the Clouds are still returning after the Rain ... Surely we have not profited by the former Dispensations, else we should not be thus exercis'd. How loud is the voice of this Rod. Therefore be ye also ready, ready for sudden death'.[93] Sarah Savage was present in Nantwich when Matthew Henry died in June 1714, on his way to London. After reflecting on the circumstances and the corpse's appearance, she puzzled over the meaning of her brother's death:

> we have no reason to weep for him, but for ourselv's, our sins have provoked God to put out this burning & shining light & as to the manner of his death (being on a journy & among strangers) I doubt not but God had wise & holy ends in so ordering it – sad, sad, sad, tydings to his poor family.[94]

If the death of an adult relative was sometimes difficult to understand, that of a child could tax the patience of the godly to the limit. The first response of a godly parent to the sickness of a child was to resign him or her to God, while beseeching his mercy.[95] When his son Philip had a bad case of measles, Matthew Henry wrote in his diary, 'I desire to give him up to my heavenly Father, yet praying – Father spare my son, my only son whom I love'.[96] Sometimes the passive obedience of parents was rewarded. When Matthew was seriously ill in 1667, Philip Henry resigned him up to God and at the same moment his condition began to improve.[97] A similar mercy was granted to Henry Newcome the younger in 1695. The physicians expressed pessimism about his son's chances:

> whereupon I went into private & resigned him to Gods disposal, & in that very act came one to the door wth a Messuage to tell me that he was better, & the Physicians coming up found such a change in a few minuits, that they gave us good hopes of him. Oh may the hearing of my resigned prayers be a happy Omen that he shall live to be a blessing to us![98]

Although the greatest sinners were not necessarily the most sick, all the sick were guilty of sin. Even children were tainted by original sin.[99] Nevertheless, it was clearly parental consciences that needed to be examined. In a lengthy letter of consolation to cousins who had lost all their children during a smallpox epidemic, Philip Henry urged patient submission to God's will, suggesting that God might be punishing them for slackness in religious duty. 'You must learn by it, as long as you live, *to keep your affections in due bounds towards creature-comforts.*' Excessive delight in the company of children, or a spouse, would lead God in his jealousy 'to remove that mercy from us, which we do thus make an idol of'.[100] Henry did not spare himself. When his elder son died, he submitted to God's will: 'He was forward every way even to admiration, but the lord that gave, or lent rather, took away & in his will I acquiesce.' He still blamed himself 14 years later.[101] Matthew Henry was continually anxious that he loved his children too dearly. When an infant daughter died in 1698, he knew the cause: 'I had set mine Affection much upon it. I am afraid too much; God is wise, and righteous, and faithful.'[102]

The fate of Matthew Henry's daughters provides a telling example of the use of the theology of affliction as an interpretative resource. A daughter born in April 1693, after a difficult labour, died within the month despite her father's prayers. He preached from Job 38, on the impossibility of questioning God's will, and wrote to his father:

> We find it hard to say w[he]n it comes to particulars Thy wil be done. I beg you wil pray hard for us, that God would shew us wherefore he contendeth with us, that he would bear up my poor disconsolate wife who finds it hard indeed now the pains of bearing and the pains of parting come so near together.

One of his nephews died during the next week, so Henry concluded that the cause was the family's having been 'too much lifted up I fear with our increase, and numbring the little ones, but God hath made them fewer'.[103] Another daughter died in November 1698 during an outbreak of measles, despite the efforts of Dr Tylston. She was almost the only child in Chester who died. Henry wrote, 'My Desire is to be sensible of the Affliction, and yet patient under it; 'tis a Rod, a smarting Rod. God calls my Sin to remembrance – the coldness of my Love to God, abuse of Spiritual Comforts'. He preached on the need for calm even in grievous affliction: 'when God by death takes away our children from us tho' it be a sore affliction yet it becomes us quietly to say It is well both w[i]th us & them'. Whereas the children went to their eternal rest, the parents benefited from the opportunity for repentance and mortification. In correspondence with his mother, he struggled to improve the affliction but he had difficulty learning the lesson: 'We are in danger of overloving the remnant that is left, whereas we should learn to sit the more loose.'[104]

Although a distinction was drawn between the interpretation of children's ailments and those of adults, the godly did not significantly differentiate between the levels of medical consumption appropriate. When his daughter needed bleeding, Henry Newcome the younger called John Catterall, a Chester surgeon, even though he was quite capable of letting blood himself. When a son was seriously ill, he called for two Chester physicians, Dr Tylston and Edward Norris MB.[105] After Tylston's death, the Henrys usually consulted two physicians when a child fell ill,

as when Esther had a fever in October 1699 and blisters were prescribed.[106] Sarah Savage's children, living in the country, received more
domestic medicine. Katherine Henry thanked God for blessing her treatment of Hannah Savage: 'the Symptoms were very Violent before they
came out, but they were kindly after. I ventured to use Laudanum for
abo[u]t 5 nights when they were at the worst w[hi]ch had very good
effect'.[107]

Age was a clearly significant influence, although more on interpretation than on treatment, but the influence of gender appears less marked,
despite the different pattern of medical consumption. The godly clearly
differentiated between male and female roles in the household but little
difference can be observed between male and female attitudes towards
health and sickness. Matthew Henry's sisters reacted to the death or
sickness of their children in the same way that he did, searching their
consciences for the cause.[108] The sickness of women was not a source of
special comment. The extremity of the dangers and pains of childbed
was recognized by the godly but, although they could not ignore the
curse laid on Eve when commenting on Genesis 3:16, they did not
otherwise lay any especial stress upon it. Although 'Naturall Births are
conceivd in pleasure and brought forth in sorrow', successful childbirth,
however worrying, was an occasion for grateful acknowledgement of
God's goodness. Birth pains, nursing difficulties, and the disappoint-
ments of child-rearing were simply examples of the affliction of all
humanity as a result of original sin, not a mark of the especial wickedness of women.[109]

To some extent, the records of godly families were consciously constructed as self-representations but it is not necessary to dismiss them as
pious fictions. The entire life of a godly man or woman was constructed
with a view to living out the Christian ideal, both for the sake of the
soul and to set a good example. The creation and preservation of these
documents merely continued a process that was daily acted out in the
self-presentation of the godly. Although one cannot penetrate beyond
their diaries and letters, it seems clear that their attitudes and behaviour
were dominated by their religious beliefs, even under the most trying of
circumstances. The Calvinist doctrine of affliction shaped the godly
understanding of everyday life, especially as regards the preservation of
health, the taking of medicine, the interpretation of sickness and preparation for death. The providentialism of the Henrys and the Newcomes
was highly developed but it was not otherwise exceptional amongst the
godly.

These two families belonged to a particular stratum of English society, on the edge of the gentry, but their friends and congregations were
drawn from all ranks. Like a patronage network, the Calvinist ideologi-

cal affinity extended across the social strata, with godly clergy and physicians acting as mediators. Through their sermons and writings, the 'illness talk' of the godly was widely diffused throughout society. Allusions to the blessing of God upon the means can be found amongst all manner of personal records, from the diaries of the aristocracy to the petitions of the poor. Their style of religion lost its formerly dominant position during the late Stuart period, partly through the political defeat of Calvinism and partly through the élite's invention of a more benevolent though remote God. Nevertheless, the Calvinist ideology remained widely influential, often appropriated in diluted or fragmentary forms, shaping English attitudes towards death, sickness and medicine.

Notes

Acknowledgement: I am grateful for the comments of Margaret Pelling and for discussion of versions of this paper at a conference on 'Medicine and the Family', organized by the Society for the Social History of Medicine at Exeter University, and at seminars in the Wellcome Unit, Cambridge and Merton College, Oxford.

The use of the letter 'y' to represent 'th' in manuscripts has been silently altered for ease of reading. Many of the sermons of Philip and Matthew Henry survive as bundles of notes so date and text will be given where possible. Matthew Henry's biblical commentary was published in many forms. References here are to the scriptural passage discussed. Quotations are from M. Henry, *An Exposition on the Old and New Testament*, 4th edn, 5 vols, London, 1737 (hereafter *Exposition*).

1. K.V. Thomas, *Religion and the Decline of Magic*, London, Weidenfeld and Nicolson, 1971, pp. 91–132.
2. For selected extracts, see L. Pollock, *A Lasting Relationship: Parents and Children Over Three Centuries*, London, Fourth Estate, 1987; R. Houlbrooke, *English Family Life, 1576–1716*, Oxford, Blackwell, 1988. For case studies, see A. Macfarlane, *The Family Life of Ralph Josselin; a Seventeenth-Century Clergyman*, Cambridge, Cambridge University Press, 1970; P.S. Seaver, *Wallington's World: A Puritan Artisan in Seventeenth-Century London*, London, Methuen, 1985; P. Crawford, 'Katharine and Philip Henry and Their Children: A Study in Family Ideology', *Transactions of the Historical Society of Lancashire and Cheshire*, **134** (1984) 39–73.
3. A. Wear, 'Puritan Perceptions of Illness in Seventeenth-Century England', in R. Porter (ed.), *Patients and Practitioners*, Cambridge, Cambridge University Press, 1985, pp. 55–99; L.M. Beier, *Sufferers and Healers: The Experience of Illness in Seventeenth-Century England*, London, Routledge, 1987, pp. 182–210, 218–39; D. Harley, 'Spiritual Physic, Providence and English Medicine, 1560–1640', in O. Grell and A. Cunningham (eds), *Medicine and the Reformation*, London, Routledge, 1993, pp. 101–17.

4. P.U. Unschuld, 'Die konzeptuelle Überformung der individuellen und kollektiven Erfahrung von Kranksein', in H. Schipperges, E. Seidler and P.U. Unschuld (eds), *Krankheit, Heilkunst, Heilung*, Freiburg, Alber, 1978, pp. 491–516; R.L. Numbers and D.W. Amundsen (eds), *Caring and Curing: Health and Medicine in the Western Religious Traditions*, New York, Macmillan, 1986. I have in mind something less theoretical than '*Weltanschauungen*' is usually taken to denote. In effect, I am arguing that the reception of ideologies leads to the formation of worldviews, which decay into *mentalités*. Sociologists of knowledge might describe this as the creation of subuniverses of meaning.

5. W.J. Sheils (ed.), *The Church and Healing*, Studies in Church History 19, 1982; D. Landy (ed.), *Culture, Disease and Healing: Studies in Medical Anthropology*, New York, Macmillan, 1977.

6. Classic studies include E. Ohnuki-Tierney, *Illness and Healing Among the Sakhalin Ainu: A Symbolic Interpretation*, Cambridge, Cambridge University Press, 1981; B. Kapferer, *A Celebration of Demons: Exorcism and the Aesthetics of Healing in Sri Lanka*, Bloomington, Indiana University Press, 1983.

7. Amongst the early Quakers, members of the gentry and those educated at university resemble Calvinists in their attitudes towards health and medicine, unlike their artisan and yeoman co-religionists. There may also have been regional differences.

8. Sketches of both families will be found in the *Dictionary of National Biography* and A.G. Matthews, *Calamy Revised*, Oxford, Oxford University Press, 1934. See also P. Crawford, 'Katharine and Philip Henry'; J.J. Bagley, *Lancashire Diarists*, Chichester, Phillimore, 1975, pp. 18–37, on Henry Newcome the elder.

9. The four daughters were Ann Hulton, Eleanor Radford, Sarah Savage and Katherine Tylston.

10. R. Parkinson, (ed.), *The Autobiography of Henry Newcome*, Chetham Society 27, 1852, p. 226; Bodleian Library (hereafter Bod.): MS Rawl.Lett.107, ff. 129–30, Z. Cawdray to Ashmole, 14 October 1681; MS Eng.misc.c.330, f. 100r–v, Matthew Henry's diary.

11. Bod.: MS Eng.th.g.4, ff. 5v–6r, undated sermon by Philip Henry (PH) on Isaiah 33:24.

12. Doctor Williams's Library (hereafter DWL): 91.16, sermons by Matthew Henry (MH) on 1 Chronicles 29:14, 22 June 1699, and on Nehemiah 2:2, 17 August 1699; MH's diary, f. 34v, 64v; Bod.: MS Eng.th.g.4, f. 5v, sermon by PH on Isaiah 33:24; Henry, *Exposition*, on Nehemiah 2:2, Chetham's Library, Manchester: Mun.A.3.114; Henry Newcome's sermons, funeral sermon no. 27, f. 183.

13. Bod.: MS Eng.misc.d.311, pp. 118–19, commonplace book of the Henry family.

14. Manchester Central Library: MS 922/3/N/21, Henry Newcome's memoranda book, p. 48; Newcome, funeral sermon no. 25, ff. 264–5; H. Newcome, *The Compleat Mother*, London, 1694, pp. 58, 67–70, 73–5, 87; D. Harley, 'The Moral Theology and Godly Practice of Maternal Breastfeeding in Stuart England', *Bulletin of the History of Medicine*, 69 (1995) pp. 198–223.

15. British Library (hereafter BL): Add. MS 42849, f. 222v, undated dis-

course by PH on 'the Duty of Christians to glorify God in or with their Bodyes'.

16. Bod.: MS Eng.th.g.4, f. 95v, sermon by PH on Psalms 116:16, 17 March 1671/2; Newcome's funeral sermon no. 26, ff. 272–3.
17. Newcome's funeral sermon no. 28, f. 194; cf. J.B. Williams, *Memoirs of ... the Rev. Matthew Henry*, London, 1828, p. 186.
18. Bod.: MS Eng.lett.e.29, f. 13, PH to Katharine Henry (hereafter KH), 8 July 1685.
19. Matthew Henry, *The Life of the Reverend Philip Henry*, J.B. Williams (ed.), London, 1825, p. 215.
20. Henry, *Exposition*, on Proverbs 17:22.
21. P. Newcome, *Peccata in Deliciis. A Discourse of Bosom Sins*, London, 1686, pp. 4–7.
22. Bod.: MS Eng. lett.e.29, ff. 1, 36r, 77, PH to MH, 16 August 1680, [25 March 1687], 7 June 1688.
23. DWL: 90.7.6, MH to PH, 18 March 1690/1.
24. Bod.: MS Eng.lett.e.29, f. 176, William Turner to PH, 22 April 1682.
25. Bod.: MS Eng.lett.e.29, ff. 6 and 32r, PH to MH, 4 May 1685 and 18 February 1686/7. The second letter expresses similar concerns re MH's aunt.
26. Bod.: MS Eng.lett.e.29, f. 5, KH to MH, 3 January 1685/6; ff. 21, 67r, 68v, PH to MH, 15 January 1685/6, 26 and 30 March 1688; f. 79r, MH to PH [June 1688].
27. Henry, *Exposition*, on Deut.28.21–35; H. Newcome, *An Help to the Duty In, and Right Improvement of Sickness*, London, 1685, sig. A3r.
28. BL: Add. MS 42849, f. 76, PH on London plagues; Bod.: MS Eng.misc.d.311, pp. 118–19.
29. Newcome, *Help to the Duty*, pp. 2, 5–6, 11.
30. Newcome's funeral sermon no. 28, f. 190.
31. DWL: 91.28.8, undated discourse by PH on the duty to be 'content with that measure of Bodily Health that wee have'.
32. Bod.: MS Eng.lett.e.29, f. 21, PH to MH [January 1685/6].
33. BL: Add. MS 45534, f. 324v, sermon by PH on Christ as 'our All', 22 May 1692. Calvin's formulation was slightly different.
34. DWL: 91.13, sermon by PH on Jeremiah 8:22, 8 October 1679.
35. Henry, *Life*, pp. 251, 375–9.
36. DWL: 91.15, sermon by PH on Hebrews 11:24–6, September 1686.
37. Henry, *Life*, pp. 240–1, 260–2; Williams, *Memoirs*, p. 205.
38. MH's diary, f. 87v. This idea of double warnings derives from Job 33:14.
39. DWL: 91.15, Sarah Savage's notes on sermon by MH on Proverbs 3:11, 2 June 1697; MH's diary, f. 11v.
40. DWL: MS 91.16, sermons by MH on 2 Chronicles 28:10, 20 July 1699, and 2 Kings 4:28, 9 February 1698/9; MH's diary, f. 12r.
41. Newcome's funeral sermons nos 40 and 41, ff. 332–45. Both texts were taken from the beginning of Luke 13.
42. Bod.: MS Eng. lett.e.29, f. 26v, PH to MH, 14/15 May 1686.
43. Henry, *Life*, p. 246; P. Henry, *Diaries and Letters*, M.H. Lee (ed.), London, 1882, pp. 159, 171; Henry, *Exposition*, on 2 Chronicles 21:20, MH's diary, ff. 5r, 33r.
44. DWL: 91.13, sermon by PH on Ezekiel 18:30, 25 June 1679; 91.26.4,

fragment of discourse by PH on Psalms 34:8; 91.26.17, monthly fast lecture by PH on Revelations 3:19, 16 September 1691.

45. Newcome's funeral sermon no. 33, f. 257; DWL: 91.16, sermon by MH on Nehemiah 2:2, 17 August 1699; Henry, *Exposition*, on Nehemiah 2:2; Bod.: MS Eng.th.c.72, f. 35, sermon by MH on Proverbs 14:32, 10 December 1693; MS Eng.th.g.4, ff. 13r–14r, sermon by PH on Hebrews 12:5, 7 January 1671/2; Newcome's sickness sermon no. 1, f. 3.

46. Bod.: MS Eng.th.g.4, ff. 6v–8r, 15r–16r, PH on Isaiah 33:24 and Hebrews 12:5.

47. Bod.: MS Eng.th.g.4, ff. 17r–v, PH on Hebrews 12:5, Henry, *Exposition*, on Job 33:25.

48. M. Henry, *A Method for Prayer*, London, 1710, pp. 192–3, 196, 198.

49. Newcome, *Help to the Duty*, p. 10; H. Newcome, 'The House of God Remembered in Sickness', in R. Slate (ed.), *Select Nonconformist Remains*, London, 1814, pp. 330–1, 333. Although nonconformists preached without permission at Gorton in the late 1660s, this was probably preached for William Leigh, ejected in 1662.

50. MH's diary, ff. 12v–13r.

51. MH's diary, f. 37r. The allusions are to Job 33:14 and Job 7:20.

52. Henry, *Exposition*, on Psalms 107:19.

53. DWL: 90.7.22, MH to PH, 27 May 1693.

54. DWL: 91.26.14, undated sermon by PH on Luke 17:17–18; cf. Henry, *Method*, pp. 17–19.

55. Henry, *Life*, p. 262.

56. T. Gipps, *Remarks on Remarks: Or the Rector of Bury's Sermon Vindicated*, London, 1698, p. 61.

57. Newcome, *Help to the Duty*, pp. 11–12.

58. Newcome's memoranda, p. 38.

59. DWL: 91.13, sermon by PH on Jeremiah 8:22, 8 October 1679; Henry, *Exposition*, on 2 Kings 20:7; cf. Newcome's funeral sermon no. 33, ff. 256–7; Newcome's sickness sermon no. 1, ff. 10–11.

60. Newcome, *Peccata*, p. 6.

61. Bod.: MS Eng.lett.e.29, ff. 118r and 119r, MH to PH, 27 December 1695 and 13 February 1695/6.

62. BL: Add. MS 42849, f. 31, MH to KH, 17 November 1699.

63. Williams, *Memoirs*, pp. 142, 144, 146; MH's diary, f. 37r.

64. Newcome's memoranda, pp. 101, 117–19, 126, 131. For a full description of Tylston, see D. Harley, 'The Good Physician and the Godly Doctor: The Exemplary Life of John Tylston of Chester, 1663–1699', *The Seventeenth Century*, 9 (1994) 93–117.

65. The strongest expression of this was that of John Sym, *Lifes Preservative Against Self-Killing*, London, 1637, pp. 92, 111, who defined both contempt for medicine and self-medication as indirect self-murder, more to be condemned than deliberate suicide.

66. Newcome's memoranda, p. 57.

67. Ibid., p. 240.

68. Henry, *Diaries and Letters*, p. 157; Newcome's memoranda, pp. 44, 54, 107, 200, 207, 220, 251.

69. Cambridge University Library: Add. MS 7338, morning lecture by PH on Genesis 8, 11 July 1658; DWL: 91.26.20, notes by PH on sermon at Whitchurch by Mr Cole on Amos 3:2, January 1662/3.

70. Newcome's memoranda, p. 41; MH's diary, f. 3v.
71. Newcome, *Help to the Duty*, pp. 13, 93; H. Newcome, *Sinners Hope*, London, 1660, pp. 53–4; BL: Add. MS 45534, ff. 191v–193v, discourse by PH on Christ as 'our Sun', 10 January 1691/2; Henry, *Exposition*, on 2 Chronicles 16:12 and Job 33:23; DWL: 91.26.20, notes on Mr Cole's sermon, January 1662/3; Newcome's funeral sermon no. 33, ff. 256–7; Newcome's sickness sermon no. 1, ff. 10–11.
72. M. Henry, *A Short Account of the Life of Lieutenant Illidge*, London, 1710, p. 93. Henry gives his friend's preparatory notes, pp. 67–92.
73. Newcome's funeral sermon no. 24, f. 251.
74. Henry, *Life*, p. 141; Henry, *Exposition*, on Job 14:22; Newcome's funeral sermon no. 31, f. 237; Newcome, *Help to the Duty*, pp. 13–15; Newcome, *Sinners Hope*, p. 46; T. Heywood (ed.), *The Diary of the Rev. Henry Newcome*, Chetham Society 18, 1849, p. 178. A sudden onset of piety in affliction was similarly suspect: DWL: 91.26.4, sermon by PH on Proverbs 15:8, January 1653/4.
75. Henry, *Exposition*, on 2 Kings 1:2.
76. D.E. Stannard, *The Puritan Way of Death*, New York, Oxford University Press, 1977; L.M. Beier, 'The Good Death in Seventeenth-Century England', in R. Houlbrooke (ed.), *Death, Ritual and Bereavement*, London, Routledge, 1989, pp. 43–61.
77. Newcome's funeral sermon no. 27, f. 181.
78. Newcome's funeral sermon no. 24, ff. 252–3; ibid. no. 31, ff. 229–30.
79. Newcome's funeral sermon no. 27, f. 183, DWL: 91.13, sermon by PH on Job 13:26, 19 November 1679; Henry, *Life*, pp. 411–16.
80. MH's diary, ff. 68v, 96r; Henry, *Exposition*, on Genesis 48:1.
81. MH's diary, f. 49r.
82. Henry, *Exposition*, on 2 Kings 13:14.
83. Add. MS 45538, ff. 19–20, PH to Henry Ashurst, 20 December 1687; Add. MS 42849, f. 6, same to same, 3 January 1687/8.
84. Henry, *Life*, p. 221.
85. Williams, *Memoirs*, pp. 159–61. This annual reckoning was a custom of Matthew Henry: ibid., pp. 81–5, 88–94, 97–8; W. Tong, *An Account of the Life and Death of the Late Reverend Matthew Henry*, London, 1716, p. 297.
86. J. Reynolds, *A Sermon Upon the Mournful Occasion of the Funeral of ... Matthew Henry*, London, 1714, p. 37.
87. A. Laurence, 'Godly Grief: Individual Responses to Death in Seventeenth-Century Britain', in *Death, Ritual and Bereavement*, pp. 62–76; Williams, *Memoirs*, p. 82.
88. Henry, *Exposition*, on Psalms 35.13; Newcome's funeral sermon no. 33, ff. 257–8.
89. Newcome's funeral sermon no. 39, f. 330; Newcome, 'The believer's rest', in Slate, *Select Non-Conformist Remains*, p. 328.
90. This evil is the 'penal evil' sent by God, not the 'moral evil' of mankind.
91. Henry, *Life*, pp. 203–4; Tong, *Account*, pp. 105–6; Williams, *Memoirs*, p. 56–7.
92. BL: Add. MS 42849, f. 21, Ann Hulton to Sarah Savage, 9 August 1697; Williams, *Memoirs*, pp. 68–70.
93. BL: Add. MS 42849, f. 31, MH to KH, 17 November 1699.
94. BL: Add. MS 42849, f. 111, transcript from diary of Sarah Savage

(hereafter SS), June 1714; see also Bod.: MS Eng.misc.e.331, pp. 4–9, diary of SS, 22–27 June 1714.

95. Henry, *Method*, p. 219; Henry, *Life*, p. 204.
96. Williams, *Memoirs*, p. 165.
97. Tong, *Account*, pp. 17–18; Williams, *Memoirs*, pp. 3–4.
98. Newcome's memoranda, p. 131.
99. Newcome's sickness sermon no. 1, f. 4; DWL: 91.26.4, sermon by PH on Mark 9:24, July 1676.
100. Henry, *Life*, pp. 138–40.
101. DWL: 91.28.1, PH's comment on death of John Henry, 12 April 1667; Bod.: MS Eng.misc.c.293, f. 45, memoranda re John Henry; Henry, *Life*, pp. 86, 109–11.
102. Tong, *Life*, pp. 113–15; Williams, *Memoirs*, pp. 59–61; Bod.: MS Eng. lett.e.29, f. 123, MH to wife, 10 May 1698.
103. DWL: 90.7.18, MH to PH, 4 April 1693; 90.7.20, MH to PH, 26 April 1693; Bod.: MS Eng. lett.e.29, MH to PH, 22 April [1693]; Williams, *Memoirs*, p. 61. The references are to Job 10:2 and to David numbering Israel, 1 Chronicles 21.
104. BL: Add. MS 42849, ff. 26–8, MH to KH, 27 October 1698, 22 November 1698, 2 December 1698; Tong, *Life*, pp. 119–20; Williams, *Memoirs*, p. 72; DWL: 91.16, sermon by MH on 2 Kings 4:26; 18 November 1698.
105. Newcome's memoranda, pp. 107, 131. Norris was later MD, FRS, MP for Liverpool and FRCP.
106. BL: Add. MS 42849, f. 30, MH to KH, 2 October 1699; Bod.: MS Eng. lett.e.29, MH to KH, 4 October 1699.
107. Bod.: MS Eng. lett.e.29, f. 165, KH to MH, 28 January, no year. This is probably a case of smallpox.
108. BL: Add. MS 42849, f. 87, transcript of comments by Ann Hulton; ibid., f. 91, transcript from Sarah Savage's notebook, July 1702.
109. Henry, *Exposition*, on Genesis 3:16 and Psalms 48:6; Henry, *Method*, pp. 153–4; Bod.: MS Eng.th.g.4, ff. 179–88, sermon by PH on Galatians 4:19, 2 December 1655; f. 209, sermon by PH on Colossians 1:21, 23 November 1656; BL: Add. MS 42849, ff. 32–3, MH to KH, 4 and 29 May 1700. There is a risk of taking such remarks out of context.

CHAPTER TWELVE

Newtonianism, Medicine and Religion

Anita Guerrini

When he wrote his *Principia* in 1687, did Isaac Newton realize that his *magnum opus* would become a battleground for contesting ideologies? In the contentious years surrounding the Glorious Revolution, political and religious debate inevitably spilled over into the discussion and interpretation of the most important English work in natural philosophy. Newton's own political and religious beliefs, not to mention the content and intent of his work, were rapidly overshadowed by individuals and groups who hastened to assume the mantle of intellectual authority and objectivity which Newton's work represented. The added appeal of patronage led many to affiliate themselves with Newton, especially after he became president of the Royal Society in 1703.

'Newtonianism' in the half-century following the publication of the *Principia* denoted no single set of doctrines, no single ideological stance. There were in fact many 'Newtonianisms', often amorphous and changeable.[1] Newton, ever fearful of controversy, held himself above the fray, giving his explicit blessing to few of his followers, and withdrawing his support with the same apparent capriciousness as he proffered it.

Medicine provided one stage for the enactment of the Newtonian melodrama. In terms of theory, Newtonian physics offered a variation on the Cartesian iatromechanical theme which increasingly dominated academic medicine in the last decades of the seventeenth century. Yet the wider issues at stake in the acceptance and definition of Newtonianism ensured that theory was not the only ground upon which Newton's ideas entered medicine. Religion, itself a battleground for competing ideologies, was one of those wider issues.

The relationship between Newtonianism, medicine and religion has been largely ignored in the modern historiography of Newton and his contemporary impact, although each of these elements has been considered separately. The most recent survey of Newton's influence on medicine does not mention religion,[2] and few of the numerous studies of Newton, Newtonianism and religion mention medicine.[3] Most recent work in the history of eighteenth-century British medicine has concentrated on the relationship between practitioner and patient,

with little attention given to medical theories.[4] The relationship between medicine and religion in this period is just beginning to be
considered.[5] Meanwhile, recent scholarship on religion in the eighteenth century has brought into question the long-standing assumption
that secularization was an inevitable consequence of enlightenment.[6]
In addition, Simon Schaffer and others have argued that mechanical
philosophy in late seventeenth-century Britain did not dismiss but
explicitly addressed the place of the soul and spirit.[7] Thus the elements
exist for an assessment of the relationship between Newtonianism,
medicine and religion. As there is no final, all-encompassing definition
of 'Newtonianism', so there is no definitive conclusion about its dia-
lectic relationship with religion and medicine in the first half of the
eighteenth century.

The relationship between Newtonianism, medicine and religion can
be approached in several ways. Robert Boyle and others had popularized the argument from design. By this argument, natural philosophy,
by providing evidence of God's design and purpose in the universe,
could support rather than undermine religious belief. The clergyman-
naturalist John Ray argued similarly in his *Wisdom of God Manifested
in the Works of Creation* (1691). Boyle endowed a series of sermons to
provide proof of Christianity against infidels and atheists, and not
surprisingly, the 'Boyle lectures', which commenced after his death in
1691, also emphasized the argument from design. Margaret Jacob has
demonstrated that some of the Boyle lectures provided an effective
outlet for the popularization and dissemination of one version of
Newtonian natural philosophy.[8]

The human body was an especially felicitous example of design.
Many physicians, such as James Keill, used Newtonian ideas simply as
a further proof of this argument from design, for Newtonian explanations of the body's workings showed it to be an even more wondrous
mechanism than Descartes had dreamed. During the early eighteenth
century, these arguments became increasingly deistic and divorced from
any specific theological doctrine.

In addition, Newtonian natural philosophy offered a critique of Cartesian mechanical philosophy by introducing the non-mechanical concept of force. This was as significant in theological terms as in scientific
terms, for as Newton himself argued, force provided a means for God
to act directly on the universe. As Boyle lecturer Richard Bentley stated,
'Universal Gravitation, a thing certainly existent in Nature, is above all
Mechanism and material Causes, and proceeds from a higher principle,
a Divine energy and impression'.[9] The failure of the mechanical philosophy to explain fully the workings of the body lent credence to this
reintroduction of immechanical forces.

Finally, mystics such as George Cheyne found in Newton's later aether theories a long-sought intermediary between matter and spirit, mind and body. Others found the aether to be more substantial, providing a material explanation for gravity. To them, Newton's God operated through material causes such as the aether rather than directly by means of immaterial forces. Newton's personal beliefs, including his rejection of the Trinity, were not generally known. But his belief in the absolute sovereignty of God, expressed in several of his works, seems at odds with such a materialist explanation.

Yet the notion that God intervened directly in the universe was diminishing even in popular belief, and the tension between providentialism and materialism steadily waned, as the works of many Newtonian physicians demonstrate. By the 1720s, providentialism was largely absent from such medical debates as the plague crisis and smallpox inoculation. While discussion of the efficacy of the 'King's Touch' carried political as well as religious implications, these implications were severely curtailed in the political atmosphere of the 1720s. Only the mind-body problem and questions of insanity still commanded theological as well as philosophical attention. Judging by the works of Newtonians such as Richard Mead, by mid-century these questions, too, seemed decided on the materialist side.

The significance of the *Principia* for medical theory was soon recognized. The Scottish physician Archibald Pitcairne (1652–1713), who learned of the *Principia* through his friend, the mathematician David Gregory (1659–1708), saw the potential of Newton's methods for medicine. He developed a theory of 'iatromathematics' which he expounded in several essays, including the public lectures he delivered during his brief tenure as professor of medicine at Leiden University (1692–93). Pitcairne emphasized the certainty and exactitude which Newtonian method gave to medicine, in contrast to the messy imprecision of chemical physicians or the hit-or-miss therapeutics of the empirics. Pitcairne's reading of Newtonian physics as an authoritarian system which was inevitably true was a product of his particular philosophical and political allegiances. As a Jacobite, he believed the absolute monarch alone could form the basis of the state; as a Scot, he viewed religious and political sectarianism as the greatest of all evils, whose only amelioration could come from a central undisputed authority; and as a physician trained in the French Cartesian tradition, he believed that mathematics was God given, immutable and inherently true.[10] Pitcairne seldom explicitly discussed religion in his works, but his God emerges as an autocrat, the supreme governor, much like Newton's description of

God, although the particulars of their theology were little in agreement. Despite their political differences, it is therefore not surprising that Pitcairne desired to have access to 'Newton's divine thoughts' about religion.[11]

Pitcairne decisively influenced the first generation of 'Newtonian' physicians in England. He directly trained many of them in Leiden or Edinburgh, and others learned his ideas through Gregory, who had been named Savilian professor of astronomy at Oxford in 1691 through Newton's influence.[12] This first generation formed an eclectic group of Scots, dissenters and Jacobites, alike mainly in being in some way outside the dominant religious and political culture.[13] The Tory and sometime Jacobite John Freind (1675–1728) and the Whig dissenter Richard Mead (1673–1754) were fast friends. While their mentors Pitcairne and Gregory were nominally Scottish Episcopalians, both were suspected of atheism or at the very least irreverence. Although Pitcairne remained a fervent Jacobite, Gregory considerably moderated his politics when he moved to England. Gregory's protégés and fellow Episcopalians James (1673–1719) and John Keill (1671–1721) were similarly not noted for excessive personal piety, although in several published works John Keill vigorously defended the High Church position. William Cockburn (1669–1739) was another Scottish Episcopalian, and a Tory later associated with Jonathan Swift. The Scottish Episcopalian George Cheyne (1671–1743), after early profligacy, experienced a conversion in 1706 and became associated with mystical circles. Easily the most overtly religious of this group, he did not, however, express his views for another decade.

In a period of intense competition among physicians for the limited élite clientele, expertise in natural philosophy could offer an additional cachet to a struggling young physician. These self-professed Newtonian physicians became so successful that by 1711 Bernard Mandeville complained bitterly about 'those Braggadocio's, who ... only make use of the Name of Mathematicks to impose upon the World for Lucre'.[14] The careers of Mead, Freind, and Cockburn particularly demonstrated that 'mathematics' could indeed be lucrative.

Even when these young men did not wholly adopt Pitcairne's interpretation of Newton's theories, they continued to investigate the problems he had identified. These included secretion and muscular motion, problems brought to the fore by Harvey's theory of circulation and given mechanical explanations by the 'Oxford physiologists' of the third quarter of the century.[15] Pitcairne and his followers reinterpreted these questions in terms of Newtonian notions of hydraulics and the theory of matter.

Although Newton did not discuss matter theory in the *Principia*, in 1692 he gave Pitcairne a copy of his seminal essay on that topic, 'De natura acidorum', in which he outlined a theory of corpuscular matter endowed with an attractive force analogous to gravity. Pitcairne questioned Newton further on the application of this theory to physiological processes. Fluids were composed of attracting particles, and Newton asserted that secretion was a function of the attraction between a fluid and its particular passage, denying the mechanistic 'strainer' explanation which proposed an identity between particular fluids and passages based on size and shape.[16]

Several physicians outlined Pitcairnean explanations of secretion in works published around 1700. These included James Keill's *Anatomy of the Humane Body* (1698); William Cockburn's *Oeconomia corporis animalis* (1695) and *Account of the Distempers that are Incident to Sea-Faring People* (1696); and George Cheyne's *New Theory of Fevers* (1701), along with many pamphlets and articles. Most of the latter were published in the *Philosophical Transactions* of the Royal Society. In his 1702 *Mechanical Account of Poisons*, Richard Mead also adopted the concept of the blood as a mixture of attracting particles.[17]

Newton had long worked on optics, and was known to be working on a book on that topic in the early 1690s, a topic of obvious medical interest.[18] In response to Pitcairne's questioning in 1692, Newton noted that in humans and in animals which focus both eyes at once, the optic nerves grow together and send one image to the brain.[19] Pitcairne briefly mentioned optics at the end of his Leiden inaugural lecture, delivered a month after he spoke with Newton.[20] Gregory had already appropriated Newton's description in his Oxford MD thesis, delivered only a week after Pitcairne's visit to Newton. Like Newton, Gregory concluded that the optic nerves separate again before reaching the brain, and that the optical image finally formed was an act of will. In query 28 of his *Opticks*, published in 1706, Newton discussed sensation as an act of will to draw an analogy between the human sensorium and the sensorium of God, which is infinite space. Gregory made no such grand metaphor; the eye was simply 'an optical mechanism made by God for the greatest good', another example of divine design.[21]

Gregory's comment rather than Newton's analogy informed Newtonian physiology. The argument from design ran throughout the works of Newtonian physicians, paralleling the work of the Boyle lecturers. The first of these, Richard Bentley (1662–1742), collectively titled three of his eight 1692 Boyle lectures *A Confutation of Atheism from the Structure and Origin of Humane Bodies*. To Bentley, 'the Organical Structure of Human Bodies ... is unquestionably the workmanship of a most wise, and powerfull, and beneficent Maker', while the atheists, he claimed, attributed 'this acknowledged Fitness of Humane Bodies ... to dead, sensless [sic] Matter'.[22]

James Keill's *Anatomy of the Humane Body* was soaked in teleology. Every part of the body had a purpose, and this purpose was obviously part of the divine plan. He commented, 'But whatever its Cause we are extremely obliged to the Maker of our Eyes, that the Optick Nerves are inserted on the inside of the Optick *Axes* rather than the outside, or our vision would be greatly impaired'.[23] Along similar lines, he argued that 'a Man has a Beard, and a Woman none', because they could not otherwise be distinguished, 'if both were dress'd in the same Habit'.[24]

Richard Mead asserted in his *Mechanical Account of Poisons* that God's design made knowledge itself possible, by ensuring that human and animal bodies were regular and orderly, and therefore knowable and not merely 'an irregular Mass, and disorderly *Jumble* of Atoms'.[25] Likewise, his 1704 *Of the Power and Influence of the Sun and Moon on Humane Bodies* 'shews the Wisdom and Goodness of the great Creator of all Things'. Even though the differences in air pressure which he described in his work had detrimental effects upon the health of some (particularly the 'weak and silly'), the Creator had not erred in giving air these effects. The climate of some parts of the world may be less pleasant than others, but Mead judged with Panglossian fervour that 'the whole ... we must own, is most carefully provided for'.[26]

Mead's emphasis in this work on the hidden powers and 'sympathys' of the sun and moon – and even the stars – kept, if at times vaguely, within the theological boundaries provided by Newton's theory of attractions, which dictated that God worked by the secondary cause of attraction. However, Mead concluded that storms were at times caused by the 'Anger of Heaven'. 'It is not my business to dispute' providential causes, he wrote, since he would not 'by any means endeavour to absolve Men's Minds from the Bands of Religion'. It was reasonable to believe that God did sometimes create calamities to keep humankind 'in a continual Sense of their Duty'.[27] One example was the storms which accompanied the death of Cromwell in 1658. Mead's Puritan upbringing (his father, Matthew Mead, was a noted Puritan divine) showed through perhaps too clearly here.[28]

While equally employing teleology, Mead's friend John Freind explicitly eschewed any hint of providentialism in his early works. In a paper published in *Philosophical Transactions* in 1701, Freind had ascribed a mysterious case of 'fits' in an Oxfordshire village to physical disturbances in the animal spirits, rejecting the 'horoscopes and sympathies' of the villagers.[29] In his *Emmenologia* (1703), a treatise on menstruation, Freind emphasized purpose rather than providence, with mechanical causes firmly at the centre of his argument, following Pitcairne's essay 'Some Observations Concerning Womens Monthly Courses' (*c.*1700).[30]

The idea of design was central to the Low Church Boyle lecturers, whose concern was to establish a broadly inclusive theology based on reasonable, agreed-upon principles. But some High Church Newtonians in the 'Church-in-danger' days of the 1690s were not content with mere design as a defence against dissenters and Catholics as well as atheists, and sought to explain the consequences of an immaterial force in nature.

In his 1693 'Dissertation upon the Circulation of the Blood in Born Animals and Embryons', Pitcairne concluded that the force of the heart, like gravity, must be directly endowed by God, since no mechanical explanation could be found for it. 'By consequence,' he stated, 'no Animal is ever produced Mechanically.'[31] In 1698 John Keill extended this argument to the ongoing cosmogonical debate sparked by Thomas Burnet's 1680 *Sacred Theory of the Earth*. In his *Examination of Dr. Burnet's Theory of the Earth*, Keill replied to what he viewed as an excessive reliance on mechanical causes by the Newtonian William Whiston (1667–1752) in his *New Theory of the Earth* (1696). Whiston's arguments, said Keill, were not only Cartesian but atheistical, since Whiston failed to acknowledge the continuous guiding hand of Providence in creation. Keill asserted that he, not the Low Church Whiston, was the true Newtonian, because like Newton, he recognized the ultimate and overriding authority of God. Characteristically, Newton gave neither view his explicit endorsement.[32]

However, the sense of urgency Keill conveyed seemed to dissipate quickly. By 1702, George Cheyne sounded very Bentleyan when he claimed that Pitcairne's works 'serve to demonstrat the *Infinit* wisdom of the CONTRIVER of the *Universe*'.[33] In his *Philosophical Principles of Natural Religion* (1705), Cheyne declared that God had given to his generation

> those great Advantages, by which the Secrets of Nature have been more happily unravell'd, than in any former Times, on purpose, to expose the Folly of a corrupt Generation of Men, who from their vitious Practices, being prone to *Atheism*, have vainly pretended, the *Oracles* of *Reason* to be on their side.[34]

Gregory recognized Bentley's influence in his derisive characterization of Cheyne's *Philosophical Principles* as an imitation Boyle lecture.[35] Like Bentley, Cheyne included examples of design drawn from the range of natural philosophy, especially the structure of human and animal bodies. Not only did the body show evidence of design, but it also clearly demonstrated that Cartesian mechanism, that crutch of atheism, was wholly inadequate to explain its workings. When, as with the animal body, 'the *complications* are infinite the Machin is altogether above the Power of *Mechanicks*, and quite impracticable by the Laws of Matter and Motion'. Cheyne concluded that 'the Production of Animals

is altogether inconsistent with the Laws of *Mechanism*', and therefore
required the existence of a conscious creator.[36]

Newton's 1706 edition of his *Opticks* included the famous query 31
(numbered query 23 in that edition) on the theory of matter, in which
Newton made explicit several points he had only hinted at in 'De natura
acidorum'. The Keills and Freind quickly seized upon this theory as the
key to both chemistry and physiology in several works published in
1708–09.

Freind and John Keill both confined their work to chemistry, but
James Keill's *Account of Animal Secretion* (1708) boldly attempted to
create a new, thoroughly Newtonian theory of physiology without any
of what he viewed to be Pitcairne's Cartesian preconceptions. Keill
wrote Hans Sloane of his book, 'It opens a new Scene in the Natural
Philosophy of Physick'.[37] Keill outlined an original theory of secretion
based on differential attractions between various particles in the blood.
However, in his preface he was careful to situate his work within the
long and ancient medical tradition, thus asserting his claim for membership in the circle of élite learned medicine while at the same time
establishing his credentials in 'mathematical physick' for another audience. Freind had stated that his highly mechanistic explanations in
Emmenologia were all 'both known and practiced by the *Ancients*', and
the *Philosophical Transaction*'s review of Mead's *Mechanical Account
of Poisons* noted 'the curious Antient and Polite Learning, with which it
is well stored'.[38] Keill argued that if the design of nature was constant,
'this Attraction of the small Particles of Matter is no Innovation in
Philosophy', but a fact which had been long known. So had Newton
himself claimed to be uncovering long-lost ancient knowledge. Keill
implied that God was somehow responsible when experiments were
correct; the 'chance' by which remedies such as cinchona bark had been
discovered was in fact 'Divine appointment'.[39]

Keill's own evidence, however, was not experimental but mathematical. Pitcairne had taught him that only mathematical knowledge is
inherently true, and if Keill consciously rejected Cartesian explanation
he none the less equated true knowledge about the body with 'Geo-
metrical Demonstration'.[40] With intricate calculations of the propor-
tionate relationships of the blood vessels, he concluded that in the
outermost branches of the vascular system the blood circulated many
times more slowly than in the main vessels. The purpose of this was to
allow secretion to take place. Keill's animal body was full of 'extraordinary Contrivance' and conscious intent. Nature's design was evident to
those who used the correct, mathematical, methods.[41]

Similarly, he determined the quantity of blood in the body not by
observing hemorrhages but by a series of calculations based on his

premise that there was a nearly infinite quantity of vessels in the body. Keill determined that a 160-pound man had about 100 pounds of blood. The intricate structure of the body was evidence not only of design but of God's omnipotence; for food could not metamorphose into the particles of the blood merely by mechanical means: 'no Matter, howsoever disposed, can at first frame these solid parts, without an Omnipotent Power immediately actuating it'.[42]

Despite certain differences, Newtonian physicians in this period reached a tenuous intellectual consensus on the outlines of a Newtonian theory of medicine, mirroring, perhaps, the tenuous Whig political consensus that had been reached in 1702. When one considers the intensity of Newton's own religious convictions and their central position in his thought, the arguments from design which dominated the works of these medical Newtonians seem weak panderings to convention. While Cheyne's *Philosophical Principles* tentatively pointed to a closer integration of religion and medical theory, his example was not followed. All of these works, including Cheyne's, were firmly within the boundaries of 'natural religion' or 'natural theology'; the laws of nature affirmed the existence of God. Revelation played little part in these ruminations.

This consensus was short-lived. James Keill's *Account of Animal Secretion* represented the peak of Newtonian physiological theory based on the notion of attracting particles. But even while Keill wrote, Newton himself was rethinking some of the foundations of his theories. The 'General Scholium' which Newton added to the second edition of his *Principia* in 1713 referred to 'a certain most subtle spirit', which he described as 'electric and elastic'. He tentatively identified this 'spirit' with the animal spirits or nervous fluid.[43] At the same time, the Low Church Whig political consensus suffered a serious setback in 1710. The case of Henry Sacheverell, convicted of sedition for an anti-government sermon, toppled the Whig government, and reminded the ruling classes how tenuous was their hold over the hearts and minds of the masses who rioted in Sacheverell's defence. In his 1709 sermon on 'False Brethren' Sacheverell had castigated 'whosoever presumes to recede the least tittle from the express word of God, or to explain the great crescenda of our Faith in new-fangled terms of modern philosophy'.[44]

George Cheyne was the first of the early group of Newtonian physicians to grasp the implications of Newton's aether theory for both medicine and religion. Cheyne's personal circumstances uniquely situated him to uncover a spiritual meaning in Newton's aether. After the publication of his *Philosophical Principles of Natural Religion* in 1705, Cheyne had experienced a religious conversion in which he came under the influence of a mystical circle. By the time he began to revise his *Philosophical Principles*, he had read deeply in mystical literature ranging from the *Imitation of Christ* to the works of contemporary French mystic Jeanne Guyon (1648–1717).[45] His new priorities were reflected in a new title, *The Philosophical Principles of Religion, Natural and Revealed* (1715).

In place of the Newtonians' earlier optimistic assessment of the inevitable progress of human knowledge, Cheyne now declared that in this 'lapsed' world, human faculties were not perhaps capable of attaining certain knowledge. Natural philosophy, he added, reaches only 'some of the grosser *Lineaments*, or more conspicuous *Out-lines* of the Works of the Almighty'.[46] In particular, it cannot prove the existence of the soul.

For Cheyne, analogy became the unifying principle between God and nature, a demonstration that natural and revealed religion were one and the same. He explained: 'The whole Foundation of *Natural Philosophy*, is *Simplicity* and *Analogy*, or a Simple, yet Beautiful *Harmony*, running through all Works of Nature in an uninterrupted Chain of Causes and Effects.'[47] Cheyne intended to echo the 'Rules of Reasoning' in the new edition of the *Principia*, which had mentioned simplicity and analogy as essential qualities of nature. But his heavily Platonized rendering of these views echoed instead the words of a much younger Newton, who in his 1675 'Hypothesis of Light' had shown himself still to be under the influence of the Cambridge Platonists.[48]

Cheyne took literally Newton's suggestion that nature was the sensorium of God. But Newton did not provide Cheyne's new explanation of gravity as analogous to God's love, 'an Essential Principle of *Re-Union*'.[49] Analogy governed the actions of both the universe and the soul, for gravity and the love of God were aspects of the same 'great and universal *Principle*'. Body and spirit occupied opposite ends of the chain of being, but both were extended and therefore capable of changing into each other. This analogical symmetry proved the existence of God as certainly 'as any *Mathematical* Demonstration infers its Proposition'. All created beings were simply the visible representations of the archetype in the mind of the Creator, a literal transformation of thought into flesh. Echoing Newton, Cheyne concluded, 'Hence *universal Space* may be very aptly called the *Sensorium Divinitatis*'. This is a far cry from the Boyle lecturers' argument from design.[50]

From this relationship Cheyne constructed an elaborate model of rational beings, who, he said, possessed three levels of consciousness: the five senses, the 'rational soul' or mind, and the 'supreme spirit', infinite in capacity, by means of which one communicated with God. In the 'due *Subordination*' of these three levels humans could reach their fullest perfection, a true imitation of Christ in which the soul is united with God by the principle of reunion. Too often, however, the sensual overrode the other two levels, leading to corruption and depravity.[51]

Cheyne expounded upon this theory of the human 'machin' in several subsequent works. In diseases such as gout, he argued that while sin did not cause illness by supernatural causation, the unhealthy behaviours associated with a sinful life certainly contributed to the onset of such maladies, which he then analysed in Newtonian terms of attracting particles. Thus his moral message intersected neatly with his therapeutic prescriptions of temperance and sober living. In him, the priestlike role of the physician is particularly evident.[52] His emphasis on behaviour echoed the message of such groups as the Societies for the Reformation of Manners, formed at the turn of the eighteenth century to combat disbelief by means of moral reform.[53]

Unlike Cheyne, James Keill remained within the framework of his earlier mechanical philosophy. While Cheyne remained deeply involved in Jacobite and mystical circles, for Keill, as for many others, the peaceful succession to power of the Hanoverian monarch George I in 1714 put an end to sectarian strife, religious or otherwise. In 1717 Keill issued a new edition of his essays on secretion, with two new essays. One of these, on the velocity of the blood, employed his usual mathematical arguments, in this case derived from his brother John's lectures on hydraulics. But in his essay on the force of the heart, he also urged the utility of 'Observation or Experiment, carefully made and duly applied'.[54] Keill's use of experimental data left him open to criticism, and a younger Newtonian physician, James Jurin (1684–1750) used Keill's data to show what he viewed as Keill's misunderstanding of Newtonian principles. Their debate continued until Keill's death in 1719.[55] The historians Frances Valadez and C.D. O'Malley noted the politeness of this debate; also missing was any mention of design.[56]

Keill issued a Latin translation of his essays in the following year, adding two new essays and a short treatise entitled *Medicina statica Britannica*. The latter work revised the popular work on 'statics' of the seventeenth-century Italian physician Sanctorius (cited frequently by Pitcairne) for British audiences and the British temperament. Like Sanctorius, Keill derived his data on human intake and excretion from his own body. His work proved sufficiently popular that Pitcairne's protégé, the apothecary John Quincy (d. 1722), translated it into English and appended it to his translation of Sanctorius's *Medicina statica*.[57]

A very different work was John Freind's 1717 *Nine Commentaries Upon Fevers*, ostensibly commentaries on certain Hippocratic works.[58] Although in the 1680s Pitcairne had written an essay denying that Hippocrates could have known about the circulation of the blood – thus demonstrating the superiority of the moderns over the ancients – Freind claimed that Hippocrates could indeed be viewed as a proto-Newtonian. The scientific basis of Hippocratic therapeutics, he argued, was made clear by the work of Newton and the Newtonian physicians. Truth, Freind explained, was eternal and God given, and God gave the privilege of understanding it to certain individuals in each generation.[59] As Julian Martin has pointed out, this view was entirely consistent with Freind's Jacobite beliefs in Divine right.[60] The Whig Mead none the less strongly supported Freind in the pamphlet war which followed, demonstrating that friendship and loyalty to Newton were, at least in this case, stronger than loyalty to politics.

Freind's *History of Physick* (1725–26) made even clearer the interconnection of politics, religion, medicine and natural philosophy. Written during his imprisonment in the Tower of London for his involvement in the Jacobite Atterbury plot of 1722, Freind intended his book to justify both his politics and his philosophy. He believed that the healer, like the monarch, was divinely ordained. These two roles came together in the 'King's Touch', a custom which, Freind wrote, was affirmed by 'undoubted authorities'.[61] However, a few years earlier John Quincy had ended his Newtonian account of the king's evil with the brusque declaration that the notion of the King's Touch was 'so remote from all good Sense, since it can take place only on a deluded Imagination, that I think it justly banished with the Superstition and Bigotry that introduced it'.[62] The earlier Newtonian consensus was long gone.

Newton's new queries in the 1718 *Opticks* complicated matters further. These developed his theory of the aether in more detail, but both in medicine and in physics, the aether created at least as many problems as it solved. There was little agreement among physicians about the aether's operation in the body, and Newtonian physicians only gradually incorporated the aether into their works.

Mead explained contagion by means of a 'volatile active Spirit' which sounded like an aether in his *Short Discourse Concerning Pestilential Contagion*, written in response to the plague scare in 1720.[63] Divine causation earned no mention; the nearest Mead came was to note that '*Fear, Despair*, and all *Dejection of Spirits* dispose the Body to receive Contagion', urging his audience to 'guard against all *Dejection of Spirits* and *immoderate Passions*'.[64] But then, even the intensely pious Puritan protagonist of Daniel Defoe's 1722 *Journal of the Plague Year* had begun to doubt divine causation by the novel's end.[65]

Soon after, James Jurin similarly discounted divine purpose in several pamphlets supporting the new technique of inoculation for the smallpox. Jurin argued that statistical evidence alone demonstrated the efficacy of inoculation, relying on 'the most Authentick Accounts' and 'well-attested Relations'.[66] Even the account of John Osborne of New England, which began by attributing the onset of smallpox in Boston to

'the Providence of God', concluded in extolling the efficacy of inoculation to avoid the consequences of that providence.[67] Against those who
argued, 'and from the Pulpit too', that inoculation was the work of the
Devil, Jurin countered that its evident benefit to mankind indicated an
attribution 'to a greater and a better Author'. This opinion 'all sober
and thinking Persons will judge and believe': a perfect expression of
rational natural religion.[68]

During the 1720s Richard Mead proved to be an important patron of
younger Newtonians, including Henry Pemberton (1697–1770) and
Nicholas Robinson (1697–1775). He commissioned Pemberton to write
a 'Discourse Upon Muscular Motion' to preface his new edition of
William Cowper's 1694 treatise *Myotomia Reformata*. Pemberton's introduction bristled with calculations and diagrams. He concluded that
Newton's aether and the animal spirits were one and the same. Newton
had not exactly concluded this in query 24, describing 'the vibrating
motion of the Aetherial Medium' along solid, not hollow, nerves.[69] In
the following year, Nicholas Robinson penned *A New Theory of Physick
and Diseases, Founded on the Principles of the Newtonian Philosophy*.
Robinson began his work with a series of queries, but unlike Newton,
he went on to answer them in a synthesis of the work of Mead and his
colleagues.[70] Both Pemberton and Robinson gave only the briefest nod
to the argument from design in their works. For them, it seems, as for
James Keill, the threat of natural philosophy to fidelity was no longer of
significance.

However, for Cheyne, the wickedness of the age was only too evident
in the health of his patients. In his 1724 *Essay of Health and Long Life*,
the Galenic 'six non-naturals' became the seven deadly sins. To Cheyne,
the body was truly God's workmanship, and to injure it wilfully by
overindulgence was a sin against God as well as against nature. The
most evident manifestation of the transgressions of the rules of health
was the great increase in nervous cases which he witnessed in his
medical practice in Bath. Cheyne's explanation of the workings of the
passions employed the analogy between spirit and Newtonian gravity
he had introduced in the 1715 *Philosophical Principles*. Both, he said,
were motive principles bestowed directly on passive matter by God.[71]

The physician and dissenting minister Thomas Morgan (d. 1743)
presented a rather unorthodox variety of Newtonian medicine in his
Philosophical Principles of Medicine (1725), which he hopefully dedicated to Sloane and the London College of Physicians. In his preface,
Morgan emphasized the argument from design, noting that the 'animal
automaton' is 'the perfect Workmanship of the almighty God', while
also asserting the usefulness of Newtonian natural philosophy as a
methodological model.[72] While his text presented a familiar hydraulic

model of the body, it also interpreted Newtonian physics as a Manichean dichotomy of expansive and contractive forces exemplified by fire and air; light, he said, was elemental fire, the original expansive force. The means of action of these forces remained unknown, but the first cause was undoubtedly 'the continued regular Operation of ... the Author of Nature, acting constantly and uniformly'.[73] In his *Mechanical Practice of Physick* a decade later, he presented himself as the only true Newtonian who would rescue medicine from the errors of the 'corpuscularian specifick Philosophy' of Pitcairne's followers.[74]

Many physicians agreed that Newton's aether was highly relevant to the mind-body problem, but few agreed where it fitted. Morgan asserted that the connection between mind and body was analogous to gravity but did not explain its operation.[75] Nicholas Robinson attempted to answer the question, 'who, from the Texture of the Parts, can account for the Juncture of Matter and Thought?' in his *New System of the Spleen, Vapours and Hypochondriack Melancholy* (1729). Robinson accounted for most mental states with a thoroughly mechanical physiology of tubes, fibres and fluids. The 'self-moving principle' known as the soul animated the matter of the body in the same way in which gravity animated matter in general. Robinson filled the gap between soul and body with a material 'animal aether' which he equated with the passions. Disturbances in this material aether accounted for mental disturbance; Robinson agreed with most of his contemporaries that insanity was a somatic disorder. His explanation left the soul, like the God of the deists, a distant actor.[76]

A few years later, the Irish physician Bryan Robinson (no relation) (1680–1754) returned to Pemberton's identification of the animal spirits as the aether. 'Muscular motion', said Bryan Robinson, 'is performed by the vibrations of a very Elastick Aether, lodged in the Nerves and Membranes investing the minute Fibres of the Muscles, excited by the Power of the Will, Heat, Wounds, the subtle and active Particles of Bodies, and other Causes'.[77] The aether acted as an intermediary between soul and body, for 'the Soul has no immediate Power over the fleshy Fibres'.[78]

Cheyne contested the materialism of both Bryan Robinson and Nicholas Robinson in his *English Malady* (1733), a treatise on 'the spleen'. Their work, he believed, implied a deism inconsistent with Newtonian principles, joining the anti-deism campaign launched by his friend, the theologian William Law (1686–1761), whose *The Case of Religion and Reason or Natural Religion Fairly and Fully Stated* had appeared in 1731. At the same time, Cheyne rejected the critique of Newtonianism offered by John Hutchinson (1674–1737) in his *Moses's Principia* (1724–27). Hutchinson believed that fire, light and air materially caused motion by direct contact, an argument which somewhat resembled Thomas Morgan's. Unlike Morgan, Hutchinson argued that Newton's reliance on God as the final cause of gravity undermined the deity's transcendent power.[79] Hutchinson's views were popular in many of the High Church circles in which Cheyne moved, making his task of defending Newton all the more urgent.

In *The English Malady*, Cheyne developed his earlier accounts of the relations among mind, body and spirit. He again described a Platonic hierarchy between matter and spirit, with Newton's aether acting as intermediary. Unlike the Robinsons, he asserted the direct and active involvement of God in the aether's action. The body, mind and spirit, and their illnesses, were therefore intimately intertwined, and each required attention to affect a cure.[80]

While Cheyne's work was very popular, his attempt to synthesize Newtonianism, medicine and religion was largely ignored. Both his supporters and his critics alike overlooked his prescriptions to piety and seized upon regimen as the key to well-being; Cheyne himself acknowledged that one could follow his rules without understanding their principles.[81] Even the clergyman Thomas Morgan omitted any mention of religion from his 1735 *Mechanical Practice of Physick*, reserving his criticism for that 'grand devouring Idol LUXURY'.[82] While John Wesley adopted Cheyne's ideas on regimen as part of the Methodist way of life, he did not adopt Cheyne's ideas on physiology.

Despite Cheyne's popularity, the most characteristic work on Newtonianism and medicine of mid-eighteenth century was not *The English Malady* but Richard Mead's *Medica sacra* (1749). While it is true that God had the power miraculously to cause or cure disease, said Mead, in fact most illnesses, including those in the Bible, could be explained by natural causes. The physician retains a priestly role because his ability to cure, as Freind had argued two decades earlier, was divinely given. But that ability worked entirely by natural causes. In his book, Mead offered natural interpretations for biblical illnesses and afflictions. The demoniacs in the Gospels, said Mead, simply needed their humours thinned out.[83]

Yet no single version of 'Newtonianism' had triumphed by 1750. Thomas Morgan referred to 'the various and contradictory Hypotheses of the Moderns', many, if not most, of which claimed some Newtonian inspiration.[84] The role of religion in these theories, however, steadily diminished. Apart from vague generalizations about secularization and enlightenment, the precise explanation for this diminution remains unclear. Much remains to be explored.

Notes

1. See Robert Markley, *Fallen Languages: Crises of Representation in Newtonian England, 1660–1740*, Ithaca, Cornell University Press, 1993, ch.5.

2. Theodore M. Brown, 'Medicine in the Shadow of the *Principia*', *Journal of the History of Ideas*, 48 (1987), 629–48.

3. See, for example, M.C. Jacob, *The Newtonians and the English Revolution*, Ithaca, Cornell University Press, 1976; Larry Stewart, *The Rise of Public Science*, Cambridge, Cambridge University Press, 1992; Markley, *Fallen Languages*.

4. N. Jewson, 'Medical Knowledge and the Patronage System in Eighteenth-Century England', *Sociology*, 8 (1974), 369–85; Malcolm Nicolson, 'The Metastatic Theory of Pathogenesis and the Professional Interests of the Eighteenth-Century Physician', *Medical History*, 32 (1988), 277–300; Roy Porter and Dorothy Porter, *In Sickness and In Health*, New York, Blackwell, 1989; Dorothy Porter and Roy Porter, *Patient's Progress*, Stanford, Stanford University Press, 1989.

5. Jonathan Barry, 'Piety and the Patient: Medicine and Religion in Eighteenth Century Bristol', in Roy Porter (ed.) *Patients and Practitioners*, Cambridge, Cambridge University Press, 1985, pp. 145–75; Roy Porter, 'Medicine and Religion in Eighteenth-Century England: A Case of Conflict?', *Ideas and Production* 7 (1987), 4–17; Andrew Wear, 'Medical Practice in Late Seventeenth- and Early Eighteenth-Century England: Continuity and Union', in Roger French and Andrew Wear (eds), *The Medical Revolution of the Seventeenth Century*, Cambridge, Cambridge University Press, 1989, pp. 294–320.

6. J.C.D. Clark, *English Society 1688–1832*, Cambridge, Cambridge University Press, 1985; for a cogent review of some recent historiography of religion, see Harry Payne, 'Review Essay: Remaking One's Maker: The Career of Religion in the Eighteenth Century', *Eighteenth-Century Life*, 9 (1984), 107–15.

7. Simon Schaffer, 'Godly Men and Mechanical Philosophers', *Science in Context*, 1 (1987), 55–85; John Henry, 'Occult Qualities and the Experimental Philosophy: Active Principles in Pre-Newtonian Matter Theory', *History of Science*, 24 (1986), 335–81.

8. Jacob, *The Newtonians and the English Revolution*.

9. Richard Bentley, *A Confutation of Atheism From the Origin and Frame of the World*, pt 3, London, H. Mortlock, 1693, p. 32. See also Jacob, *Newtonians*; Michael Hunter, *Science and Society in Restoration England*, Cambridge, Cambridge University Press, 1981, pp. 182–5.

10. Anita Guerrini, 'Archibald Pitcairne and Newtonian Medicine', *Medical History*, 31 (1987), 70–83; Simon Schaffer, 'The Glorious Revolution and Medicine in Britain and the Netherlands', *Notes and Records of the Royal Society*, 43 (1989), 167–90.

11. Pitcairne to Robert Grey, 24–25 October 1694, in W.T. Johnston (ed.), '*The Best of our Owne': Letters of Archibald Pitcairne*, Edinburgh, Saorsa Books, 1979, pp. 19–20.

12. See R.S. Westfall, *Never at Rest*, Cambridge, Cambridge University Press, 1980, pp. 499–500.

13. For a more detailed account of the following, see Anita Guerrini, 'The

Tory Newtonians: Gregory, Pitcairne and their Circle', *Journal of British Studies*, **26** (1986), 288–311.

14. B. Mandeville, *A Treatise of the Hypochondriack and Hysterick Diseases*, 2nd edn, London, J. Tonson, 1730, p. 182. First edition 1711.

15. See Robert G. Frank, *Harvey and the Oxford Physiologists*, Berkeley, University of California Press, 1980.

16. Isaac Newton, 'De natura acidorum,' in H.W. Turnbull, J.F. Scott, A.R. Hall and L. Tilling (eds), *The Correspondence of Isaac Newton*, 7 vols, Cambridge, Cambridge University Press, 1959–77, vol. 3, pp. 202–14.

17. William Cockburn, *Oeconomia corporis animalis*, London, H. Newman, 1695; W. Cockburn, *An Account of the Nature, Causes, Symptoms and Cure of the Distempers That Are Incident to Sea-Faring People*, London, Hugh Newman, 1696; W. Cockburn, 'A Discourse of the Operation of a Blister When It Cures a Fever', *Philosophical Transactions*, **21** (1699), 161–82; George Cheyne, *A New Theory of Continual Fevers*, London, H. Newman and J. Nutt, 1701; G. Cheyne, *An Essay Concerning the Improvements in the Theory of Medicine*, Edinburgh, 1702; James Keill, *The Anatomy of the Humane Body Abridg'd*, London, William Keblewhite, 1698; Richard Mead, *A Mechanical Account of Poisons in Several Essays*, London, R. South, 1702.

18. Westfall, *Never at Rest*, 520–4.

19. Newton, 'De natura acidorum', p. 212.

20. Archibald Pitcairne, 'An Oration Proving the Profession of Physic Free of Any Sect of Philosophers', trans. George Sewell and J.T. Desaguliers in A. Pitcairne, *The Works*, London, E. Curll, 1715, pp. 7–24.

21. David Gregory, *Tres lectiones cursoriae*, University Library Aberdeen, MS 2206/8, ff. 3, 26–7; Isaac Newton, *Opticks*, 4th edn (1730), reprinted New York, Dover, 1952; Schaffer, 'Glorious Revolution and Medicine', pp. 174–5; Martin Tamny, 'Newton, Creation, and Perception', *Isis*, **70** (1979), 48–58, at 54–55.

22. Richard Bentley, *A Confutation of Atheism From the Structure and Origin of Humane Bodies. Part 1.*, London, Tho. Parkhurst and H. Mortlock, 1692, pp. 8–10.

23. Keill, *Anatomy of the Humane Body Abridg'd*, 3rd edn, London, J.B. for Ralph Smith and William Keble, 1708, p. 162.

24. Ibid., p. 16.

25. Mead, *Mechanical Account of Poisons*, Preface.

26. Richard Mead, *Of the Power and Influence of the Sun and Moon on Humane Bodies*, London, Richard Wellington, 1712 (1st publ. in Latin, 1704), pp. xxii, 25–6.

27. Richard Mead, *Of the Power and Influence*, pp. 86–9.

28. Ibid., p. 86. On Matthew Mead, see *DNB*.

29. John Freind, 'Epistola de spasmi rarioris historia', *Philosophical Transactions*, **22** (1701), 799–804. For a fuller account of this work, see Anita Guerrini, 'Ether Madness: Newtonianism, Religion, and Insanity in Eighteenth-Century England', in Paul Theerman and Adele Seeff (eds) *Action and Reaction*, Newark, DE, University of Delaware Press, 1993, pp. 232–54.

30. John Freind, *Emmenologia*, trans. Thomas Dale, London, T. Cox, 1729; Archibald Pitcairne, 'Some Observations Concerning Womens Monthly Courses', in *Works*, pp. 221–37.

31. Pitcairne, *Works*, p. 167.
32. John Keill, *An Examination of Dr Burnet's Theory of the Earth. Together With Some Remarks on Mr Whiston's New Theory of the Earth*, Oxford, 1698; see David Kubrin, 'Providence and the Mechanical Philosophy', PhD diss., Cornell University, 1968; J.E. Force, *William Whiston, Honest Newtonian*, Cambridge, Cambridge University Press, 1985.
33. George Cheyne, *Remarks on Two Late Pamphlets Written by Dr Oliphant, Against Dr Pitcairn's Dissertations*, Edinburgh, 1702, p. 2.
34. George Cheyne, *Philosophical Principles of Natural Religion* London, G. Strahan, 1705, Dedication.
35. David Gregory, memorandum, ?3 June 1705, in W.G. Hiscock (ed.), *David Gregory, Isaac Newton, and Their Circle*, Oxford, 1937, p. 25.
36. Cheyne, *Philosophical Principles* (1705), pt II, pp. 17, 22–3.
37. James Keill to Hans Sloane, 16 May 1708, British Library, Sloane MS 4041, ff. 140–1.
38. Freind, *Emmenologia*, p. 215; 'Accounts of Books', *Philosophical Transactions*, 23 (1703), 1327.
39. James Keill, *An Account of Animal Secretion, the Quantity of Blood in the Humane Body, and Muscular Motion*, London, George Strahan, 1708, Preface, pp. ix, xxvii.
40. Ibid., p. v.
41. Ibid., p. 146–7.
42. Ibid., p. 153.
43. Isaac Newton, *Mathematical Principles of Natural Philosophy*, trans. Andrew Motte, revised Florian Cajori, Berkeley, University of California Press, 1934, pp. 543–7.
44. Henry Sacheverell, *The Perils of False Brethren, Both in Church and State*, London, Henry Clements, 1709, pp. 9–10, quoted in Geoffrey Holmes, *The Trial of Doctor Sacheverell*, London, Eyre Methuen, 1973, p. 65.
45. On these issues, see my forthcoming biography of Cheyne.
46. George Cheyne, *The Philosophical Principles of Religion, Natural and Revealed*, London, George Strahan, 1715, pt 1, pp. 2, 46.
47. Ibid., pt 1, p. 42.
48. See Westfall, *Never at Rest*, pp. 303–8; J.E. McGuire, 'Neoplatonism and Active Principles: Newton and the *Corpus Hermeticum*', in R.S. Westman and J.E. McGuire, *Hermeticism and the Scientific Revolution*, William Andrews Clark Memorial Library, UCLA, 1977), pp. 95–142.
49. Cheyne, *Philosophical Principles* (1715), pt 1, p. 47.
50. Cheyne, *Philosophical Principles* (1715), pt 2: pp. 3, 39–40, 53; Newton, *Opticks*, query 28. For other similar arguments about attraction, see Geoffrey Bowles, 'The Place of Newtonian Explanation in English Popular Thought, 1687–1727', D.Phil. thesis, Oxford University, 1977, pp. 225–7.
51. Cheyne, *Philosophical Principles* (1715), pt 2, pp. 61–6.
52. George Cheyne, *Observations on the Nature and Method of Treating the Gout*, London, G. Strahan, 1720 (subsequent editions retitled *An Essay on the Gout*); on the physician as priest, see Porter, 'Medicine and Religion'.
53. T.C. Curtis and W.A. Speck, 'The Societies for the Reformation of Manners: A Case Study in the Theory and Practice of Moral Reform', *Literature and History*, 3 (1976), 45–64.

54. James Keill, *Essays on Several Parts the Animal Oeconomy*, 2nd edn, London, G. Strahan, 1717, p. 82.

55. James Jurin, 'De potentia cordis', *Philosophical Transactions*, 29, (1718), 863–72 and 30 (1719), 929–38; James Keill, 'De viribus cordis epistola,' *Philosophical Transactions*, 30 (1719), 995–1000; James Jurin, 'Epistola ... qua doctrinam suam De potentia cordis ... defendit', *Philosophical Transactions*, 30 (1719), 1039–50.

56. F.M. Valadez and C.D. O'Malley, 'James Keill of Northampton: Physician, Anatomist and Physiologist', *Medical History*, 15 (1971), 317–35, at 331.

57. John Quincy, *Medicina Statica ... As Also Medico-Physical Essays*, 4th edn, London, J. Osborn, T. Longman, and J. Newton, 1728, first published 1720. See Valadez and O'Malley, 'James Keill', pp. 331–3.

58. John Freind, *Nine Commentaries Upon Fevers; and Two Epistles Concerning the Small-Pox, Addressed to Dr. Mead*, trans. Thomas Dale, London, T. Cox, 1730.

59. Archibald Pitcairne, *Solutio problematis de historicis: seu de inventoribus dissertatio* (1688), trans. in *Works*, pp. 135–63; Freind, *Nine Commentaries*, preface.

60. R.J.J. Martin, 'Explaining John Freind's *History of Physick*', *Studies in History and Philosophy of Science*, 19 (1988), 399–418.

61. John Freind, *The History of Physick*, 2 vols, 4th edn, London, J. Walthoe and M. Cooper, 1744–50), vol. 2, pp. 274–5. See Martin, 'John Freind's *History of Physick*'.

62. Quincy, *Medicina Statica*, p. 456.

63. Richard Mead, *A Short Discourse Concerning Pestilential Contagion, and the Methods To Be Used To Prevent It*, London, Sam. Buckley and Ralph Smith, 1720, p. 11.

64. Ibid., pp. 34, 49.

65. Daniel Defoe, *A Journal of the Plague Year*, Paula Backscheider (ed.), New York, Norton, 1990.

66. James Jurin, *An Account of the Success of Inoculating the Small Pox in Great Britain. With a Comparison Between the Miscarriages in that Practice, and the Mortality of the Natural Small Pox*, London, J. Peele, 1724, p. 2. See also his *A Letter to the Learned Caleb Cotesworth, M.D.*, London, W. and J. Innys, 1724; Deborah Brunton, 'Pox Britannica: Smallpox Inoculation in Britain, 1721–1830', PhD diss, University of Pennsylvania, 1990; Andrea Rusnock, 'The Quantification of Things Human: Medicine and Political Arithmetic in Enlightenment England and France', PhD diss., Princeton University, 1990.

67. Jurin, *Letter to Caleb Cotesworth*, pp. 19–22.

68. Jurin, *Account*, pp. 32–3.

69. William Cowper, *Myotomia Reformata*, revised edn, London, R. Knaplock et al., 1724, introduction; Newton, *Opticks*, query 24.

70. Nicholas Robinson, *A New Theory of Physick and Diseases, Founded on the Principles of the Newtonian Philosophy*, London, C. Rivington, J. Lacy, and J. Clarke, 1725.

71. George Cheyne, *An Essay of Health and Long Life*, London, G. Strahan, 1724.

72. Thomas Morgan, *Philosophical Principles of Medicine in Three Parts*, London, J. Osborne et al., 1725, pp. ix, xxxv. On Morgan see *DNB*.

73. Morgan, *Philosophical Principles*, pp. 95–110, 373.
74. Thomas Morgan, *The Mechanical Practice of Physick*, London, T. Woodward, 1735, pp. xv–xvi, 1–2, 59.
75. Morgan, *Philosophical Principles of Medicine*, p. 372.
76. Nicholas Robinson, *A New System of the Spleen, Vapours and Hypochondriack Melancholy*, London, 1729.
77. Bryan Robinson, *A Treatise of the Animal Oeconomy*, Dublin, George Grierson, 1732, pp. 82–3.
78. Ibid., p. 98.
79. For Hutchinson, see C.R. Wilde, 'Hutchinsonianism, Natural Philosophy and Religious Controversy in Eighteenth-Century Britain', *History of Science*, 18 (1980), pp. 1–24; C.R. Wilde, 'Matter and Spirit as Natural Symbols in Eighteenth-Century British Natural Philosophy', *British Journal for the History of Science*, 15 (1982), 99–131.
80. George Cheyne, *The English Malady*, London, G. Strahan and J. Leake, Bath, 1733, pp. 69–89.
81. Cheyne, *English Malady*, pp. 2–4. For responses to Cheyne, see my forthcoming book.
82. Morgan, *Mechanical Practice of Physick*, p. 313.
83. Richard Mead, *Medica sacra*, trans. in *The Medical Works of Richard Mead, M.D.*, London, C. Hitch et al., 1762, pp. DLXXX–629. Mead originally published this work in Latin, he explained, to keep it from the eyes of the 'profane or vulgar' (p. DLXXXIV).
84. Morgan, *Mechanical Practice of Physick*, p. xii.

CHAPTER THIRTEEN

Quackery and Enthusiasm, or Why Drinking Water Cured the Plague[1]

Mark Jenner

'We are a people strangely given to quackery and novelty,' wrote a commentator in *The Grub Street Journal* in August 1733,

> and I make no doubt but the cry would run ... in praise of hasty-pudding, or ... of cow-heels, if half a dozen leading people, with a medicaster at the head of them, did but bellow out the wonderful cures they had perform'd. A few years ago, the whole nation, run a madding after the reverend Doctor *Hancock's* practice of drinking cold water, in almost every distemper ... Till at last up starts some merry fellow, by the name of *Gabriel John*, and exposed the Doctor and his practice, in such a ludicrous, but witty manner, that from that time, the customs dwindled, and grew out of use.[2]

Little more has been heard of the reverend John Hancocke's book *Febrifugum Magnum: Or Common Water the Best Cure for Fevers, and Probably for the Plague* (1722) in the intervening 250 years. In this chapter I explore the brief celebrity of Hancocke's publication, asking why a Low Church London clergyman and one time Boyle lecturer should publish a work recommending the drinking of cold water as a remedy for the plague. I discuss why the book warranted frequent reprinting, how it sparked off a brief controversy and conclude by elucidating the wider historiographical issues raised by this pamphlet literature.

For the debates provoked by *Febrifugum Magnum* reveal connections between late seventeenth- and early eighteenth-century anxieties about enthusiasm and the contemporaneous indictments of quacks. This raises questions about how the subject of quackery in this period should be approached. Historians discussing irregular medical practitioners between *c.*1650 and *c.* 1770 have concentrated upon the economic aspects of their subject, emphasizing themes such as commercialization and the medical market-place. I argue that they have consequently paid insufficient attention to the content and structure of condemnations of irregular medicine and to the discursive constructions of 'the quack'. In particular they have failed to discuss the importance of religious, and especially ecclesiological, discourse in the framing of much medical debate in the late seventeenth and early eighteenth centuries.

In November 1722 John Hancocke, rector of St Margaret Lothbury in London and chaplain to the Duke of Bedford, published what was to turn out to be his most popular though also his most criticized book.[3] In *Febrifugum Magnum* Hancocke announced that if you drank cold water early in a fever and then retired to bed, the water would act as a sudorific, promoting perspiration and taking off the disease. The author explained that the origin of this therapy was 'a chance and accidental Experience'.[4] Twenty-seven or 28 years before he had suffered terribly from jaundice, attended by 'a great *Fever*'. The physicians despaired of his recovery, indeed of his survival, for he was racked by an appalling cough that injured his lungs and led him to expectorate blood and phlegm that was 'as black as my Hat'. A friend recommended that he take yellow amber in cold water and this swiftly relieved his next attack. Reasoning that the amber could not have worked so quickly, when he was next afflicted by his jaundice he simply drank water. A gentle sweat resulted and he found that he recovered.[5]

Hancocke then described how he had successfully employed cold water to treat serious fevers and other diseases which had afflicted his children. Perhaps the most dramatic of these cures was when his youngest daughter was sick with measles. She had been attended by an apothecary, but at three o'clock in the morning Hancocke's wife woke him to say that their child was grievously ill. The clergyman concluded that she was unlikely to live more than a few more hours. Reckoning that the apothecary could do little or nothing to relieve her and doubting whether he would arrive in time so late at night, Hancocke persuaded his wife 'to leave her to me, and to submit to God's Providence, whatever might happen'. A wine-glass full of water, followed by three more worked wonders. The blisters which had sunk into the child's body erupted, expelling the poison. She slept peacefully and recovered.[6] Unsurprisingly such medical successes became known in Hancocke's neighbourhood. He described how the wife of a local coffee-house keeper had succumbed to a deadly fever, but when her spouse was afflicted with the same disease, he followed the advice of a clerical acquaintance of Hancocke's, drank water and recovered.

In the remainder of the book Hancocke described other ways in which drinking cold water could improve or preserve health. It was good for asthma and was 'the best Cure for Colds, and soonest sweetens and digests those Humours into a thick, white, sweet Phlegm'. When a curate in a large parish, he had found that an infusion of toast in water was a far better way of relieving tiredness than more usual tonics such as canary or small beer. Water might be combined with other therapies such as exercise.

> If any one that is troubled with a Fit of the Cholick, would drink a
> Quart of cold Water, and keep himself in a moving Posture, now
> sit, now lye, ... lean forward, lean backward, tumble on a Bed, and
> if he can sometimes stand on his Head; or ... get into a Coach, and
> ride on the Stones ... ; the Water ... would set the Peristaltick
> Motion of the Bowels on work, so as to take off the Fit.[7]

He was finally moved to publish his remarkable findings after a conversation with 'a worthy Dignitary of our Church ... talking, as most
People have been apt to do, of the Plague in *France*'. Hancocke outlined
his fever therapy and how he reasoned that it would prove a useful
remedy for the plague. His clerical superior concurred and encouraged
him to publish.[8]

Hancocke is not one of the great names of early eighteenth-century
religion, science or medicine. He warrants no entry in the *Dictionary of
National Biography*. Ginnie Smith has styled him a 'cold-water empiric'.[9] Steven Shapin and Margaret Jacob have described him as a
representative Low Church Newtonian alarmed about the the threat
posed to the Established Church by deists and free-thinkers such as
Toland, Collins and Blount.[10] When he appeared in a satire of Bishop
Berkeley's tar water he was introduced as the reverend doctor whose
'Method of curing the Cholic' was to 'advise the Patient to swallow a
quart of cold Water, and then to stand upon his Head'.[11] He was,
however, not a complete nonentity. During the 1690s he preached before the Society for the Reformation of Manners in St Mary le Bow.[12] In
1706 he preached the Boyle sermons against atheism, meeting Newton
at Archbishop Wake's house that year;[13] he took up his pen in theological dispute with Whiston and the non-juror George Hickes.[14] Charles
Trimnell, Whig Bishop of Norwich and a trustee of the Boyle sermons,
singled out Hancocke's refutation of Hickes in his charge to the diocese's clergy.[15] In 1719 he was made a canon of Canterbury Cathedral
and dined regularly at Lambeth Palace with the Archbishop of Canterbury, William Wake, through the following decade.[16] Hancocke was
Low Church in sympathy, entertaining hopes of comprehension for
Presbyterians. In print he angrily repudiated the suggestion by one
anonymous pamphleteer that Low Church men were no churchmen and
opposed Tory attempts to ban occasional conformity.[17]

In *Febrifugum Magnum* Hancocke made no great claims to medical
expertise. 'It may (and perhaps justly)', he announced, 'be wonder'd,
that I who am not a Physician, should pretend to give ... Directions
about the Cure of any Distemper'.[18] Indeed, he told his readers that
when he came to draw up his book, he found he 'had forgotten the
most common Terms in Physick ... and that I should be forced to talk
more like a Fool than a Physician, unless I took some Time to read a

little'. During the first seven years of his studies he had, he explained, read as many medical books as 'most did that never had a Thought of making a Business' of medicine, but some 30 years before he had given all his books of physick to his son who had become a doctor.[19] So in order to prepare for publication and to establish the novelty of his findings he explained he had 'looked into a great many Physick Books, both Antient and Modern, so far as Indexes will carry me (for I cannot be supposed to have read many of 'em in a few Months time) ... '.[20]

Such statements were to prove a gift for satirists, but Hancocke's bluff declarations of comparative ignorance had a rhetorical purpose. His method, he argued, was based on experiment not arcane medical philosophy. 'I am no Physician', he declared, 'and but a Smatterer in any kind of Philosophy. Only I think my self capable of judging of a plain Experiment, and of Reasoning a little upon it.'[21] Such relatively unambitious intellectual work was, Hancocke argued, appropriate to the state of medical knowledge. He ridiculed the Helmontian

> fanciful Account of the Cause of Fevers, his *Archeus* that inhabits in the upper Orifice of the Stomach, and when any Thing offends him, like a surly Master, or a scolding Mistress ... sets all in a Flame, and ... causes a Fever. But if there be such a testy old Gentleman in the Mouth of the Stomach, I have found, if you put him to bed, and pour a Pint of cold Water on his Head, he will be as quiet as a Lamb.[22]

There had, Hancocke further noted, 'been several very ingenious Books wrote of late about the Animal Oeconomy, about Animal Secretion, &c. We have Mechanical Accounts of Fevers, of the Non-naturals, &c. but these are not enough to raise Physick to a demonstrative Science, equal to Geometry'. He wished 'the Mechanical Men good Success; ... But ... [was] afraid we must still be content to depend upon now and then a little Experiment'.[23]

Several years later Hancocke returned to the subject with another (larger) volume recounting the numerous cures by cold water of which a variety of people had informed him. In the words of its subtitle, the book was 'An ESSAY, to make it probable, that common Water is good for many Distempers that are not mentioned in Dr. Hancocke's *Febrifugum Magnum*'. These included 'Phrensy, Madness, ... Scurvy, Apoplexy, ... Falling-Sickness, ... Diarrhea, Dystentery, ... Piles' and so on. The work was less autobiographical and more systematically organized than Hancocke's first venture into medicine, being arranged according to the conditions for which water therapy was effective. However, the author's empiricism was as pronounced as ever and took on an anti-Newtonian flavour unusual in a former Boyle lecturer.

> We may see by the various Accounts of the Causes of Diseases, given by the best Physicians, how short and dark our Reasonings are of the Causes of Things, and that *Materia subtilis*, Gravitation, Attraction, Specifick Gravity, the Laws of Motion, old or new, when applied to form a Hypothesis to salve the *Phenomena* of Nature, or to lead us to the intimate Nature and Causes of Things are but new Names for the old occult Qualities. And I think experimental Physick too ought to be encouraged, for I doubt there is little Knowledge *a priori* to be had by Dint of Reason, either of the Causes of many Diseases, or the Medicines that will cure them.[24]

Regardless of the physiological theory to which one subscribed (and he maintained a modified scepticism about them all), water was, Hancocke maintained, an excellent form of therapy.

Febrifugum Magnum caused quite a stir. It was republished five times in 1723 and twice more in 1724 and 1726. He was clearly widely read. One obvious attraction of the book was that it offered a cheap therapy for the plague at a time of great anxiety about the disease because of the catastrophic outbreak in Marseilles during 1719–21.[25] This epidemic provoked the government to draw up a draconian and widely criticized quarantine act with the power to enforce military cordons sanitaires.[26] The Church of England ordered official days of fasting; members of the College of Physicians formed a committee to advise Parliament about precautionary measures; the *Philosophical Transactions* (1722–23) reported the results of experiments introducing the bile of dead human plague victims into previously healthy dogs.[27] The magistrates of Middlesex and London established committees to supervise the cleaning of the streets and to take precautions about possible sources of miasma.[28] The press was full of possible panaceas for the disease – including coffee, a variety of tonic drinks, an 'Cephalick and Opthalmick TOBACCO ... impregnated with the Quintessence and Virtues of ... Herbs and Chymical Oils' and a brand of sugar plums.[29] Publishers competed to produce histories of the plague, elaborate comparisons between the outbreak in Marseilles and the 1665 plague in London, as well as debates about its origin and whether it was contagious or not.[30]

Yet this cannot wholly explain the controversy which Hancocke's work provoked. *Febrifugum Magnum* appeared as the danger of infection from France was receding; his harshest critics published their pamphlets after the official days of thanksgiving for the nation's escape from pestilence. Hancocke won a wide readership because his work engaged with earlier debates about therapeutics and became embroiled in long-standing disputes about the nature of medical and religious authority. The appropriate treatment of fevers was one of the most controversial areas of early eighteenth-century medicine, and there was a Europe-wide debate about the therapeutic efficacy of water in such cases. Hancocke's suggestion that water might cure the plague had some plausibility as many commentators saw it as a form of fever,[31] but in the words of the chemist and author, Peter Shaw, '*Whether cold Water may be safely administred in Fevers, is a Question of great Antiquity*'.[32]

During the 1690s Edinburgh had seen a particularly bitter dispute about the proper treatment of fevers. This controversy between partisans of Newton and of Sydenham became (like the one that followed *Febrifugum Magnum*) bound up with issues of politics and religion. Hancocke's scepticism about overarching theory and his emphasis upon therapeutic success and experiment resembled the approach of Thomas Sydenham who, like Hancocke, preferred those who could cure people to those who discoursed learnedly about disease.[33] The London clergyman acknowledged this similarity and stated how pleased he had been to read Sydenham's writings when he was composing his book. Furthermore, Hancocke concurred with the overall thrust of the doctor's approach to therapeutics, stating that 'My Design is only to carry on, and a little improve the cool *Regimen*', which Sydenham had thought best in acute diseases.[34] Hancocke's Low Church sympathies and Whig politics resemble those of Sydenham's protagonists in Edinburgh which have been discussed by Andrew Cunningham.[35]

More generally, water cures were far from a total innovation in the 1720s. Water gruel had long been used as a form of ascetic purification of the body.[36] One contemporary pamphleteer noted that he had been using water as a therapy for over 30 years;[37] in the *Curiosities of Common Water* (London 1723) John Smith claimed more than 40 years experience of the healthful benefits of water drinking. At the turn of the century Sir John Floyer and Edward Baynard had described the virtues of cold bathing and water drinking. In the fifth edition of their *Ancient Psychrolousia Revived* (1722) Baynard claimed that very few inhabitants of London Bridge had died during the 1665 epidemic due to the proximity of cool water.[38]

Like other hydrotherapeutic works, Hancocke's book appealed to sections of opinion anxious about the impact of luxury. As one might expect from a former partisan of the Society for the Reformation of Manners, he lamented plebeian preference for gin over water.[39] In another work Hancocke summarized the arguments in favour of water drinking advanced by the French Jansenist teetotaller and physician, Phillippe Hecquet, though he emphasized that unlike the Frenchman he did not abstain completely from wine.[40] (Interestingly Hancocke's work was considered significant enough on the Continent to be translated into French, Dutch and Italian by the middle of the eighteenth cen-

tury.[41]) Sharing the late seventeenth- and early eighteenth-century pre-
occupation with the correct upbringing of children, he criticized unduly
tight swaddling and excessive parental diet as a prime cause of rickets.[42]
Terrifyingly, in the light of what we know about the infant death rate in
London due to gastro-enteritic disorders, Hancocke recommended cold
water as a remedy for teething children. 'When Children breed their
Teeth they often have a Fever, and sometimes a Diarrhea', he wrote.
'When Parents perceive this, if they would give the Child Water often,
'tis not unlikely it might cure the Fever, and stop the Diarrhea, ...'
Water was, he also maintained, good for young children while they
breast fed. It would be 'good to keep the Milk from coagulating upon
their Stomachs, which many Physicians think is the Original of many ...
Diseases in Children'.[43]

His publications and his reputation as a clergyman encouraged like-
minded people to enter print. During February 1723 Ralph Thoresby
FRS finished Hancocke's pamphlet and reckoned it 'an useful and excellent piece for cure of fevers'.[44] In April of that year Thoresby noted
meeting Hancocke, 'yᵉ pious Author of several learned tracts in divinity
& lately of *Febrifugum Magnum*' and that he was 'pleased with his
conversation'. The following day he went to St Margaret Lothbury and
heard Hancocke preach. He found the sermon 'not very modish', but
one that (unlike the one he heard in the afternoon) 'wil bide ruminating
on'.[45] Indeed Thoresby was moved to advocate hydrotherapy, assisting
the distinctively named clock maker, John Smith, to compile a volume
of water cures.[46] *The Curiosities of Common Water* provided a comprehensive catalogue of doctors' recommendations of cold water therapy
drawing not only upon Hancocke, but upon a wide array of medical
authorities ranging from Sir Thomas Elyot's *Castel of Helthe* to
Boerhaave, Gideon Harvey and John Floyer. The compendium was
further swollen by Smith's extensive personal experience of using water
cures, and cures of which he had learnt from Thoresby and 'by Word of
Mouth'. This work too met with considerable success.[47]

Hancocke's piety and sound theology clearly attracted men such as
Thoresby, while his clerical position lent weight to his opinions.[48] One
critic alleged that his work gained credence because of 'the Influence
which the Canonic Robes constantly obtains over the Minds of the
Populace, and the Air of Candor, and regard for the Safety of Mankind,
with which the Doctor ... communicated his Method'.[49] Yet such clerical influence was controversial. What was the basis of Hancocke's
claims? Was it appropriate for a clergyman to put forward medical
recommendations? Hancocke recognized the difficulty. 'I confess', he
wrote,

> it is a little out of my Way to write in Physick; but I am not the first
> Man that has writ a Book of a Subject he knows little of. And if
> any of the Profession, that censure me for this, will write a good
> Book in Divinity or Morality (as some of 'em have lately done,
> very good ones) I shall not think they intrude upon my Profession,
> I will buy it, and read it, and thank 'em for it.[50]

Not all his contemporaries were so ready to gloss over the demarcation
lines of intellectual and sacerdotal authority. Issues of religion quickly
came to the fore in the pamphlet controversy which *Febrifugum Magnum* provoked. Many of Hancocke's critics interpreted his opinions as
an assault upon their ideal of a society regulated by powerful but
separate clerical and medical professions. As will become clear, religion
(especially ecclesiology) was central to the articulation of these concerns.

One of the first critiques of his work, ostensibly written by one James
Gardner MD, appeared in spring 1723. As 'trifling' as Hancocke's essay
was, Gardner announced, it 'has found a surprizing Acceptance, nor are
there wanting some whose Education might have given them a better
Taste, that defend our Author's Notions'. He sought to demonstrate
that 'the Doctor [i.e. Hancocke] is entirely unqualified to dictate in
Physick', and that his recommendations ought therefore 'to be very
much suspected'.[51] 'There is indeed a Possibility', he acknowledged,
'that cold Water, when duly administred by a prudent Physician, in
proper Circumstances, may be very serviceable.'[52] Galen, Alpinus and
other ancient physicians had on occasions recommended water drinking. Hancocke 'instead of advancing natural Philosophy, or the Practice
of Physick ... has only said what has been often ... practised before'.[53]
But if water was 'not prescrib'd under proper Limitations, what will be
the Consequence but certain Death, a lingering Sickness, or a ruin'd
Constitution?'[54] Hancocke should stick to theology.

> Let him leave Physick to those Gentlemen whose Province it is, and
> cease to be solicitous to *kill for God's Sake*. For I assure him, that a
> Discourse upon Faith and Repentance would have been abun-
> dantly more becoming his Character than a silly Treatise upon the
> Use of Water, and that Dr. *Waterland*'s Defence of his Queries will
> be read with Applause when ... *Febrifugum Magnum* will be hissed
> at with Scorn, and condemn'd to discharge such Duties ... as are
> necessary in the Jakes.[55]

Hancocke, he continued, was neither philosopher nor physician enough
to profer sage medical advice. Gardner repeatedly compared the divine
with notorious quacks such as 'the wonderful Mr *Wiggins*, the Shoe-
Maker of *Leaden-Hall-Street*', whose 'Diet Drink, seems to be abun-
dantly superior to ... *common Water*'. Indeed he concluded his *Remarks* with six pages comparing passages from the two authors in order

to show that they were 'much upon an Equality, in regard to Language and Physick'.[56]

In his prefatory dedication to the College of Physicians, Gardner spelt out general recommendations for medicine. The College ought to regulate medical practice properly, prosecuting unlicensed practitioners rather than countenancing them. They should persuade the Justices of the Peace of Westminster and the Mayor and Aldermen of London to initiate prosecutions for nuisance against the posting of bills for quack cures. They should revert to Latin – 'let him be for ever esteem'd a QUACK,' he declared, 'who presumes to discover the Art of Physick in an English Stile'.[57]

The next and more damaging response to Hancocke's pamphlet was pseudonymous and like most anonymous writing of the 1720s has been attributed to Defoe. Gabriel John's *Flagellum: Or, A Dry Answer to Dr Hancock's Wonderfully Comical Liquid Book, Which He Merrily Calls Febrifugum Magnum ... (a Book Proved Beyond Contradiction, To Be Wrote When the Doctor Was Asleep)*, was published in April 1723, with a second edition a couple of months later. He attacked Hancocke on several fronts. First, like Gardner, 'Gabriel John' emphasized the variety of fevers, of colics and other afflictions and argued that Hancocke's universal recommendation was thus dangerous as it did not distinguish between the varieties of disease. Furthermore, water was not a single substance. There were as many sorts of it as there were kinds of disease.

His satirical technique was to deconstruct Hancocke's arguments, juxtaposing passages from different sections of *Febrifugum Magnum* in order to make it appear nonsensical. 'Gabriel John' seized upon individual words and launched into a series of associative, punning diatribes. He noted that the reason which Hancocke had given for the uncertainty as to when to bleed a fever patient was 'because *Fevers are such tickle Things*'. (Judging by the *Oxford English Dictionary*, 'tickle' was an acceptable, if perhaps unusual term, meaning 'uncertain'.) But then he went on to explore frenetically the possible meanings of the word. 'Now here', he wrote, 'the Doctor wants an *Expositor*, for our *English ones* have no such word; – tickle Things! – the word *tickles* my Fancy strangely! and is really *a ticklish Point*. I fancy the Doctor still remembers a fragment of an old Song (common when he was a Boy) *of* John *come tickle me &c*'.[58]

In other passages he burlesqued the clergymen's claims. He turned Hancocke's jocular remedy for the Helmontian *archeus* of fever into the Hudibrastic patter of a juggling fairground mountebank or a parody of an exorcism.

> Gentlemen, do you see this *thirsty*, red-hot *Phantom*? Gentlemen, this is what we call a *Fever*; now Gentlemen, *you* shall see, how by

my Art of *hocus pocus*, I'll make this Tyrant run away, like a Dog
that has burnt his Tail. In the name of cold Water: Hey! pass!
presto! arise Blunderbuss! *Hixius Doxius*! Be gone! – look ye Gentlemen! ... where's the Fever? Gone! fled! and dead as a Door-
Nail.[59]

Gabriel John did not simply ridicule Hancocke; he attacked the epistemological foundations of his work and associated his claims with those
of religious sectaries. He portrayed the cleric as claiming illumination,
direct inspiration. *Febrifugum*, he maintained, contained '*many things
hard to be understood*, some that have *no meaning* at all, and others
that have a *very good meaning*, but it is not to be come at without very
deep Learning or *Revelation*'.[60] This 'revelation', he suggested, had
come in a dream after eating stewed prunes. Gabriel John was referring
to one (admittedly bizarre) passage of *Febrifugum Magnum* where
Hancocke described how he overcame consumption. He suffered so
badly from this disease that Dr Charleton despaired of his recovery.
One night, however, he ate some stewed prunes that his wife had
cooked and thereafter recovered his health and vitality.[61]

Gabriel John did not simply suggest that Hancocke's experiments
lacked method and that his findings were ill digested. He argued that
Hancocke's utterances were the unwanted results of digestion – in this
case of stewed prunes. By attributing the cleric's text to physiological
(indeed purgative) causes, the satirist's polemic resembled Swift's account in *A Tale of a Tub* of enthusiastic preaching as misdirected
flatus,[62] and echoed many of the descriptions of the French Camisard
prophets as enthusiasts.[63] For one of the most important developments
in English religious and intellectual life during the second half of the
seventeenth century was the emergence and wide dissemination of the
category of 'enthusiasm'. A variety of emotional or ecstatic religious
behaviour, ranging from the Quakers to St Teresa of Avila, was reinterpreted as being the result of physiological and psychological
misfunction.[64]

Gardner too employed this line of argument. Hancocke, he main-
tained, should remember that 'there is in *Physick*, as well as in Matters
Theological, what we call a *Zeal* without knowledge, and that such a
Zeal is very often of fatal Consequence'. The divine was 'in a Passion'.[65]
His prefatory dedication spelt out this link with enthusiasm at greater
length.

> There is not any Profession so much abused as that of Physick, nor
> is there any Nation ... so stupid as to give Encouragement to every
> silly Pretender to Physick as *England*. Should any Enthusiast fancy
> himself gifted, and dare to mount a Pulpit, in order to communi-
> cate his Knowledge to the Populace, the Clergy immediately stand

upon their Guard, take due Care to oppose the bold Attempt, and speedily suppress the presumptuous Invader of their Rights.[66]

Gabriel John and Gardner were not idiosyncratic. The critique of Hancocke's work which was appended to the second edition of the surgeon-turned-physician Daniel Turner's *The Modern Quack* adopted a similar line of argument. It should not 'appear strange', the author maintained, that he had numbered Hancocke 'amongst those *Quacks*, since I find you are, however one of more Letters, yet, in *Physick* as ignorant, and a more dangerous *Empirick* than any of them all'. By working 'under Shew of *godly Simplicity*, abstracted from all sinister Views of Profit', Hancocke, he argued, worked 'more on the unthinking Part of Mankind, and may be said to lay a Snare for their Ruin'.[67] For Hancocke 'to make [water] ... the grand *Febrifuge*', his opponent continued,

> must be surely the Effect of a *Delirium*, or the Result of *Dotage*: Which Belief of ours is farther countenanc'd by some *Enthusiastick* Strains in other Places ... ; such ... as ... *where you are persuading the good Woman to leave your Child to the cold Water and Providence: and committing your self to the stew'd Prunes* ... .[68]

As Philip Wilson has noted, Turner's attacks upon quackery were not simply designed to assist his professional advancement. They were consonant with his alarm about the irreligious implications of Newtonian natural religion. Turner's private devotions reveal that he meditated upon the religious history of mid-seventeenth-century England, including such episodes as James Naylor's entry into Bristol. He felt that the Established Church was in danger from sectaries and those who decried the alleged formality of Anglican services, basing their worship upon their own 'Experience'.[69] In Wilson's words, 'Turner's description of the contemporary "prophets" as pretenders who claimed themselves privileged with divine inspiration was consistent with his characterization of the medical pretenders who claimed themselves privileged in holding cures'.[70]

In Defoe's *Journal of the Plague Year* (published like *Febrifugum* in 1722) we see this same collocation of quacks and enthusiasts. Defoe's depiction of London in 1665 noted how 'the Posts of Houses, and Corners of Streets were plaster'd over with Doctors' Bills, and Papers of ignorant Fellows; quacking and tampering in Physic', while many frightened Londoners were 'wearing Charms, Philters, Exorcisms, Amulets, and I know not what Preparations'. Amidst the plague-stricken city's despair he noted also 'the famous Soloman Eagle, an Enthusiast ... [who] went about denouncing of Judgement upon the City in a frightful manner; sometimes quite naked, and with a Pan of burning Charcoal on his Head'.[71]

The parallels between doctors and the Church, between quackery and enthusiasm, were a particularly live issue in the early 1720s. For in these years medicine was the object of unusual public concern. As we have seen, doctors were in dispute over plague and the quarantine act; the clergy were preaching on the lessons of plague. In addition the introduction of inoculation during these years provoked fierce public criticism in sermons and medical texts.[72] As Gardner noted, Hancocke was not the first clergyman at the time to instruct the public on medical matters.

> Has not his Reverend Brother, ... Mr. *Massey*, dabbl'd in the same Way? Has he not made the Method of managing the Small Pox, the subject of a Sermon, and wittily ... inform'd us ... the Devil *inoculated Job*, in order to deter us from a *laudible* Practice? Has not *Tanner*, the Popish Priest, oblig'd the World with a *Practical Scheme*, a Treatise on the Plague, which he has had the Insolence to dedicate to the *President* of the College ... .[73]

He was referring to the corruscating attack upon inoculation by the London vicar Edward Massey, who in 1722 denounced the practice as impious and dangerous – tempting God by introducing disease into the bodies of the healthy.[74]

However, the relation between religion and medicine in seventeenth- and early eighteenth-century England should not simply be discussed with reference to the piety or theology of individuals like Massey or Turner. Religion was social and structured discussions of the social. As Boyd Hilton has argued, 'Before 1850, especially, religious feeling and biblical terminology so permeated *all* aspects of thought (including atheism) that it is hard to dismiss them as epiphenomenal'.[75] In the late seventeenth and early eighteenth centuries arguments about the organization of knowledge and society almost inevitably spilled over into ecclesiology because 'religion' was not the individual matter that it is today in Western Europe. It was collective, concerned above all with public expression, with issues of authority and the organization of consent.[76]

Commentators moved swiftly from discussions of physicians of the body to physicians of the soul and vice versa. Hancocke's supporters turned naturally to arguments about religious duty and the proper domain of priestly authority when replying to critics of *Febrifugum Magnum*. Thomas Taylor used biblical examples like the cure of Naaman to justify Hancocke's hydrotherapy and seized upon the religious implications of attacking the publication of medical texts in English.

> Tis a mighty Crime, indeed, to translate or write Physick Books in English, 'twas and is so with the Bible in the *Roman* Church, and their Laws against it are as strong as any in *Warwick-Lane*, ... how

can these ... Men condemn the *Roman* Clergy of Barbarity, when they are Guilty of the same Barbarity themselves and would engross the Art of Physick, as the *Papists* do the Bible, only for the use of Language-mongers.[77]

In May 1723 *Pasquin*, a Whig paper fond of summarizing anti-clericalists like John Trenchard, drew the same moral from Gardner's intellectual exclusivity. That month it published a letter to Francis Atterbury, the Bishop of Rochester, supposedly from one 'Passive Bigot'. The latter recommends that in order to win the voice of the populace, the clergy should 'give out that the WHIGS are *inoculating* new Heresies' and use the flaming sermons of Massey to stir up the nation. It further commends the recent words of the clergyman, 'Dr. *Wealthy*' near London, who preached that monastic lands should be restored and '"We have had no good Times ... since the *Bible* has been *translated into English*."' A footnote pointed up the parallel between this caricature of High Church Tory clericalism and Gardner's recent defence of a physician's monopoly.[78]

In contrast, by emphasizing experiment Hancocke and Smith, like Sydenham and many mid-seventeenth-century radicals, said that anyone could make useful innovations in therapy. In the words of one of Hancocke's defenders, 'the liberty of finding out and using those things for the good of others' was 'every Man's Right, whom it shall please God to enable, as is plain from the Sacred Text'.[79] Such an inclusive attitude to medical practice accorded with what we know of Hancocke's notion of the ministry, a topic on which he had debated with the non-juror George Hickes a decade previously. In a volume asserting that the celebration of the sacrament was an authentic sacrifice, Hickes had greatly elevated the function and status of the priest. In Hancocke's eyes such sentiments were not only based upon a misreading of the Scriptures, but smacked of the Roman Catholic mass. He outlined a far less exclusive account of functions of a Church of England minister. He welcomed lay works of piety; he showed himself to be sympathetic to proposals to revise the prayer book in ways which would facilitate the re-entry of dissenters into the Church of England.[80] There was thus a parallel between his relatively comprehensive churchmanship and his attitude towards the medical profession.

The debates about *Febrifugum Magnum* should alert us to developments of broader significance in the representation of quackery. The remainder of this chapter seeks to explore the wider historiographical themes broached in this case study. It will seek first to elucidate the implications of this apparent link between 'quackery' and 'enthusiasm' for the ways in which historians can approach the 'quack'. Secondly, it will explore the origin of the association between these terms and outline how the reaction against enthusiasm in the later seventeenth century altered the ways in which the figure of the quack was represented.

In recent years historians of medicine, religion and science have emphasized how in the late seventeenth and early eighteenth centuries many members of the Church of England reacted against the emotional and illuminist forms of Protestantism supposedly practised by the Quakers and other sects. Such perceived excesses of zeal were labelled as enthusiasm. For Simon Schaffer and Steve Shapin, Boyle's construction of a delimited physical and intellectual space for experiment was in part at least a reaction to the epistemological challenge of the Quakers. Schaffer has further demonstrated how when the Scottish Jacobite physician, Archibald Pitcairne, reduced medicine to Newtonian principles he was building a buttress against the social upheavals which in his opinion were the result of the enthusiasm and levelling principles of Whig Presbyterians.[81] Michael MacDonald has argued convincingly that a crucial reason for the marginalization of the belief in demonic possession and the efficacy of exorcism was that during the late seventeenth and early eighteenth centuries such beliefs became tarred with the brush of enthusiastic religion. Similarly, Mary Fissell has suggested that the repudiation of enthusiasm was a central theme in the élite retreat from popular forms of medical care over the eighteenth century and that this reaction against the 'enthusiastic' was most marked during times of political anxiety such as the 1740s and 1790s.[82]

However, historians discussing seventeenth- and eighteenth-century irregular medicine have downplayed such religious and political themes. The literature on quackery in the long eighteenth century is not particularly extensive; Roy Porter's *Health for Sale* is the most important recent survey of the topic.[83] Porter's account of irregular practice is dominated by the market. Unfettered commercial medicine manipulating the resources of print gave every eighteenth-century doctor a potentially quackish aura. The cash nexus liberated more affluent patients from the strictures of their physicians, permitting them to consult freely across the diverse range of practitioners as their whims and their wallets permitted.

A similar account of the medical market in the sixteenth and seventeenth centuries can be found in Lucinda Beier's work. She offers a largely commercial analysis of the sixteenth- and seventeenth-century texts attacking empirics. '[M]otivated partly by a desire to raise medical standards ... and partly by the wish to protect and increase their own practices, incomes and social status, licensed medical practitioners launched what might be described as an advertising campaign to sell their own point of view.'[84] Although she has written extensively of how religion structured individual responses to illness and death,[85] her account does not link such ideological themes and religious tropes with the representations and workings of the medical market.

H.J. Cook's surveys of the professional status of learned physic bear many similarities to Porter's account of the long eighteenth century. He emphasizes the professional status and self-consciousness of learned physicians in the sixteenth and seventeenth centuries, bringing out the striking similarities with the self-image of the clergy; it was the physicians' prudence and good moral character that were their essential qualities and qualifications. However, he argues that the increasingly commercial nature of late seventeenth- and eighteenth century society, coupled with the 'alternative notions of virtue' articulated by, for example, medical chemists, dissolved the respect and social connections upon which learned physic depended.[86]

This historiography admirably integrates the history of medicine into a broader picture of England's social and economic experience, but I find its account unsatisfyingly economistic. Many historians would now argue that political and class identities in the eighteenth and nineteenth centuries were not a simple reflection of economic transformation but were culturally and discursively constructed.[87] By contrast many historians continue to treat the terms denoting the social identity of eighteenth-century medical practitioners as if they simply reflected market forces. In Porter's words, 'Quackery was the capitalist mode of production in its medical face'.[88]

Yet as Porter's work also demonstrates, such an economic framework is singularly unhelpful if you wish to discuss the contemporary meanings of the term. The 'quack' was above all an imaginative construct, a label which you applied to others, a phantasm which haunted medical jeremiads.[89] Practitioners such as William Read, the occulist, or Joshua Ward, purveyor of his celebrated pills, were hailed as quacks by some and as orthodox and efficacious by others. Unlike the names 'Sydenham', 'Hippocrates', and 'Galen', or the labels 'ancient' or 'learned', the word 'quack' was not one around which social or professional solidarities were constructed. Economic changes, such as the so-called 'consumer revolution',[90] can provide an explanation for the increase in the sale of drugs and the number of doctors in late seventeenth- and early eighteenth-century England, but they do not account for the ways in which 'quacks' were denounced in the same period.[91] In particular the relevant historiography underestimates the extent to which late Stuart and early Hanoverian systems of authority were articulated with reference to religious discourse; it suggests that 'commercial society' was somehow isolated from the Societies for the Reformation of Manners, the Society for Promoting Christian Knowledge and 'Church in Danger' riots.

It is revealing that the one time Porter acknowledges the association which contemporaries drew between quacks and enthusiasts, he denies that the congruence of these tropes had any significance. In his words,

> Enthusiastic religion and radical politics spelt danger in post-Restoration England because they presented alternative, critical metaphysics that rocked the boat of oligarchic consensus. Not so with quack medicine. The 'Enthusiast in Physick' was not a schismatic or a revolutionary but an entertainer; radical, if radical at all, only as radical chic.[92]

This denial of a significant religious dimension to the question of quackery and to the discursive structure of medicine after 1660 is historiographically perplexing.[93] Although Christopher Hill, Charles Webster and Peter Elmer disagree with each other, they concur on the centrality of religion for many mid-seventeenth century advocates of empirical medicine.[94] Furthermore, as Porter has noted, there is a burgeoning literature on the intersection between the various forms of Victorian fringe medicine and nonconformist or spiritualist sects.[95] Simon Schaffer has shown the epistemological divisions which surfaced around electrical therapy and showmanship in the mid-eighteenth century. Jonathan Barry has shown the links between the religious beliefs of the Bristol accountant, William Dyer, and the forms of treatment which he found conducive.[96] There is a substantial literature about the religious dimensions of the medical work of, for instance, Cheyne and Berkeley.[97] If we are to develop a fuller account of the construction of regular and irregular medicine in the long eighteenth century we need to incorporate these kinds of therapies and these kinds of cosmologies into our image of the period and also into our examination of the ways in which the categories 'regular' and 'irregular', 'quack' and 'orthodox' were constituted.

For the parallel between the physicians and the priest or godly minister was an ancient one in late Stuart England,[98] as was the more specific analogy between mechanic preachers and empirics in medicine. However, the polemical link between medical and religious *enthusiasm* was really forged in the anti-chemical and anti-illuminist discourses of the 1640s and 1650s. Just as the political language of the 1720s revolved around the events of the civil war and Interregnum with Tory election crowds in Westminster accusing their Whig opponents of following the Rump, so some of quackery's role in the language of medical dispute can be traced back to the mid-seventeenth century.[99]

In the middle decades of the seventeenth century there was, I would suggest, a shift in the representations of the unlicensed practitioner, the 'other' of learned medicine.[100] Previously denunciations of the 'quacksalver' or empiric were structured either by the Calvinist notion of the calling, as in John Hart's 1625 denunciation of piss-prophets,[101] or were related to the anxieties expressed in the 'coney catching' literature of the time, purporting to expose the fraud and deceit of a highly organized underworld. The poor law legislation of the sixteenth century was highly suspicious of cunning folk and itinerant healers; generically many denunciations of the mountebank were related to the texts denouncing masterless men. Thus in 1564 Thomas Gale wrote of empirics as the 'dross of the earth', 'minstrels, souters, horseleeches, jugglers ... and a rabble of that sect', who turned to healing 'when they cannot otherwise live'.[102]

During the mid-seventeenth century there were, as is well known, bitter attacks upon the alleged élitism, profiteering and incompetence of learned medicine from advocates of chemical medicine, state-sponsored training and Baconian empiricism. Regardless of whether more or less Antinomian sects or Calvinist Puritans were the main source of such medical innovation in the mid-seventeenth century, the anti-sectarian and anti-Puritan stereotypes generated during the 1650s structured the representations of unorthodox medicine for the next half century and beyond. You 'may call him an Enthusiast in Physick, or a Gifted Brother in the knack of healing', wrote a 1676 satirist of a quack-doctor. In 1667 George Castle, a former fellow of All Souls' College, Oxford, who sought to reconcile chemical and Galenist medicine along mechanist lines, lamented that 'Our Nation is of late grown as fond of Enthusiasts in *Physick*, as they were of those in *Divinity*; and Ignorance (amongst some men) is become as necessary a qualification for the practise of *Physick*, as it us'd to be for *Preaching*'.[102]

A couple of years earlier the physician, Nathaniel Hodges, sought to enlist Archbishop Sheldon to the cause of the college of physicians and a system of medical regulation by playing on episcopal memories of the interregnum. '*The neer alliance between* DIVINITY *and* MEDICINE,' he wrote,

> whose relation is as intimate as the Union of SOUL and BODY, hath setled such a Sympathy in both Professions, that they necessarily partake of the Infelicity and Prosperity happening to each other; and thence it was, that when the REVEREND CLERGY (during the late Rebellion) suffered according to their sworn Enemies implacable Fury, the Professors of PHYSICK also by the prevailing INVASION of Empericks shared in the common Calamity.

However, he spelt out still further the implications of this relation in a post-revolutionary society:

> since the Restitution of our RELIGION and CLERGY, Physicians do justly congratulate the Success of both, and do most heartily

wish that the CHURCH may never fall again into the hands of
Emperical Divines who as rudely treated peoples Souls, as the
present Quacks in Physick do their Bodies, their crude and extemporary Effusions directly answering the others unskilful and dangerous Medicaments.

And although the condition of Physick ... [he continued] is very
little bettered, as if it were to be quite excluded from the benefits of
the PUBLICK DELIVERANCE, yet we despair not by reason particularly of your GRACES Readiness ... to Patronize LEARNING,
that the Profession of PHYSICK and legitimate Physicians will
after a long Confusion be separated ... from the Dregs of illiterate
Practisers: Such it seems is the boldness both of our common
Empericks and upstart Pseudochymists, that they presume to entertain as great hopes of their prevailing over all ACADEMICKS, as
the CHURCHES Enemies impatiently expect a Revolution.[104]

Hodges was appealing to Sheldon in an attempt to head off the Archbishop's sponsorship of the Society of Chemical Physicians established
in London at the time of the 1665 plague.[105] Moreover, Paracelsians
and Helmontians (often associated with forms of extreme and sectarian
Protestantism) were also most frequently tarred with the brush of enthusiasm. Chemists were one of the varieties of enthusiast identified by
Henry More in *Enthusiasmus Triumphatus*, and this label was regularly
reused up into the early eighteenth century and revealingly resurfaced in
the 1720s when the authority of learned physick was once again implicitly under challenge by the possible spread of plague. Thus Sir Richard
Blackmore's discussion of plague spoke of 'THE *Paracelsians,
Rosycrusians* and *Helmontian Chymists*, those *Mystical Philososphers*
and *Enthusiasts* in *Physick*'.[106]

More generally, the hostile representations and constructions high-
lighted three themes common to quacks and enthusiasts. The first was
their shared extravagance of language. Both quacks and the enthusiast
were accused of making grandiloquent and universalizing claims, of
breaking textual authorities (be they Biblical or classical) into fragments, invoking their authority while not interpreting their overall sense
correctly.[107] During the 1690s a critic of Sir John Colbatch's treatise on
gout complained how Colbatch 'got into a Cant of *Experimental knowledge, Experiments* upon the *Blood*, and such things you understand,
and use the very same way that *Enthusiasts* do the Scripture'.[108] As we
have seen in the case of Hancocke, hostile portrayals of unofficial
healers often tortured their texts into incoherence. Secondly, the
demonized others of religion and medicine – the tub preacher and the
mountebank – were itinerant, without a fixed or properly appointed
place in which to perform their services. Thirdly, they were alike in
ignorance. They denied the need for formal education, particularly
university education, invoking unstructured and unregulated authority.

More generally, hostile commentators saw the claims to inspiration imputed to quacks and enthusiasts, (and which can be seen in much seventeenth- and eighteenth-century medical advertising) as indicating a loss of the rational faculties. For Henry More enthusiasm resulted from the excess of the passions; similarly the credence given to quackery or godly simplicity like drinking water was attributed to the temporary triumph of the passions. James Sedgwick, an apothecary of Stratford le Bow, in a sensible book recommending the medicinal virtues of warm beer and good wine, argued that the credence given to Hancocke's 'preposterous' assertions showed that 'SUCH is our unhappy Frailty, when our Passions are hoisted, whatever is predominant, becomes suasive and prevailing, hood-winks our Reason so, as ... to deprive us of its true Exertion'. 'Mankind', Peter Shaw concluded, 'are not less ready to be abused about their Bodies, than their Souls; nor did Priest-craft ever run ... to greater Extravagancies ... than Physick-craft'.[109]

However, there was a symmetry in the use of these terms of abuse. If quacks were medical enthusiasts, then enthusiasts were spiritual mountebanks and religious quacks. In the press of the 1650s Quakers quacked as well as quaking. Meric Casaubon worried that the Cartesian cultivation of doubt would 'raise the expectations of the credulous, and ... send them away pure Quacks or arrand Quakers', [110] while more popular pamphlets like The Quacking Mountebanck, or The Jesuite Turn'd Quaker (1655) made the association even more explicit.

Later in the seventeenth century Anglicans frequently termed Roman Catholics religious mountebanks and their nonconformist and sectarian rivals spiritual quacks. 'There are Quacks in Divinity, as well as in Physick', noted The Entertainer in 1717.[111] Jonathan Swift parodied papal pronouncements by turning Peter's projects in A Tale of a Tub into quacking advertisements.[112] In a sermon on the use of words, Robert South termed church fanatics 'mountebanks and quacks'.[113] In his assault on enthusiasm delivered in Oxford in 1680 George Hickes styled the Quakers 'Spiritual Mountebanks', while 40 years later Thomas Lewis described the canting tones of a conventicle meeting and concluded that he had no wonder that there were such throngs at mountebanks' stalls when one saw the ways in which enthusiasts played upon the foolish sensibilities of emotional women susceptible to the influence of rhetoric.[114] Later in the century London debating societies argued about the relative danger posed by Methodist teachers, trading justices and quacks in medicine.[115]

It is striking how often in the late seventeenth and early eighteenth centuries this language – describing enthusiasts as quacks and vice versa – was associated with High Churchmen. They are not the attacks on unlicensed practitioners made by early seventeenth-century Calvinists.

Later seventeenth-century critics of quackery tended to be sacramentalist in their ecclesiology and thus wished to elevate the status of the clergy and to stress the virtues of university scholarship. The sociological fit between this rhetoric and a particular wing of the church was far from perfect – the language of quackery was far too protean and and adaptable for that, but it is clear that one cannot disassociate religious authority from the workings and representations of the medical market-place.

Notes

1. A version of this paper was presented to a seminar at All Souls' College, Oxford in March 1994. I am grateful to the organizers and audience for their comments. I have learnt much from conversations with Justin Champion, Mary Fissell, David Harley and Rob Illiffe. My thanks also to Roger Cooter, Ludmilla Jordanova, Margaret Pelling, Adrian Wilson and especially to Patricia Greene for their comments on drafts of this article. I wish to acknowledge the financial assistance of the Wellcome Trust which supported the research for this paper.
2. I quote from the reprint in *The Gentleman's Magazine*, III (1733), 418.
3. For an announcement of publication, see *The Post-Boy* No. 5202, 22–24 November 1722.
4. *Febrifugum Magnum: Or, Common Water the Best Cure for Fevers, and Probably for the Plague*, London, 1723, p. 8.
5. Ibid., pp. 19–21.
6. Ibid., pp. 40–42. Quotation p. 41. For a discussion of the relationship between the doctrine of Providence and godly understandings of disease, see D. Harley, 'Spiritual Physic, Providence and English Medicine, 1560–1640', in O.P. Grell and A. Cunningham (eds), *Medicine and the Reformation*, London, 1993.
7. Hancocke, *Febrifugum*, pp. 47–58, quotations pp. 54 and 58.
8. Ibid., p. 28.
9. V. Smith, 'Physical Puritanism and Sanitary Science: Material and Immaterial Beliefs in Popular Physiology, 1650–1840', in W.F. Bynum and R. Porter (eds), *Medical Fringe and Medical Orthodoxy 1750–1850*, London, 1987, p. 179; V. Smith, 'Prescribing the Rules of Health: Self-Help and Advice in the Late Eighteenth Century', in R. Porter (ed.), *Patients and Practitioners*, Cambridge, 1985, p. 261. Hancocke's advocacy of cold water is also noted in C.F. Mullett, *The Bubonic Plague and England*, Lexington, KY, 1956, p. 296.
10. S. Shapin, 'Of Gods and Kings:', *Isis*, 71 (1981), 197; M.C. Jacob, *The Newtonians and the English Revolution*, Hassocks, 1976, p. 158. Hancocke died in 1728: Public Record Office, PROB11/623/209.
11. *Siris in the Shades: A Dialogue Concerning Tar Water*, London, 1744, p. 20. Some other commentators were more respectful; T.H. Croker, T. Williams and S. Clark (eds), *The Complete Dictionary of Arts and Sciences*, 3 vols, London, 1765–66, s.v. water.
12. J. Hancocke, *A Sermon Preach'd at the Church of St. Mary le Bow ... December 26. 1698*, London, 1699. He was appointed to St Margaret

Lothbury six months before preaching this sermon, Guildhall Library, MS 9550, entry under St Margaret Lothbury.

13. Hancocke, *Sermon*; Jacob, *Newtonians*, p. 158.
14. J. Hancocke, *Arianism not the Primitive Christianity*, London, 1713; J. Hancocke, *An Answer to Some Things Contain'd in Dr. Hick's Christian Priesthood Asserted*, London, 1709; J. Hancocke, *Patres Vindicati*, London, 1709.
15. J. Johnson, *The Propitiatory Oblation in the Holy Eucharist Truly Stated, and Defended*, London, 1710, p. 110.
16. Lambeth Palace Library MS 1770 f. 223v and *passim*. For a letter from Hancocke to Wake, see, Christ Church, Oxford, Wake MS 21 no. 291.
17. J. Hancocke, *The Low-Church-Men Vindicated From the Unjust Imputation of Being No-Church-Men*, London, 1705, esp. pp. 14–26.
18. *Febrifugum Magnum*, p. 3.
19. Ibid., p. 16.
20. Ibid., p. 18. Hancocke was a learned man and possessed an extensive library which was sold in 1730. Unfortunately, the sale catalogue amalgamated his books with two other collections and it is thus impossible to say what books he owned, *A Catalogue of the Libraries of ... William HEWER, ... Thomas Hobart M.D. And the Reverend JOHN HANCOCKE D.D.*, London, 1730.
21. *Febrifugum Magnum*, p. 15.
22. Ibid., pp. 12–13.
23. Ibid., pp. 9, 10–11.
24. J. Hancocke, *Febrifugum Magnum, Morbifugum Magnum*, London, 1726, pp. 28–9. Although the sale catalogue including Hancocke's library (see n. 20 above) contains copies of Newton's *Opticks*, *Principia* and *Chronology* there is no evidence to suggest that they belonged to Hancocke.
25. C. Carrière, M. Courdurié and F. Rebuffat, *Marseille, ville morte. La peste de 1720*, Marseille, 1968; J.B. Bertrand, *A Historical Relation of the Plague at Marseilles in the Year 1720*, trans. A. Plumptre, London, 1805; reprinted with an introduction by J.N. Biraben, n.p., 1973.
26. For this episode, see P. Slack, *The Impact of Plague in Tudor and Stuart England*, London, 1985, pp. 326–37; L. Stewart, 'The Edge of Utility: Slaves and Smallpox in the Early Eighteenth Century', *Medical History*, 29 (1985), 54–7; C.F. Mullett, 'The English Plague Scare of 1720–23', *Osiris*, 2 (1936), 484–516.
27. Mullett, *Bubonic Plague*, ch. 12; *Philosophical Transactions*, 370 (January–March 1722/3), 20–32; R. Williamson, 'The Plague of Marseilles and the Experiments of Professor Anton Deidier on its Transmission', *Medical History*, 2 (1958), 237–52.
28. S. Webb and B. Webb, *English Local Government From the Revolution to the Municipal Corporations Act: The Parish and the County*, London, 1906, p. 402.
29. Anon., *Of the Use of Tobacco, Tea, Coffee, Chocolate and Drams*, London, 1722, p. 6 and *passim*; Anon., *The Late Dreadful Plague at Marseilles Compared with that Terrible Plague in London, in the Year 1665*, London, 1721.
30. Mullett, 'The English Plague Scare'.

31. Some Marseilles physicians initially insisted that the disease afflicting their city 'was only a putrid fever', Bertrand, *Historical Relation*, p. 59.

32. P. Shaw, *The Juice of the Grape*, London, 1724, p. 1n. As Jan Golinski has pointed out, in the 1720s Shaw was heavily dependent upon the patronage of élite London physicians, 'Peter Shaw: Chemistry and Communication in Augustan England', *Ambix*, 30 (1983), 19–29.

33. The best available study of Sydenham is A. Cunningham, 'Thomas Sydenham: Epidemics, Experiment and the "Good Old Cause"', in R. French and A. Wear (eds), *The Medical Revolution of the Seventeenth Century*, Cambridge, 1989, pp. 164–90.

34. Hancocke, *Febrifugum Magnum*, pp. 17–19, quotation p. 19. Fundamental for discussions of the cool regimen, is Smith 'Physical Puritanism'.

35. A. Cunningham, 'Sydenham Versus Newton: The Edinburgh Fever Dispute of the 1690s Between Andrew Brown and Archibald Pitcairne', in W.F. Bynum and V. Nutton (eds), *Theories of Fever, Medical History*, Supplement 1 (1981), 71–98. For further discussion of this dispute, see, A. Guerrini, '"A Club of Little Villains": Rhetoric, Professional Identity and Medical Pamphlet Wars', in M.M. Roberts and R. Porter (eds), *Literature and Medicine during the Eighteenth Century*, London, 1993.

36. E.g. the reference in Sir Charles Sedley's poem, 'The Doctor and His Patients', printed in V. de Sola Pinto, *Restoration Carnival*, London, 1954, p. 62; or *The Tatler*, D.F. Bond (ed.), 3 vols, Oxford, 1987, vol. iii p. 236.

37. T. Taylor, *Remarks on Remarks*, London, 1723, pp. 22–3. This work (which is not on the ESTC CD-Rom) is to be found in the Guildhall Library in London, Pamphlet 8369.

38. J. Floyer and E. Baynard, *Ancient Psychrolousia Revived*, pt II, pp. 232–5. See also, pp. 293–4 and pp. 431–2, 'The *Country Parson's* Verses on *Cold-bathing*, &c'. One should, however, also note that most early modern water cures were surrounded by pamphlet disputes.

39. Hancocke, *Febrifugum Magnum*, 8th edn, London, 1726, p. 112.

40. *The Physical Use of Common Water, Recommended from France*, London, 1726, esp. pp. 17–18. For Hecquet, see L. Brockliss, 'The Medico-Religious Universe of an Early Eighteenth-Century Parisian Doctor: The Case of Philippe Hecquet', in French and Wear (eds), *The Medical Revolution of the Seventeenth Century*.

41. *Traité des Vertus Medicinales de l'eau Commune*, Paris, 1725; *Verhandeling van de genezende kragten van't gemeene water*, Amsterdam, 1726; *Trattato delle virtu' medicinali dell'acqua comune*, Venice, 1749.

42. On this see, M. Jenner, 'Bathing and Baptism: Sir John Floyer and the Politics of Cold Bathing', forthcoming in K. Sharpe and S. Zwicker (eds), *Refiguring Revolutions*, Berkeley and Los Angeles, 1997.

43. Hancocke, *Febrifugum Magnum, Morbifugum Magnum*, pp. 230, 280.

44. *Diary of Ralph Thoresby*, J. Hunter (ed.), 2 vols, London, 1830, vol. ii p. 354. Thoresby may well have discussed the work with his friends and acquaintances. The next month the Leeds schoolmaster, John Lucas, wrote to him, mentioning that his wife 'fell very ill that morning you set out; wee thought 'twas a fever; she drank water, swet profusely, and the

fever abated', *Letters Addressed to Ralph Thoresby F.R.S.*, W.T. Lancaster (ed.), Thoresby Society, **21** (1912), 256.

45. Yorkshire Archaeological Society (hereafter YAS), MS 25 p. 179. Thoresby met Hancocke nearly a decade before, styling him 'a moderate & pious divine' and noting his publications against Hickes and Whiston, York Minster Library, Add. MS 21 p. 393.

46. YAS, MS 25 p. 178. Several decades earlier Smith published tracts on the barometer and on painting with oils: *A Compleat Discourse of the Baroscope*, London, 1688; *The Art of Painting in Oyl*, 2nd impression, London, 1687.

47. *The Curiosities of Common Water*, London, 1723, ran to 12 editions by 1740. The Wellcome Institute Library contains a copy of the third edition with Thoresby's ownership signature, (MST.162.9).

48. Shortly after his return from his stay in London Thoresby berated himself for not making more of Hancocke's pious company, YAS MS 25 p.194.

49. J. Gardner, *Remarks Upon the Reverend Dr. Hancocke's Febrifugum Magnum*, London, 1723, p. 8.

50. *Febrifugum*, p. 108. Hancocke singled out Sir Richard Blackmore's religious writing for praise. For the latter's contemporary reputation, see R.C. Boys, *Sir Richard Blackmore and the Wits* London, 1949; repr. New York, 1969.

51. J. Gardner, *Remarks*, sig. A2v–3. Gardner's identity is mysterious; the name almost certainly a pseudonym; see, *A Counterfeit Detected*, London, 1723.

52. Ibid., p. 45.

53. Ibid., pp. 14–20, quotation p. 14–15.

54. Ibid., p. 45.

55. Ibid., pp. 12–13. Daniel Waterland was a highly influential divine who wrote widely read critiques of Arianism during the 1710s and 1720s.

56. Ibid., pp. 5, 62–8.

57. Ibid., Preface.

58. Gabriel John, *Flagellum: Or, A Dry Answer to Dr Hancocke's Wonderfully Comical Liquid Book, Which He Merrily Calls Febrifugum Magnum ... (a Book Proved Beyond Contradiction To Be Wrote When the Doctor Was Asleep)*, London, 1723, p. 42–3. Hearne noted both Hancocke's work and Gabriel John's 'comical' response, *Remarks and Collections of Thomas Hearne VIII (1722–1725)*, Oxford Historical Society, **50** (1907), 73.

59. *Flagellum*, p. 25.

60. *Flagellum*, p. 12.

61. Hancocke, *Febrifugum Magnum*, pp. 44–5.

62. For the intellectual genealogy of Swift's satire from Burton and Henry More, see C.M. Webster, 'Swift and Some Earlier Satirists of Puritan Enthusiasm', *PMLA* **48** (1933), 1141–53; M.V. DePorte, *Nightmares and Hobbyhorses*, San Marino, 1974, ch. 2; P. Harth, *Swift and Anglican Rationalism*, Chicago, 1959.

63. H. Schwarz, *Knaves, Fools, Madmen, and that Subtile Effluvium*, Gainsville, FL, 1978, ch. 2. For a full account of the prophecies of these French Protestant refugees and their reception in late seventeenth- and

early eighteenth-century London, see H. Schwarz, *The French Prophets*, Berkeley and Los Angeles, 1980.

64. G. Rosen, 'Enthusiasm: "a Dark Lanthorn of the Spirit"', *Bulletin of the History of Medicine*, 42 (1968), 393–421; G. Williamson, 'The Restoration Revolt Against Enthusiasm', *Studies in Philology*, 30 (1933), 571–603; M. Heyd, 'The Reaction to Enthusiasm in the Seventeenth Century: Towards in Integrative Approach', *Journal of Modern History*, 53 (1981), 258–80.

65. Gardner, *Remarks*, pp. 2, 44. For the contemporary interpretation of frenzy as zeal unrestrained by reason, Rosen, 'Enthusiasm: "a Dark Lanthorn of the Spirit"', pp. 400–1.

66. Gardner, *Remarks*, sig. [A3]. Gardner also compared the situation in medicine with that in the law. 'The Gentlemen of the long Robe are under proper Restrictions, and none can be admitted to the Bar, but by a just Observance of the Circumstances previously necessary for the obtaining of such an Honour.'

67. D. Turner, *The Modern Quack; or Medicinal Impostor*, 2nd edn, London, 1724, p. 155.

68. Ibid., p. 157.

69. British Library, Add. MS 14, 404 ff. 5–6v.

70. P. Wilson, 'Surgeon "Turned" Physician: The Career and Writings of Daniel Turner (1667–1741)', PhD, London University, 1992, p. 161.

71. D. Defoe, *A Journal of the Plague Year* L. Landa (ed.), with a new introduction by D. Roberts, Oxford, 1990, pp. 30, 32, 103. Cf. S. Schaffer, 'Defoe's Natural Philosophy and the Worlds of Credit', in J. Christie and S. Shuttleworth (eds), *Nature Transfigured*, Manchester, 1989, pp. 30–4.

72. See G. Miller, *The Adoption of Inoculation for Smallpox in England and France*, Philadelphia, 1957; D. Brunton, 'Pox Britannica: Smallpox Inoculation in Britain, 1721–1830', PhD, University of Pennsylvania, 1990, esp. chs 1–2; A. Wilson, 'The Politics of Medical Improvement in Early Hanoverian London' in A. Cunningham and R. French (eds), *The Medical Enlightenment of the Eighteenth Century*, Cambridge, 1990, pp. 24–34; Stewart, 'The Edge of Utility'.

73. Gardner, *Remarks*, pp. 4–5.

74. E. Massey, *A Sermon Against the Dangerous and Sinful Practice of Inoculation*, London, 1722.

75. B. Hilton, *The Age of Atonement*, Oxford, paperback edn, 1991, p. ix. For the importance of religious and Biblical rhetorics in early nineteenth-century radicalism, see I. McCalman, *Radical Underworld*, Cambridge, 1988.

76. For a perceptive commentary on these issues, see J. Champion, 'Europe's Enlightenment and National Historiographies: Rethinking Religion and Revolution (1649–1789)', *Europa*, I, i (1993), 73–93.

77. *Remarks on Remarks*, pp. 32–3.

78. *Pasquin*, 31, 3 May 1723.

79. Taylor, *Remarks*, pp. 4–5.

80. J. Hancocke, *An Answer to Some Things Contain'd in Dr. Hick's Christian Priesthood Asserted*, London, 1709; *The Low-Church-men Vindicated*, London, 1705, p. 26.

81. S. Shapin and S. Schaffer, *Leviathan and the Air Pump*, Princeton, 1985;

S. Schaffer, 'Anglo-Dutch Medicine and the Glorious Revolution', *Notes and Records of the Royal Society*, **43** (1989), 174–7.

82. M. MacDonald, 'Religion, Social Change and Psychological Healing in England 1600–1800', in W.J. Sheils (ed.), *The Church and Healing*, Oxford, 1982; M. Fissell, *Patients, Power and the Poor in Eighteenth-Century Bristol*, Cambridge, 1991, esp. ch. 9.

83. R. Porter, *Health for Sale*, Manchester, 1989.

84. L.M. Beier, *Suffers and Healers*, London, 1987, p. 33.

85. Ibid., esp. chs 6–8; L.M. Beier, 'The Good Death in Seventeenth-Century England', in R. Houlbrooke (ed.), *Death, Ritual and Bereavement*, London, 1989.

86. H.J. Cook, 'Good Advice and Little Medicine: The Professional Authority of Early Modern English Physicians', *Journal of British Studies*, **33** (1994), 1–31; quotation p. 23. See also H.J. Cook, 'The New Philosophy and Medicine in Seventeenth-Century England', in D.C. Lindberg and R.S. Westman (eds), *Reappraisals of the Scientific Revolution*, Cambridge, 1990.

87. Notable in this historiography are G. Stedman Jones, 'Rethinking Chartism', in his *Languages of the People*, Cambridge, 1983; P. Joyce, *Visions of the People*, Cambridge, 1991; J. Epstein, 'Understanding the Cap of Liberty: Symbolic Practice and Social Conflict in Early Nineteenth-Century England', *Past and Present*, **122** (1989), 75–118; A. Clark, 'The Rhetoric of Chartist Domesticity', *Journal of British Studies*, **31** (1992), 62–88.

88. Porter, *Health for Sale*, p. 43.

89. E.g. R. Porter, '"I think Ye Both Quacks": The Controversy Between Dr Theodore Myersbach and Dr John Coakley Lettsom', in Bynum and Porter (eds), *Medical Fringe and Medical Orthodoxy*.

90. The classic text on these themes is N. McKendrick, J. Brewer and J.H. Plumb, *The Birth of a Consumer Society*, London, 1982.

91. Cf. Andrew Wear's thorough discussion of the rhetorical uses of Christian ethics and the law in the physicians' writings in Tudor and early Stuart England, 'Medical Ethics in Early Modern England', in A. Wear, J. Geyer-Kordesch and R. French (eds), *Doctors and Ethics*, Amsterdam and Atlanta, 1993, pp. 98–130.

92. Porter, *Health for Sale*, p. 48.

93. Some of Porter's more recent writings moderate this emphasis upon the market: 'Historians have been so concerned with questions such as the secularization of the medical world-view that they have neglected to study the continuing religious motivations for medical practice', R. Porter, 'Thomas Gisborne: Physicians, Christians and Gentlemen', in Wear, Geyer-Kordesch and French (eds), *Doctors and Ethics*, p. 267.

94. C. Hill, *The World Turned Upside Down*, London, 1972, ch. 14; C. Webster, *The Great Instauration*, London, 1975, esp. ch. 4; P. Elmer, 'Medicine, Religion and the Puritan Revolution', in French and Wear (eds), *Medical Revolution*.

95. Porter, *Health for Sale*, pp. 231–35; L. Barrow, *Independent Spirits*, London, 1986; J.V. Pickstone, 'Establishment and Dissent in Nineteenth-Century Medicine' in Sheils (ed.), *The Church and Healing*.

96. S. Schaffer 'The Consuming Flame: Electrical Showmen and Tory Mystics in the World of Goods', in J. Brewer and R. Porter (eds), *Consump-*

tion and the World of Goods, London, 1993, pp. 489–526; J. Barry, 'Piety and the Patient: Medicine and Religion in Eighteenth-century Bristol', in Porter (ed.), *Patients and Practitioners*.

97. G. Rousseau, 'Mysticism and Millenarianism: "Immortal Dr. Cheyne"', in R.H. Popkin (ed.), *Millenarianism and Messianism in English Literature and Thought*, Leiden, 1988; A. Guerrini, 'Isaac Newton, George Cheyne and the "Principia Medicinae"', in French and Wear (eds), *Medical Revolution*; M. Benjamin, 'Medicine Morality and the Politics of Berkeley's Tar-Water', in Cunningham and French (eds), *Medical Enlightenment*.

98. See D.N. Harley, 'Medical Metaphors in English Moral Theology, 1560–1660', *Journal of the History of Medicine*, 48 (1993), 396–435.

99. For a particularly vivid example of this, see *The Flying-Post*, 29–31 March 1722. Recent discussions of the enduring importance of the religious and political issues of the Civil War and Interregnum in Restoration and Augustan society can be sampled from the essays in T. Harris, P. Seaward and M. Goldie (eds), *The Politics of Religion in Restoration Society*, Oxford, 1990.

100. I here borrow my terminology from A.K. Lingo, 'Empirics and Charlatans in Early Modern France: The Genesis of the Classification of the "Other" in Medical Practice', *Journal of Social History*, 19 (1985–86), 583–603.

101. J. Hart, *The Anatomie of Urines*, London, 1625; Wear, 'Medical Ethics', p. 114.

102. Quoted in Beier, *Sufferers and Healers*, p. 39.

103. C.J.S. Thompson, *The Quacks of Old London*, London, 1928, p. 78; G. Castle, *The Chymical Galenist*, London, 1667, sig. A6.

104. N. Hodges, *Vindiciae Medicinae and Medicorum: Or An Apology for the Profession and Professors of Physick*, London, 1665, sigs. A3–4.

105. See H.J. Cook, *The Decline of the Old Medical Regime in Stuart London*, Ithaca and London, 1986, pp. 145–62.

106. H. More, *Enthusiasmus Triumphatus*, Augustan Reprint Society, 118 (1966), 29–36; Sir R. Blackmore, *A Discourse Upon the Plague*, London, 1721, Preface. Cf. also, C. Goodall, *The Colledge of Physicians Vindicated*, London, 1676, p. 157.

107. They thus violated the proprieties increasingly expected of civil intellectual prose. For this see, Williamson, 'The Restoration Revolt Against Enthusiasm'; P. Dear, 'Totius in Verba: Rhetoric and Authority in the Early Royal Society', *Isis*, 76 (1985), 145–61; P.B. Wood, 'Methodology and Apologetics: Thomas Sprat's *History of the Royal Society*', *British Journal for the History of Science*, 13 (1980), 1–26.

108. S.W., *An Examination of a Late Treatise of the Gout*, London, 1697, Preface. In the Bodleian Library copy of this pamphlet there is a marginal MS emphasis at this passage.

109. H. Sedgwick, *A New Treatise on Liquors*, London, 1725, p. i; Shaw, *Juice of the Grape*, pp. iii–iv.

110. Quoted by J. Henry, 'The Scientific Revolution in England', in R. Porter and M. Teich (eds), *The Scientific Revolution in National Context*, Cambridge, 1992, p. 195.

111. Quoted in Wilson, 'Surgeon "Turned" Physician', p. 164.

112. J. Swift, *A Tale of a Tub*, A.C. Guthkelch and D. Nichol Smith (eds), Oxford, 1958, pp. 107–9.
113. G. Reedy, *Robert South (1634–1716)*, Cambridge, 1992.
114. G. Hickes, *The Spirit of Enthusiasm Exorcised*, London, 1680, p. 42; T. Lewis, *English Presbyterian Eloquence*, London, 1720, p. 113.
115. *London Debating Societies, 1776–1799*, D.T. Andrew (ed.), London Record Society, 30 (1994), nos 877, 1087, 1147, 1374, 1940.

Index